Drug and Device Selection in Heart Failure

Drug and Device Selection in Heart Failure

Editors

Prakash C Deedwania MD FACC FACP FASH FAHA
Professor of Medicine and Chief, Division of Cardiology
Department of Medicine
Veterans Affairs Central California Health Care System
University of California, San Francisco
Fresno, CA, USA

Paul J Mather MD FACC FACP
Professor of Medicine
Director, Advanced Heart Failure and Cardiac Transplant Center
Jefferson Heart Institute, Jefferson Medical College,
Thomas Jefferson University
Philadelphia, PA, USA

Foreword

Marvin A Konstam

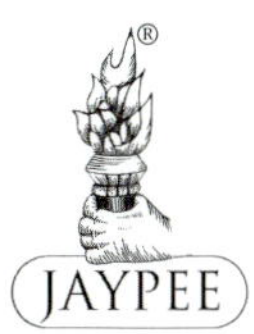

JAYPEE BROTHERS MEDICAL PUBLISHERS (P) LTD.

New Delhi • London • Philadelphia • Panama

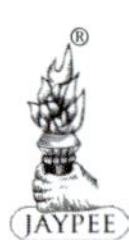

Jaypee Brothers Medical Publishers (P) Ltd

Headquarters

Jaypee Brothers Medical Publishers (P) Ltd
4838/24, Ansari Road, Daryaganj
New Delhi 110 002, India
Phone: +91-11-43574357
Fax: +91-11-43574314
Email: jaypee@jaypeebrothers.com

Overseas Offices

J.P. Medical Ltd
83, Victoria Street, London
SW1H 0HW (UK)
Phone: +44-2031708910
Fax: +02-03-0086180
Email: info@jpmedpub.com

Jaypee-Highlights Medical Publishers Inc
City of Knowledge, Bld. 237, Clayton
Panama City, Panama
Phone: + 507-301-0496
Fax: + 507-301-0499
Email: cservice@jphmedical.com

Jaypee Medical Inc
The Bourse
111 South Independence Mall East
Suite 835, Philadelphia, PA 19106, USA
Phone: + 267-519-9789
Email: joe.rusko@jaypeebrothers.com

Jaypee Brothers Medical Publishers (P) Ltd
17/1-B Babar Road, Block-B, Shaymali
Mohammadpur, Dhaka-1207
Bangladesh
Mobile: +08801912003485
Email: jaypeedhaka@gmail.com

Jaypee Brothers Medical Publishers (P) Ltd
Shorakhute, Kathmandu
Nepal
Phone: +00977-9841528578
Email: jaypee.nepal@gmail.com

Website: www.jaypeebrothers.com
Website: www.jaypeedigital.com

Inquiries for bulk sales may be solicited at: jaypee@jaypeebrothers.com

Drug and Device Selection in Heart Failure

First Edition: **2014**

ISBN 978-93-5090-723-8

Printed at : Samrat Offset Pvt. Ltd

Dedications

I will like to dedicate this book to my mother Paras Devi who has constantly taught me that faith and humility are essential components for a peaceful and harmonious life.

Prakash C Deedwania

Dedicated to Pia, Nick, and Chris

"Knowledge belongs to humanity, and thus science knows no country and is the torch that illuminates the world."

–Louis Pasteur

Paul J Mather

Contents

Contributors

EDITOR

Prakash C Deedwania MD FACC FACP FASH FAHA
Professor of Medicine and Chief, Division of Cardiology
Department of Medicine
Veterans Affairs Central California Health Care System
University of California, San Francisco
Fresno, CA, USA

Paul J Mather MD FACC FACP
Professor of Medicine
Director, Advanced Heart Failure and Cardiac Transplant Center
Jefferson Heart Institute, Jefferson Medical College,
Thomas Jefferson University
Philadelphia, PA, USA

CONTRIBUTING AUTHORS

Kariann Abbate MD
Cardiology Fellow
Jefferson Heart Institute, Jefferson
Medical College,
Thomas Jefferson University
Philadelphia, PA, USA

Jagroop S Basraon DO
Physician
Cardiology Fellow
University of California, San Francisco
Fresno, CA, USA

Raphael E Bonita MD ScM FACC
Assistant Professor of Medicine
Advanced Heart Failure and Cardiac
Transplant Center
Jefferson Heart Institute, Jefferson
Medical College,
Thomas Jefferson University
Philadelphia, PA, USA

Anne P Canny RN MSN
Heart Failure Nurse Coordinator
Jefferson Heart Institute, Jefferson
Medical College,
Thomas Jefferson University
Philadelphia, PA, USA

Enrique Carbajal MD
Associate Clinical Professor of Medicine
Division of Cardiology, Department of
Medicine
Veterans Affairs Central California

Health Care System
University of California
San Francisco, Fresno Medical
Education Program
Fresno, CA, USA

Kanu Chatterjee MBBS FRCP (London) FRCP (Edin) FAHA FCCP FACC MACP
Clinical Professor of Medicine
Division of Cardiology
The Carver College of Medicine
University of Iowa
Iowa City, Iowa, USA
Emeritus Professor of Medicine
University of California
San Francisco
California, USA

Sumeet K Chhabra MD
Cardiology Fellow
Jefferson Heart Institute, Jefferson
Medical College
Thomas Jefferson University
Philadelphia, PA, USA

Daniel R Frisch MD
Director, Atrial Fibrillation Program
Assistant Professor of Medicine
Jefferson Heart Institute, Jefferson
Medical College
Thomas Jefferson University
Philadelphia, PA, USA

Mihai Gheorghiade MD FACC
Professor of Medicine and Surgery
Director of Experimental Therapeutics
Center for Cardiovascular Innovation
Northwestern University Feinberg
School of Medicine
Chicago, IL, USA

Manjunath C Harlapur MD
Fellow, Division of Cardiology
Department of Medicine
University of California, San Francisco
Fresno, CA, USA
Paul J Hauptman MD
Professor of Internal Medicine
Saint Louis University Hospital
Saint Louis University School of
Medicine
Saint Louis, MO, USA

Reginald T Ho MD
Associate Professor of Medicine
Division of Cardiac Electrophysiology
Jefferson Heart Institute, Jefferson
Medical College,
Thomas Jefferson University
Philadelphia, PA, USA

Patrick McCann MD
Division of Cardioloy
Department of Medicine
Saint Louis University School of Medicine
Saint Louis, MO, USA

Toshimasa Okabe MD
Cardiology Fellow
Jefferson Heart Institute, Jefferson
Medical College,
Thomas Jefferson University
Philadelphia, PA, USA

Behzad B Pavri MD
Associate Professor of Medicine
Director, CCEP Fellowship
Jefferson Heart Institute, Jefferson
Medical College,
Thomas Jefferson University
Philadelphia, PA, USA

Gordon R Reeves MD MPT
Cardiology Fellow
Jefferson Heart Institute, Jefferson Medical College,
Thomas Jefferson University
Philadelphia, PA, USA

Muthiah Vaduganathan MD MPH
Resident Physician
Department of Medicine
Massachusetts General Hospital,
Harvard Medical School
Boston, MA, USA

Andrew Yin MD
Cardiology Fellow
Jefferson Heart Institute, Jefferson Medical College,
Thomas Jefferson University
Philadelphia, PA, USA

Foreword

Marvin A Konstam MD
Chief Physician Executive
CardioVascular Center, Tufts Medical Center
Professor of Medicine
Tufts University School of Medicine
Boston, MA 02111, USA

There has never been more focus and interest in the field of heart failure than there is today. The number of patients with this condition is inexorably increasing, expected to rise in the US from 5.8 million to 8.5 million over the next 20 years,[1] owing principally to the aging of our population. Assuming continuation of current patient management models and continued technical and pharmaceutical advances, annual direct costs for this condition are conservatively estimated to rise from $21 billion to $53 billion, and annual total costs from $31 billion to $70 billion, over that same time frame.[1]

It is no surprise that the Centers for Medicare and Medicaid Services have placed great focus on heart failure in their policy initiatives, including penalties for quality deficiencies and excess readmission rates and exploration of bundled payments models for patients with this condition. At the same time, major advances in drug and device therapy for heart failure have emerged over the past 2 decades. Recognition of the increased complexity of heart failure management options sparked the Heart Failure Society of America to launch a multi-year effort culminating in designation, by the American Board of Internal Medicine, of Advanced Heart Failure and Transplant Cardiology as an official secondary subspecialty.

It is mandatory that the next generation of clinicians, including physicians advanced care providers, and nurses approach the care of patients with heart failure well-schooled in several critical tenets. These include: (i) delivering drug, device, and advanced therapies in the most evidence-based and cost-effective manner possible; (ii) melding technical competency with keen cognitive skills, including awareness of the psychosocial needs of this vulnerable population; (iii) balancing delivery of complex, expensive diagnostic, and therapeutic modalities with attention to patient preference and end-of-life considerations.

It is in this context that Mather and Deedwania (editors) provide clinicians with this timely resource. They have assembled an outstanding group of experts to generate a clear and well-organized compendium of the evidence behind drug and device therapy for heart failure. The authors go further, offering thoughtful approaches to the selection of these therapies in patients with disease severity ranging from mild to the most severe. This contribution will serve as a valuable guide to current therapeutic evidence, as we advance toward more system-oriented, cost-effective approaches to managing our expanding population of patients with heart failure.

REFERENCE

1. Heidenreich PA, Albert NM, Allen LA, Bluemke DA, Butler J, Fonarow GC, et al. Forecasting the impact of heart failure in the United States: a policy statement from the American Heart Association. Circ Heart Fail. 2013;6:606-19.

Preface

Heart failure is a major public health problem that is growing across the world and has become a leading cause of hospitalization in the elderly with more than 1 million admissions every year in the US medicare population. Clinicians frequently encounter patients with heart failure in their everyday practice. The prognosis of heart failure, although much improved (in recent years), still remains worse than many cancers. Appropriate treatment designed to prevent and treat heart failure can significantly reduce the associated high morbidity and mortality. However, with the expanding pharmacopeia of drug therapy and the use of various devices, selection of an appropriate therapeutic strategy for a given patient has become quite challenging. This comprehensive monograph on Drug and Device Selection in Heart Failure is designed to provide a series of state-of-the-art reviews on the most important topics that will help educate and equip the clinician with the appropriate knowledge-base to select the best evidence-based therapy for patients with heart failure.

As it is critical to understand the pathophysiologic processes involved in various stages of development of heart failure before appropriate therapy can be chosen, the book begins with a chapter on renewed understanding of the pathophysiology of heart failure. Subsequent chapter discuses the use of old and newer diuretics. It is emphasized in this chapter that diuretics need to be used only in the setting of fluid overloaded state and that excessive and unnecessary use of diuretics can lead to further activation of neurohormonal axes and in some cases the development of cardiorenal syndrome.

The following chapter describes the evidence based therapies with renin-angiotensin-aldosterone system blocking drugs and includes a detailed review behind the rationale for the use of angiotensin converting enzyme inhibitors and angiotensin receptor blockers, as well as recent evidence emphasizing the role of aldosterone blockade in early as well as advanced stages of heart failure. The role of inotropic therapy has been a subject of constant debate and even though the evidence does not support routine use of inotropes, the clinician sometimes is left with little choice but to consider their use, even if for a short period, and for palliative reasons to keep the patient out of hospital. A critical appraisal comparing various old and newer inotropic drugs has been described in detail in the subsequent chapter. Acute decompensated heart failure (ADHF) leading to frequent visits to the emergency rooms or hospital has become a new specialty and requires fundamental understanding of the different pathophysiologic processes involved and varying therapeutic strategies accordingly. The chapter on ADHF provides an exhaustive review on these aspects and provides the clinician with tools to individualize therapy in a variety of patients with ADHF with the goal of reducing future recurrent hospitalizations, which has now become a new yardstick by which many organizations now evaluate the quality of care given to patients with heart failure. Subsequent chapters discuss the concept of disease management strategy including the need for a team based approach consisting of the physician specialist, nursing staff, pharmacist, nutritionist, and a social worker. The importance of including the patient and family members/care-givers on the team is also emphasized.

It is well known that many patients with heart failure have concomitant atrial and ventricular arrhythmias that can lead to both adverse hemodynamic consequences and life threatening arrhythmias. Even more challenging is the fact that many anti-arrhythmic agents are poorly tolerated and can have pro-arrhythmic effects. This has been discussed in subsequent chapters including appropriate use and limitations of the automatic implantable cardioverter defibrillators and cardiac resynchronization therapy. Final chapters describes the role of cardiac assist devices and cardiac transplantation including the emphasis on the need for proper selection and a team approach as well as psychological and social support system without which such interventions cannot be successful.

The chapters included in this book have been written by clinicians who have considerable expertise in the given areas and have made a lot of efforts in synthesizing complex and extensive literature to prepare their reviews. Finally, both of us would like to thank all our residents and fellows for their ongoing support as well as patients who have been a constant source of inspiration to us.

Prakash C Deedwania
Paul J Mather

CHAPTER

1

Renewed Understanding of the Pathophysiology of Heart Failure

Kanu Chatterjee

INTRODUCTION

Heart failure is a common clinical syndrome which can be caused by many pathophysiologic conditions. It can be caused by valvular, myocardial, and pericardial diseases. It can be acute and of recent onset or chronic and may be present for several months or years. It can be caused by primarily by left ventricular systolic or diastolic dysfunction. In this chapter, heart failure due to myocardial disease has been discussed. Heart failure resulting from left ventricular myocardial systolic dysfunction is referred as systolic heart failure (SHF). It is also called heart failure with reduced ejection fraction (HFREF). When it is primarily due to diastolic dysfunction, it is termed diastolic heart failure (DHF). It is also called heart failure with normal ejection fraction (HFNEF). In this chapter, primarily the pathophysiology of systolic and diastolic heart failure has been discussed. The epidemiology has been briefly discussed.

INCIDENCE, PREVALENCE, AND RISK FACTORS

The incidence of heart failure caused by myocardial disease is high. The lifetime risk of developing heart failure due to myocardial disease is about 20% at all ages older than 40 years.[1] In the United States, the prevalence of heart failure is approximately 2.4% of the adult population. It was estimated that in 2011, 5.7 million people had established diagnosis of heart failure.[2] By the year 2040, it is expected that 10 million people will have heart failure in the United States of America. Approximately, 23 millions of people have heart failure worldwide. The estimated incidence of heart failure in the United States presently is approaching 10 per 1,000 population older than 65 years of age.[3]

The prevalence of DHF is very similar to that of SHF. Heart failure due to diastolic dysfunction (HFNEF) is diagnosed in approximately 50% of patients with heart failure.[4] DHF is more frequent in women than in men. In the cardiovascular health study, the prevalence of DHF was 67% in women and 42% in men.[5-7]

The risk factors for developing SHF and DHF are also similar.[6] In both SHF and DHF, older age, hypertension, diabetes and obesity are the major risk factors. The incidence of coronary artery disease appears to be higher in SHF than in DHF. However, the incidence of coronary artery disease in DHF is still considerable, about 54% as compared to 63% in SHF. The patients with SHF are relatively younger than patients with DHF. The average age of patients with SHF is 70 years and with DHF, 74 years.[6]

COST OF MANAGEMENT

The management of established symptomatic heart failure is expensive. In many developed countries, the cost of management of heart failure is 1–2% of the health care budget. In 2007, the cost of management of heart failure exceeded 35 billion dollars in the United States. Presently, it remains unknown about the cost of management of heart failure in underdeveloped countries.

PATHOPHYSIOLOGY OF HEART FAILURE

During the last two decades, there have been considerable advances in the understanding of the pathophysiology of both SHF and DHF. Our knowledge of left ventricular morphology, remodeling, and molecular features in SHF and DHF has improved.

Morphologic Changes in Systolic and Diastolic Heart Failure

In SHF, there is eccentric left ventricular hypertrophy with left ventricular dilatation. There is a substantial increase in left ventricular end-diastolic volumes (LVEDV) and left ventricular end-systolic volumes (LVESV).[8,9] The magnitude of increase in end-systolic volume is greater than that of end-diastolic volume. Thus, left ventricular ejection fraction declines. Left ventricular ejection fraction is the ratio of left ventricular total stroke volume (LVTSV) and LVEDV. LVTSV is the difference between LVEDV and LVESV. In patients with SHF, ejection fraction can be reduced due to disproportionate increase in LVEDV with unchanged LVTSV. Left ventricular ejection fraction may also decline when there is marked decrease in LVTSV without any increase in LVEDV. In SHF, there is usually both decrease in LVTSV and an increase in LVEDV.

Left ventricular cavity size is markedly increased in SHF. Left ventricular mass is also increased. However, as the cavity size increases by a greater magnitude than the mass, the cavity/mass ratio is increased. Left ventricular wall thickness remains normal or even decreases despite myocyte hypertrophy. Increased cavity size with normal or decreased wall thickness is associated with increased wall stress (La Place Relation). As wall stress represents left ventricular afterload, increased wall stress is associated with decreased ejection fraction. There is also an increase in myocardial oxygen consumption due to increased wall stress.

Table 1	Systolic heart failure-remodeling
•	Usually eccentric hypertrophy
•	Disproportionate increase in ventricular cavity size
•	Increased ventricular mass
•	Wall thickness-decreased or unchanged
•	Increased wall stress
•	Reduced ejection fraction
•	Altered ventricular shape and geometry
•	Frequent mechanical dyssynchrony with or without electrical dyssynchrony

In SHF, there are considerable changes in left ventricular shape and geometry. Normally, left ventricle is ellipsoidal. In SHF, left ventricle becomes globular and spherical. The transverse diameter of left ventricle increases by greater magnitude than the longitudinal diameter. The distance between anterolateral and posteromedial papillary muscles increases causing misalignment of the papillary muscles, chordae, and mitral valve leaflets which produces secondary mitral regurgitation.

In patients with advanced SHF, dyssynchrony of left ventricular wall motion is observed in over one-third of patients. Normally, left ventricular septum contracts and relaxes before the lateral and posterior walls. In SHF, lateral and posterior walls contract and relaxes before interventricular septum. Mechanical dyssynchrony is frequently associated with electrical dyssynchrony, particularly left bundle branch block (LBBB). The morphologic changes in systolic heart failure are summarized in table 1.

In DHF, there is concentric left ventricular hypertrophy without any cavity dilatation. LVEDV and LVEDVs remain normal. There is increased wall thickness. As the cavity size remains normal, wall stress decreases which contributes to maintain normal ejection fraction. Left ventricular mass is increased but as the cavity size remains normal, left ventricular cavity/mass ratio is increased. In DHF, there is little or no change in left ventricular shape and geometry. Left ventricular shape remains ellipsoidal and the transverse axis is shorter than the long axis. There is little or no secondary mitral regurgitation. In approximately one-third of patients with DHF, there is mechanical dyssynchrony.[10] The morphologic changes in DHF are summarized in table 2.

Hemodynamic Abnormalities in Systolic and Diastolic Abnormalities

In SHF, the primary hemodynamic abnormality is reduced ejection fraction. Reduced ejection fraction is associated with reduced stroke volume and an increase in LVEDV and LVESV. Increased left ventricular diastolic volumes is associated with increased left ventricular diastolic pressures, a passive increase in left atrial

Table 2	Diastolic heart failure remodeling
•	Ventricular hypertrophy-usually concentric
•	Increased left ventricular mass
•	Increased left ventricular wall thickness
•	Little or no change in left ventricular volumes
•	Decreased left ventricular wall stress
•	Maintained ejection fraction
•	Little or no change in ventricular shape
•	Mechanical dyssynchrony with or without electrical dyssynchrony is present in approxmately 30% of patients

and pulmonary venous pressure. Increased pulmonary venous pressure causes symptoms and signs of pulmonary venous congestion. When there is increased pulmonary venous pressure, there is also an obligatory increase in pulmonary artery pressure which is right ventricular afterload. This secondary pulmonary hypertension may precipitate right ventricular failure. Right ventricular failure is manifested by elevated systemic venous pressure and dependent edema. In advanced SHF, stroke volume decreases; but reflex increase in heart rate may maintain normal cardiac output.

In DHF, the primary functional abnormality is increased left ventricular stiffness which is associated with increased left ventricular diastolic pressure, a passive increase in left atrial and pulmonary venous pressure which causes signs and symptoms of pulmonary venous congestion. There is also an obligatory increase in pulmonary artery pressure when there is increase in pulmonary venous pressure. This secondary pulmonary hypertension may precipitate right ventricular failure manifested by elevated systemic venous pressure and peripheral edema. When there is marked impairment of left ventricular filling, stroke volume is decreased. However, a reflex increase in heart rate may maintain normal cardiac output.

Functional Changes in Systolic and Diastolic Heart Failure

In SHF, the major functional abnormality is impaired contractile function. The indices of contractile function, such as left ventricular dP/dt is decreased. The velocity of contraction is also dereased. When left ventricular pressure volume loops are constructed and end-systolic pressure volume relation is determined, in SHF the end-systolic pressure-volume line shifts downwards and to the right (Fig. 1). End-systolic pressure volume relation is a reliable index of contractile function. Left ventricular stroke volume declines resulting from decreased contractility. In SHF, diastolic pressure volume relation remains unchanged. However, in patients with advanced SHF, left ventricular filling may be abnormal.

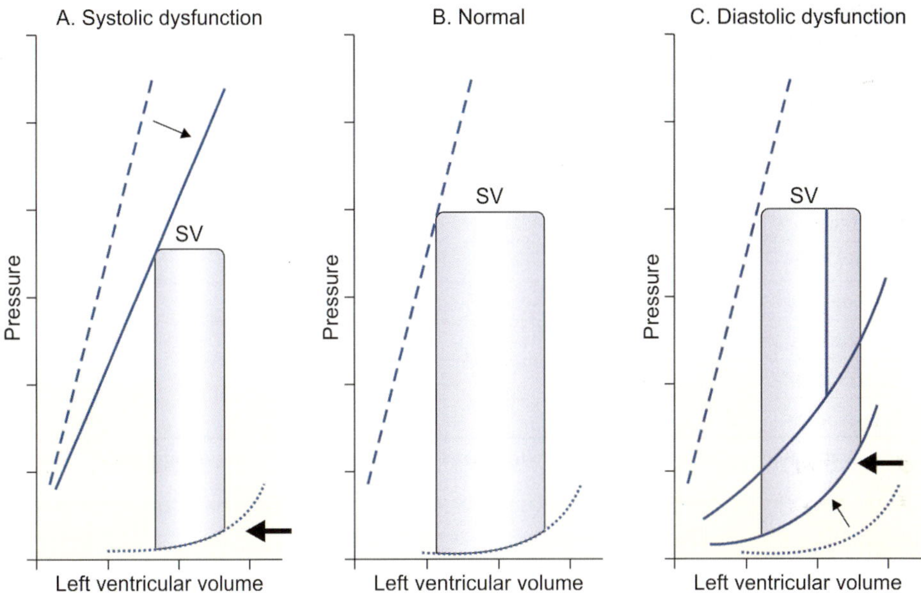

Figure 1: Schematic illustration of pressure-volume loops in normal, systolic, and diastolic dysfunction. SV, stroke volume.

In DHF, left ventricular contractile function remains normal. Diastolic dysfunction is the primary functional abnormality in DHF. Diastolic pressure volume relation shifts upwards and to the left. As discussed earlier, left ventricular stiffness is increased which is the primary mechanism for this shift of diastolic pressure volume curve. Left ventricular end-diastolic pressure increases. If there is a further upward shift of the diastolic pressure volume curve, there is a reduction in stroke volume resulting from marked impairment of left ventricular filling (Fig. 1).

Long-term follow-up studies have demonstrated that, in patients with DHF without coronary artery disease, left ventricular dilatation does not occur. Ejection fraction remains normal. Left ventricular stiffness increases.[11]

Myocyte and Myocardial Structure in Systolic and Diastolic Heart Failure

In SHF, myocyte length is increased without any change in myocyte diameter. There is increased myosine degradation. There is myocyte hypertrophy, apoptosis and necrosis. Myocardial architecure is abnormal. There is disruption of extracellular matrix. There is disintegration of collagen fibers. The collagen bundles are thinner than normal. The collagen cross links are decreased. There is increased myocardial fibrosis (Table 3).

Calcium regulation is abnormal in SHF. The ratio of matrix metalloproteinases and tissue inhibitor of metalloproteinases is increased in SHF. The ratio of titin isoforms N_2BA/N_2B is increased in SHF.

Table 3 **Myocyte and myocardial structural changes in systolic and diastolic heart failure**

	Systolic heart failure	*Diastolic heart failure*
Myocyte		
• Hypertrophy	+	+
• Apoptosis	+	+
• Necrosis	+	+
Fibrosis	+	+
Collagen cross-links	–	+
Calcium regulation	–	+
MMPs/TIMPs	+	–
Titin isoforms N_2BA/N_2B	+	–

(+), increased; (–), decreased; MMPs, matrix metalloproteinases; TIMPs, tissue inhibitor of metalloproteinases

In DHF, myocyte is thicker than normal and there is no change in myocyte length. In DHF, there is increased synthesis of myosin.

As in SHF, there is myocyte hypertrophy, apoptosis, and necrosis. There is also disorganized extracellular matrix. The collagen bundles are thicker than normal. The collagen volume is increased. The collagen cross links are increased.

In DHF, there is also calcium dysregulation. The ratio of matrix metalloproteinases and tissue inhibitor of metalloproteinases is decreased. The ratio of titin isoforms N_2BA/N_2B is decreased in DHF.[12,13]

The solid line represents end-systolic pressure-volume line which shifts downwards and to the right in SHF. Diastolic pressure-volume relation is also illustrated. In DHF, there is an upward and leftward shift.

Neurohormonal Changes in Systolic and Diastolic Heart Failure

In both SHF and DHF, a significant neurohormonal abnormalities occur.[14] There is increased norepinephrine levels which reflect activation of sympathetic activity. There is also increased in muscle sympathetic nerve activity. There is also increased renal sympathetic activity which is associated with renal vascular constriction and deterioration of renal function. Increased sympathetic activity promotes myocyte and vascular remodeling. There is also increased systemic vascular resistance which increases left ventricular afterload which contributes to adverse ventricular remodeling. Increased adrenergic activity is associated with vascular remodeling as well. There is hyperplasia of vascular smooth muscle cells. There is also enhanced inflammatory responses which also promote atherothrombosis.

In SHF, there is activation of renin-angiotensin system. Activation of renin-angiotensin also produces ventricular, myocyte, and vascular remodeling.

Ventricular remodeling is characterized by ventricular dilatation and reduction of left ventricular ejection fraction. There is an increase in both end-diastolic and end-systolic volumes as has been discussed earlier. Angiotensin II increases renal efferent arteriolar tone which initially can maintain glomerular filtration rate.

The myocyte remodeling is characterized by increase in myocyte length without an increase in myocyte width. There is increased myosin degradation. Vascular remodeling is associated with smooth muscle cell hyperplasia, thickening of internal, and external elastic lamina.

There is also activation of aldosterone system as evident from increased serum levels of aldosterone. Stimulation of aldosterone system also promotes ventricular and vascular adverse remodeling. There is increased myocardial fibrosis, increased collagen synthesis, and decreased collagen break down.

In SHF, arginine vasopressin levels are increased.[14] The level of vasopressin is higher in symptomatic patients than in asymptomatic patients with left ventricular dysfunction. Vasopressin is released from pituitary glands. Vasopressin stimulates both vasopressin 1 and 2 receptors.[15] Vasopressin 2 receptors are primarily concentrated in renal collecting ducts. Normally, the major stimulus for vasopressin release is increased plasma osmolality. However, in heart failure, vasopressin is released irrespective of changes in plasma osmolality. Stimulation of renal vasopressin 2 receptors is associated with inappropriate release of vasopressin and hyponatremia. Activation of vasopressin 1 receptors is associated with myocyte hypertrophy, myocardial fibrosis, and coronary vasoconstriction. It also increases systemic vascular resistance which increases left ventricular afterload and produces adverse remodeling.

In SHF, endothelins are also increased.[16] Endothelins are produced by vascular smooth muscle cells and they are potent vasoconstrictors. Endothelin is produced by conversion of big endothelin-1 by a converting enzyme. Endothelin synthesis and release are promoted by norepinephrine, angiotensin II, and oxidized low density lipoproteins.[17]

In DHF, plasma norepinephrine levels are increased indicating activated adrenergic system. It is not clear whether renin-angiotensin-aldosterone system is activated or not in DHF. However, it appears that neurohormonal abnormalities are very similar in DHF and SHF. Characteristics of ventricular remodeling in SHF and DHF are different. Adverse effects of neurohormonal abnormalities in SHF are summarized in table 4.

Counter-regulatory vasodilating and antimitogenic neurohormones are also elevated both in systolic and diastolic heart failure. Plasma brain natriuretic peptide levels and vasodilating prostacyclins are also increased. However, the effects of these hormones in attenuation of ventricular remodeling appear inadequate.

Table 4	Adverse effects of neurohormonal activation
•	Adverse hemodynamic effects
•	Vascular remodeling
•	Ventricular remodeling
•	Myocyte hypertrophy
•	Extracellular matrix changes
•	Pomotes atherothrombosis
•	Increased oxidative stress
•	myocardial necrosis
•	Apoptosis

CONCLUSIONS

In this chapter, the pathophysiology of SHF and DHF is discussed. The functional, morphologic, and remodeling features are discussed. Features of ventricular remodeling are distinctly different in SHF and DHF. Changes in myocyte and myocardial architecture are also described, and the differences in SHF and DHF are discussed. Abnormalities in neurohormonal profile in these two clinical subsets are also discussed in details.

REFERENCES

1. Roger VL, Go AS, Lloyd-Jones DM, et al. Heart disease and stroke statistics--2011 update: a report from the American Heart Association. Circulation. 2011;123:e18-209.
2. Rosamond W, Flegal K, Friday G, et al. Heart Disease and stroke statistics--2007 update: a report from the American Heart Association Statistics Committee and Stroke Statistics Subcommittee. Circulation. 2007;115:e69-71.
3. Lloyd-Jones D, Adams RJ, Brown TM, et al. Executive summary: Heart Disease and stroke statistics--2010 update: a report from the American Heart Association. Circulation. 2010;121: e259.
4. Gary R, Davis L. Diastolic heart failure. Heart Lung. 2008;37:405-16.
5. Gottdiener JS, Arnold AM, Aurigemma GP, et al. Predictors of congestive heart failure in the elderly: the cardiovascular health study. J Am Coll Cardiol. 2000;35:1628-37.
6. Sweitzer NK, Lopatin M, Yancy CW, et al. Comparison of clinical features and outcomes of patients hospitalized with heart failure and normal ejection fraction (> or = 55%) versus those with mildly reduced (40% to 50%) and moderately to severely reduced (<40%) ejection fractions. Am J Cardiol. 2008;101:1151-6.
7. McKee PA, Castelli WP, McNamara PM, et al. The natural history of congestive heart failure: the Framingham study. N Engl J Med. 1971;285:1441-6.
8. Konstam MA. "Systolic and diastolic dysfunction" in heart failure? Time for a new paradigm. J Card Fail. 2003;9:1-3.
9. Aurigema GP, Zile MR, Gaasch WH. Contractile behavior of the left ventricle in diastolic heart failure with emphasis on regional systolic function. Circulation. 2006;113:296-304.
10. Chatterjee K, Massie B. Systolic and diastolic heart failure: differences and similarities. J Card Fail. 2007;13:569-76.

11. Handoko ML, van Heeerbook L, Bronzwaer JG, et al. Does diastolic heart failure evolve to systolic heart failure? Circulation. 2006;114(Suppl II): 816.
12. Katz AM, Zile MR. New molecular mechanism in diastolic heart failure. Circulation. 2006;113:1922-5.
13. Kitzman DW, Little WC, Brubaker PH, et al. Pathophysiological characterization of isolated diastolic heart failure in comparison to systolic heart failure. JAMA. 2002;288:2144-50.
14. Francis GS, Benedict C, Johnstone DE, et al. Comparison of neuroendocrine activation in patients with left ventricular dysfunction with and without congestive heart failure. A substudy of the Studies of Left Ventricular Dysfunction (SOLVD). Circulation. 1990;82:1724-9.
15. Schrier RW, Abraham WT. Hormones and hemodynamics in heart failure. N Engl J Med. 1999;341:577-85.
16. MacMurray JJ, Ray SG, Abdullah I, et al. Plasma endothelin in chronic heart failure. Circulation. 1992;85:1374-9.
17. Levine ER. Endothelins. N Engl J Med. 1995;333:356-63.

CHAPTER 2

New Diuretics in Heart Failure

Jagroop S Basraon, Prakash C Deedwania

INTRODUCTION

Treatment with diuretic therapy is an essential component of treatment for a wide spectrum of heart failure presentations. This chapter discusses the role of newer and older diuretic agents that are currently used in heart failure by focusing on different classifications and mechanism of action. Pharmacodynamic and pharmacokinetic properties of diuretics are elucidated. Different methods of utilizing this therapy in different settings along with a comprehensive review of the side effect profile are highlighted. Special situations necessitating adjustment and the phenomenon of diuretic resistance are explained.

Diuretics are commonly used as the first-line therapy for treatment of acute decompensation as well as chronic treatment of heart failure to help maintain a euvolemic state. Practitioners in every specialty of medicine are exposed to patients with chronic heart failure for management of comorbid conditions; therefore, an in-depth understanding of diuretic therapy is essential in optimizing patient care.

Additionally, with development of newer agents, understanding the mechanism of action of each class of diuretics is necessary to prevent complications and enhance effectiveness.

MECHANISM OF ACTION

Diuretics that utilize different modes of action are available for heart failure therapy. They are classified based on different sites of action within the nephron. In older diuretics, pharmacological effect is achieved because of their inhibition of electrolyte transporters which causes corresponding hemodynamic effect due to alteration of the interstitial tonicity and loss of fluid due to osmotic gradients (Fig. 1). Diuretics are tightly bound to plasma proteins, and therefore, restricted to the intravascular space. They are actively secreted into the proximal tubular lumen.

Loop diuretics inhibit the $Na^+/K^+/Cl^-$ symporter in the ascending loop of Henle, while thiazide-type diuretics affect the Na^+/Cl^- in the distal convoluted tubules.

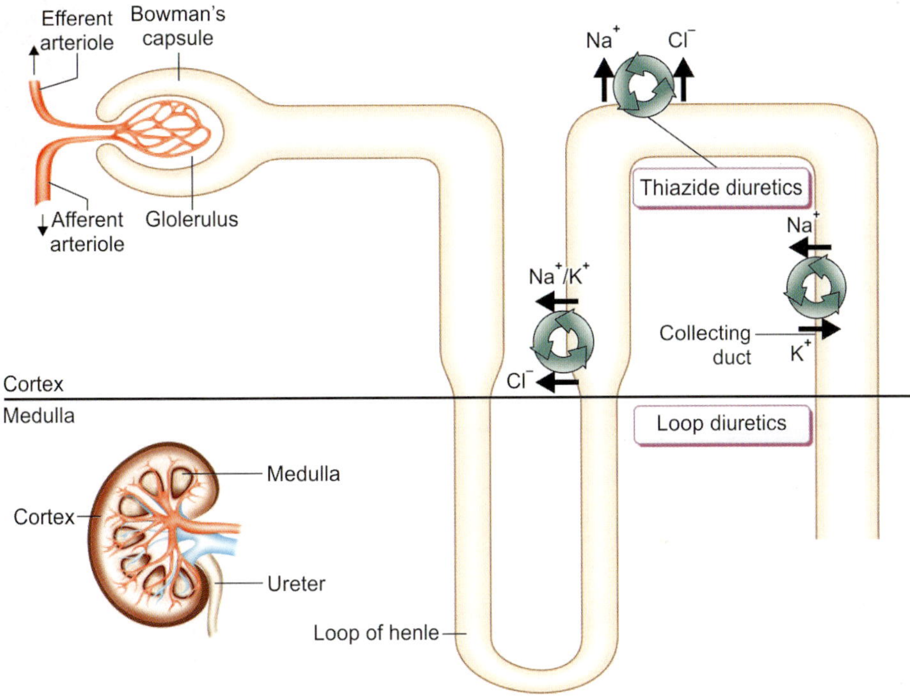

Figure 1: Mechanism of action.

Potassium sparing diuretics and mineralocorticoid receptor antagonists, which are utilized more for concomitant therapeutics as renin-angiotensin-aldosterone system (RAAS) blocking agents and reduction of diuretic-induced hypokalemia instead of control of edema, work at sites in the collecting duct to inhibit the Na^+/K^+ transporter.

Two newer agents have recently been evaluated which have targeted vasopressin and adenosine receptors in the kidneys to enhance volume control. The vaptans, which block the action of hormone vasopressin, help in controlling the retention of water by the kidneys. Pathological adenosine receptor activation in heart failure often leads to reduction in glomerular filtration rate (GFR) and sodium retention. The adenosine receptor blocker rolofylline is currently under investigation, and preliminary data indicates that it can improve kidney function and achieve net diuresis.

PHARMACOKINETICS

Loop diuretics have different pharmacokinetic properties depending on the diuretic used and patients' underlying comorbidities (Table 1). Particularly, patients with kidney and liver disease can be challenging to manage due to varied elimination

Table 1 Pharmacology of diuretics

	Oral bioavailability (%)	*Dosing (mg)*	*Half-life (hours)*	*Elimination*
Loop				
Furosemide	0–100	80–160	2	Renal
Torsemide	80–100	5–10	1	Liver
Bumetanide	80–100	2–4	3	Liver
Others				
Hydrochlorothiazide (HCTZ)	65–75	12.5–100	6-15	Renal
Metolazone	70–85	2.5–10	14	Renal
Vaptans				
Tolvaptan	40	15–60	6–8	Liver
Conivaptan	44%	40–80 (Intravenous only)	3–8	Liver

and altered metabolisms. Orally dosed furosemide typically has 50% bioavailability; however, significant variability has been reported with a range from 10% to 100% in patients with heart failure.[1] Bumetanide and torsemide, the newer agents are absorbed more completely with 80% bioavailability after oral dosing.[2,3] Furosemide is eliminated by the kidneys while torsemide and bumetanide are metabolized by the liver. Metolazone and thiazides are all eliminated by renal mechanisms.[4] Loop diuretics typically have short half-lives with Bumex at about 3–4 hours, 1–2 hours for torsemide, and 2–3 hours for furosemide.

Hydrochlorothiazide (HCTZ) and thiazide-type diuretic metolazone have reported bioavailability of 60–70%.[4] Thiazides typically stay in the system longer with average half-life of 10–15 hours.[5]

Tolvaptan, the vasopressin antagonist, has oral bioavailability of 40% with half-life of 6–9 hours. Conivaptan is available as an intravenous (IV) formulation with half-life of 3–8 hours. Both are metabolized in the liver and are administered once a day.

PHARMACODYNAMICS

Pharmacodynamics of diuretics can be evaluated by an indirect measurement of the rate of excretion within the urine. Typically, this relationship is represented by a sigmoidal curve, where a minimal amount of diuretic is required to achieve a renal response with an upper level for maximal effect (Fig. 2).[3,6] These dose response curves have helped established the optimal dose limits of the commonly used diuretics.[2,7-9] Therefore, it is important to keep in mind that clinical application

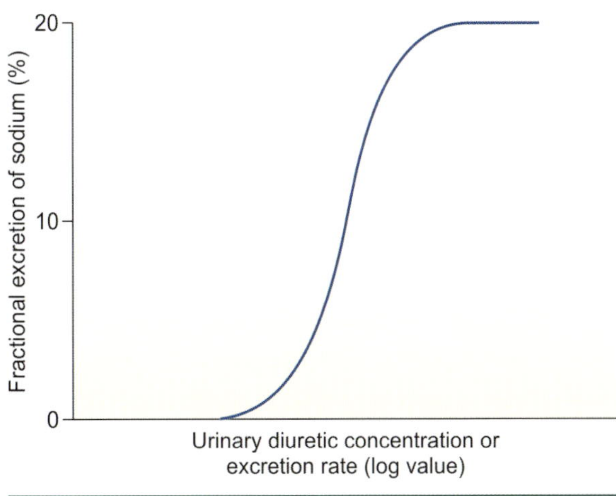

Figure 2: Pharmacodynamics of loop diuretics.[13]

of the diuretic usually requires a minimal dose before an effective diuresis can be established.

DOSING

Diuretics are typically administered on a schedule which accounts for their different half-lives. Loop diuretics are dosed twice a day because of typical (1–4 hour) half-lives. Thiazides and metolazone typically have longest half-lives and, therefore, are dosed daily. Patients presenting with evidence of volume overload are typically started on 40 mg of furosemide twice a day and observed for diuretic response. In case of inadequate diuresis or those on chronic therapy, the patients' basal dose is adjusted to increase urine output. Tolvaptan is dosed daily with dose range of 15–60 mg and conivaptan has dose of 40–80 mg and also administered daily as an IV formulation.

DIURETICS IN RENAL AND LIVER DISEASE

These characteristics have an important impact in management of patients with hepatic or renal disease. Presence of renal dysfunction due to underlying kidney disease or secondary to hypoperfusion because of chronic heart failure can lead to altered pharmacokinetics, which requires adjustment of the diuretic dose to ensure adequate dose response.

In patients with renal disease, there is decreased renal flow and often decreased production of urine in the later stages. Physiological alterations also lead to decreased renal conjugation. Irrespective of the specific kidney disease, the functioning nephrons remain responsive to diuretic therapy. These changes necessitate the use of higher doses of the loop diuretic to achieve adequate concentration in the tubular fluid to be effective. Additionally, this results in the increased half-life of furosemide which is renally excreted; however, bumetanide and torsemide are not affected due to their hepatic metabolism.[10]

The predominant diuretic used in patients with liver disease without heart failure is spironolactone. This is because of the fact that the volume problems are manifestations of state of hyperaldosteronism.[11] The response of the loop diuretics is reduced in patients with liver disease with heart failure.[12] Typically, spironolactone is used with additional low-dose HCTZ or intra-abdominal procedures, such as paracentesis to control fluid status. These patients can often suffer from intravascular fluid depletion; therefore, the addition of loop diuretic has to be carefully utilized. In these patients, the amount of fluid excretion is lower due to shift of the natriuretic curve to the right and cannot be overcome with larger doses. Lastly, the frequency of the response is not affected and thus multiple doses may be utilized to increase urine output.[13] Therefore, frequent dosing or combination therapy can overcome some of this decrease.

INTRAVENOUS THERAPY

Intravenous loop diuretics are the most commonly used medication during acute decompensated heart failure. Intravenous dosing forms of certain diuretics are available for therapy and are usually equivalent in efficacy to the oral form with the exception of furosemide, where half of the oral dose should be used in the IV format because of bioavailability differences.

BOLUS VERSUS CONTINUOUS DOSING

There has been a contentious debate over the effectiveness of different methods of administering IV diuretics. Additionally, there had been concerns over adverse effects of utilizing high doses of diuretics in patients with heart failure.[14] Comparison of bolus versus continuous dosing in several older studies did not clearly establish superiority of either method.[15-17] However, recently, a randomized clinical trial has provided further information in this regard.

In the Diuretic Optimization Strategies Evaluation (DOSE) trial, which was a prospective randomized controlled trial, different strategies of applying diuretic therapy in patient with clinical heart failure were evaluated.[18] Patients were evaluated at low dose versus high dose which was defined as 2.5 times their usual daily therapeutic dose both in an IV and continuous infusion methods during acute decompensated heart failure. There was no difference in the kidney function and in the overall assessment of heart failure symptoms between the two treatment strategies (Figs. 3A and B). Therefore, based on the results of this study, either mode of administration can be utilized with appropriate clinical monitoring.

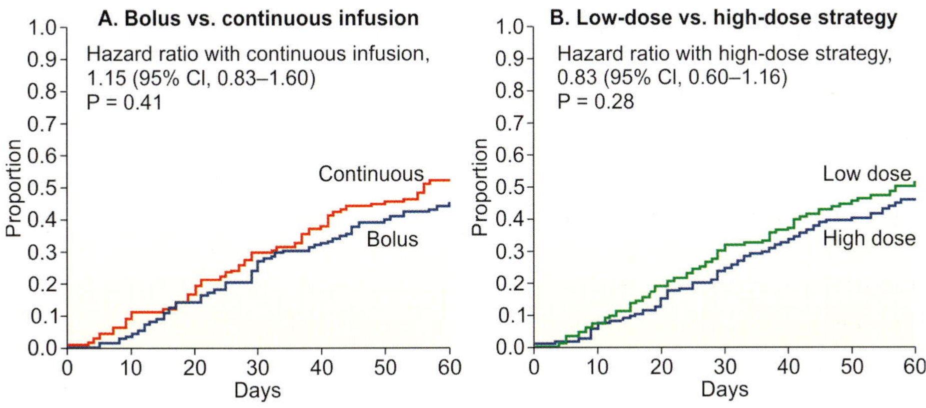

Figure 3A and B: Diuretic Optimization Strategies Evaluation (DOSE) trial[18]

COMBINATION THERAPY

In patients with high-dose diuretic requirements or worsening response due to diuretic resistance, combination therapy can be employed to increase diuretic efficacy. Commonly, metolazone or HCTZ is added as a single dose to the scheduled loop diuretic dosing.[19] This combination has proved efficacious in multiple conditions including heart failure, liver disease independent of age.[20],[21] This strategy employs a sequential blockade of the electrolyte transporters which counteracts the chronic adaptions of the nephrons to previously prescribed diuretic therapy. Although this strategy has never tested in large randomized clinical trials, smaller studies of up to 300 patients have demonstrated positive outcomes.[22]

Optimal candidates for combination therapy include those with advanced kidney disease, high oral dose requirements of loop diuretics, and those with advanced heart failure with multiple repeated hospitalizations as well as those with acute decompensation refractory to IV diuretics. Such combination therapy also requires consideration of patients' electrolyte status as arrhythmogenic complications from hypokalemia can occur and are preventable with adequate supplementation or use of potassium-sparing diuretic therapy.[23]

ADVERSE EFFECTS

Diuretics are effective agents for volume control in patients with heart failure. However, this potent effect comes at the cost of several common side effects. In addition to the expected volume depletion, several electrolyte perturbans are commonly identified. These include difficulty with maintenance of adequate serum potassium concentration. Hyponatremia which is often multifactorial in patients with heart failure can be exacerbated. Additionally, magnesium and calcium irregularities can also occur. Uric acid levels leading to hyperuricemia, which can exacerbate underlying crystalloid arthritides (gout) has also been identified as a potential complication. Lastly, dose-related ototoxicity is a well-known complication which requires careful monitoring due to potential for permanent damage.

As expected, any agent that results in the net loss of fluid will result in the reduction of intravascular volume with associated clinical findings. Overdiuresis can frequently lead to states of hypoperfusion, especially in the elderly or patients who are dependent or debilitated. Clinical sequelae from the organ affected due to hypoperfusion can lead to some very common presentations. These include acute renal failure, hypotension with altered mentation which is often compounded if patient is on concurrent antihypertensive therapy. Additionally, factors such as limited fluid intake, fluid loss from diarrhea, or other systemic illness can further compromise the normal intravascular volume. Also, initiation and/or uptitration of RAAS blocking drugs can be associated with hypotension, especially in certain patients who have an overactive RAAS phenomenon secondary to diuresis. This scenario can be easily remedied with the use of gentle fluid hydration with isotonic saline or increased oral intake.

Hypokalemia is one of the most frequent complications of diuretic therapy.[24] Physiological design of the nephron and the effect of aldosterone are responsible for this finding. Decreased absorption of the sodium establishes an increased sodium gradient in the nephron which leads to increased potassium secretion when this sodium load reaches the distal part of the nephron. Additionally, volume depletion leads to increased secretion of aldosterone in an attempt to retain sodium and that leads to further potassium loss.[25] Loss of chloride ion has also been implicated as potential reason for hypokalemia. Higher doses of diuretics are generally associated with lower potassium levels. However, a direct dose response cannot be clearly established because of variability in diet, effect of other concurrent factors, such as medication and other active disease processes.

The threshold of treatment of hypokalemia in patients with diuretic therapy is often determined by a number of factors. These include serum potassium concentration, where generally potassium level less than 3.5 mmol/L indicates significantly decreased potassium stores. Additionally, cardiac arrhythmogenic complications due to hypokalemia especially in patients on digitalis glycosides often require acute and chronic treatment to maintain adequate levels. Another option depending on compelling indication is an addition of potassium-sparing diuretic or aldosterone-blocking agent which can counteract the expected potassium loss. Irrespective of the strategy, close clinical monitoring of the patient is required to achieve the desired diuresis and to minimize electrolyte complications.

Uric acid levels can be adversely affected by use of diuretic therapy.[26] Although most patients with diuretic-induced hyperuricemia are asymptomatic, an attack of gout can be precipitated on the initiation of diuretic therapy.[27] Diuretic therapy can often be continued with acute treatment of the gout episode and monitoring of uric acid level trends.

Hyponatremia in patients treated with heart failure is associated with adverse outcome.[28] No single factor can be identified and it is likely a result of multiple systems acting on the kidney that interfere with fluid excretion. Diuretics can exacerbate hyponatremia because alterations in concentration gradient can impair urinary diluting ability.

Ototoxicity is another serious complication of high-dose loop diuretic therapy and failure to recognize can lead to permanent sensory damage. Toxicity is presumed to be mediated by alteration in the electrochemical gradients in the lymphatics of the inner ear. Toxicity is directly related to the level and rate of accumulation of the diuretic in the serum. Rapid bolus injection or large amounts of daily dosing increases the likelihood of ototoxicity. Empirical data indicates that this damage is most often reversible if it is recognized in a timely fashion and the diuretic held or reduced. Additionally, it is much more common with older diuretic ethacrynic acid instead of furosemide or bumetanide.

DIURETIC RESISTANCE

Diuretic use is associated with two important physiological phenomena which are important to understand when utilizing diuretics for chronic therapy. These include the diuretic braking phenomenon and the development of diuretic resistance with longer duration of therapy. These are not independent mechanisms, but likely a combination or interrelated adaptation in response to the diuretic therapy.[29]

After initial diuretic treatment, the repeated dose of the diuretic results in the retention of sodium in order to compensate for the volume contraction. This results in decreasing natriuresis following each administration with an eventual return to preadministration levels. Additionally, over the long-term, many adaptations in the tubular microchannels result in decreasing efficacy of the diuretic with requirements for higher dosing and the need for continuous or concurrent administration of the another diuretic to maintain effective response.[30] Therefore, patients on stable doses who begin to require titration of their current therapy may be candidates for the above-mentioned combination therapy or with alternative approaches for maintenance of euvolemic state.

CARDIORENAL SYNDROME

Adverse effects on kidney function in patients with heart failure have led to an emerging concept of cardiorenal syndrome. It is considered to be a complex process that is likely multifactorial in etiology.[31] Several of these factors can be attributed to concurrent diuretic use. Experimental studies have indicated that use of diuretics is associated with increased stimulation of the renal-angiotensin syndrome with increased levels of aldosterone. Animal studies have demonstrated that these changes can lead to increased renal fibrosis.[32] Additionally, other physiological factors, such as anemia, increased sympathetic tone, oxidative stress, and endothelial dysfunction are under investigation as potential therapeutic targets for reduction in cardiorenal syndrome, because they are associated with detrimental vascular changes within the kidneys in patient with heart failure.[33,34] Therefore, neurohormonal consequences of diuretics need to be understood and appropriate therapy with RAAS blocking agents needs to be implemented concurrently with diuretic use to mitigate the chronic and often irreversible deterioration of the renal system, which is essential in maintaining volume control in patients with heart failure.

VAPTANS

Continued investigation has led to development of several newer classes of diuretics which will likely play a significant role in the future management of patients with heart failure. predominant among these is the development of vasopressin antagonists known as the vaptans.[35] Additionally, active research has led to development of adenosine receptor antagonists, which have been evaluated in clinical trials.[36]

Arginine vasopressin is released from the neurohypophysis in response to changes in plasma tonicity and volume and plays a key role in regulation of total body water content.[37] There are three types of vasopressin receptors: (1) V1a on the vascular smooth muscle, (2) V1b which has a general distribution, and (3) V2 which is expressed predominantly on the principal cells of the renal-collecting-duct system.[38] Stimulation of the V2 receptor leads to addition of aquaporin channels, which increases free water absorption and decreases osmolarity.[39] Pathological activation of this mechanism plays a significant role in development of hyponatremia in patients with heart failure. This has been associated with adverse outcomes in patients with chronic heart failure.[40,41] Recently, vasopressin antagonist tolvaptan and conivaptan have been approved for use in patients with congestive heart failure and hyponatremia.[42]

Tolvaptan has been evaluation in several randomized clinical trials/studies in patients with heart failure. The first double blind randomized trial in 254 patients demonstrated decreased edema and reduction in body weight and improvement in serum sodium levels without any significant adverse effects.[43] Tolvaptan demonstrated similar results in a follow-up trial where 319 patients with acute exacerbation of congestive heart failure requiring heart failure were treated in addition to standard therapies.[44]

These encouraging results led to a large multicenter phase III Efficacy of Vasopressin Antagonist in Heart Failure: Outcome Study With Tolvaptan (EVEREST) trial in which 4,133 patients were evaluated for short-term and long-term outcomes after treatment with 30 mg tolvaptan within 48 hours of admission of heart failure.[45] In short-term assessment on day 7 and at the time of discharge, patients receiving tolvaptan had greater reduction in weight loss (average 0.8 kg) and better improvement in patient assessed dyspnea. Serious adverse events were similar in both groups with no effect noted on heart rate or blood pressure.[46] In the long-term analysis with median follow-up of 9.9 months, tolvaptan did not result in any long-term mortality or morbidity benefit in patients with heart failure.[47]

Effect of tolvaptan on left ventricular remodeling and function in patient with heart failure were also assessed in the Multicenter Evaluation of Tolvaptan Effect On Remodeling (METEOR) trial.[48] However, there was no improvement in left ventricular volumes or ejection fraction over 1 year. Lastly, use of tolvaptan to correct hyponatremia from cirrhosis, heart failure, or Syndrome of Inappropriate Antidiuretic Hormone Secretion (SIADH) in euvolemic or hypervolemic patients of any causes have been evaluated in the Study of Ascending Levels of Tolvaptan in Hyponatremia 1 and 2 (SALT 1-2) trials.[42] This trial demonstrated normalization of hyponatremia in higher percentage of patient taking tolvaptan versus placebo (55% vs. 25%). Also, small improvements were noted in patients' mental health. Whether this improvement in sodium level leads to long-term benefit in heart failure patients is unknown.

An IV form of vasopressin antagonist conivaptan is also available. It antagonizes both V1a/V2 receptors.[49] Conivaptan has been studied in a several trials in heart failure patients.[50] In this study dose, patients with New York Heart Association (NYHA) class III/IV with acute decompensated heart failure had a dose dependent decrease in pulmonary capillary wedge pressure and right atrial pressure. In more recent trial, conivaptan did not show any improvement in respiratory status after 48 hours of therapy, but was associated with increased urine output.[51] Additional vaptans, such as satavaptan and lixivaptan are under development to enhance specific pharmacological properties (i.e., half-life's) for future treatment of heart failure.[52,53]

The most common side effects of the vaptans include thirst, dry mouth, hypernatremia, and polyuria. Rapid improvement in hyponatremia can lead to a fatal complication known as osmotic demyelination syndrome.[54] This results for damage to neuronal cells from rapidly changed volume shifts due to plasma tonicity. Presentation can range from subtle neurological defects to generalized seizure with permanent neurological sequelae.[55] As per the recommendation of an expert panel, patients' serum potassium levels should be monitored to ensure slow correction, with ideal rate of 8–10 mmol/L per 24 hour.[56]

Currently, the role of vaptans continues to evolve in treatment of heart failure. In chronic heart failure patients, the only acceptable indication for treatment is difficult to control hyponatremia (<115–120 mmol/L) despite standard therapy. There is no clear benefit for treatment of acute symptoms or for chronic therapy to reduce cardiovascular end-points in heart failure patients. One benefit that was noted in *ad hoc* analysis was the reduction in the amount of diuretic dose required to achieve a euvolemic state, but this needs to further validated in future trials.[46]

ADENOSINE RECEPTOR ANTAGONIST

Adenosine is an important regulator of renal blood flow and glomerular filtration rate. It also has direct effects on the luminal absorption of sodium in the proximal tubules.[57] Goal of blocking this receptor led to development of a novel A1 receptor antagonist rolofylline. This was shown to have diuretic and natriuretic properties in animal models as well as renoprotective effect in ambulatory patients.[58,59] A small phase II pilot study showed 22% increase in urine output and trend towards reduction in 60-day mortality and readmission for heart failure.[36] Another study also showed improvement in pulmonary artery pressure with no change in renal function and improvement in diuresis.[60]

The pivotal phase III study to further evaluate rolofylline was the Placebo-Controlled Randomized Study of the Selective A1 Adenosine Receptor Antagonist Rolofylline for Patients Hospitalized with Acute Decompensated Heart Failure and Volume Overload to Assess Treatment Effect on Congestion and Renal Function (PROTECT) trial.[61] Rolofylline did not have a favorable effect for the composite end-point of treatment success as defined by patient reported improvement in dyspnea 24–48 hours after administration of the medication. Additionally, it did not improve renal function or 60-day outcomes. It was also associated with higher incidence of seizures and stroke. Therefore, at this time, there is no role for this medicine in treatment of heart failure.

GUIDELINES

Clear recommendations for diuretic therapy have been issued in the guidelines from the Heart Failure Society of America regarding use in acute and chronic heart failure. In chronic care, loop diuretics are recommended as the class I agents to control fluid and relieve congestion with level of evidence A for oral and IV therapy. Thiazide-type diuretics are described as the second-line agents with class I and level of evidence B. Combination therapy carries a class II and level of evidence C. In cases of acute decompensation, the society recommends IV therapy with loop diuretic as class I with level of evidence B.

CONCLUSION

Diuretic therapy is an essential component for control of heart failure symptoms and to prevent the morbidity and mortality associated with this condition. They are effective agents which cause diuresis by altering the osmotic gradients in the kidney and help to generate net fluid loss. Newer agents indirectly counteract regulatory hormones or directly block the receptor sites in the kidneys. Liver and kidney disease can affect the pharmacological properties and patients profile needs to be evaluated prior to their application.

Different routes of administration are available depending on the clinical presentation and no particular type of administration has been shown to be superior to others in patients with heart failure. Prolonged use can result in resistance and requires application in combinations and the titration of dosing to get the desired effect.

These agents are not risk-free and close patient monitoring is necessary for successful application. Hypokalemia is the most frequent electrolyte abnormality which can be associated with significant mortality due to risk of arrhythmia if not properly recognized. Additionally, improvement of hyponatremia by newer agents requires close monitoring to prevent pontine myelinosis. Over time, the effectiveness of the diuretic therapy is diminished due to adverse remodeling of the renal system from hormonal disturbances due to heart failure. This entity known as the cardiorenal system can make it difficult to control patients volume status with diuretics. However, proper use of diuretic therapy with concurrently aggressive heart failure treatment with RAAS blockade can ensure effectiveness of diuretics.

Newer agents, such as vasopressin antagonist tolvaptan are now available to help treat hyponatremia from chronic fluid overload states in heart failure. The clinical practice guidelines have also recognized the use of diuretics of different combinations and in different scenarios and have given strong and specific recommendations to advance evidence-based care of heart failure patients.

In summary, diuretics were the first agents to be utilized in the care of patients with heart failure. Proper understanding of their role and applying them in an evidence-based manner will help reduce the burden of heart failure for our society.

REFERENCES

1. Vargo DL, Kramer WG, Black PK, et al. Bioavailability, pharmacokinetics, and pharmacodynamics of torsemide and furosemide in patients with congestive heart failure. Clin Pharmacol Ther. 1995;57(6):601-9.
2. Brater DC, Leinfelder J, Anderson SA. Clinical pharmacology of torasemide, a new loop diuretic. Clin Pharmacol Ther. 1987;42(2):187-92.
3. Brater DC, Chennavasin P, Day B, et al. Bumetanide and furosemide. Clin Pharmacol Ther. 1983;34(2):207-13.
4. Welling PG. Pharmacokinetics of the thiazide diuretics. Biopharm Drug Dispos. 1986;7(6):501-35.
5. Beermann B, Groschinsky-Grind M, Rosén A. Absorption, metabolism, and excretion of hydrochlorothiazide. Clin Pharmacol Ther. 1976;19(5 Pt 1):531-7.

6. Chennavasin P, Seiwell R, Brater DC. Pharmacokinetic-dynamic analysis of the indomethacin-furosemide interaction in man. J Pharmacol Exp Ther. 1980;215(1):77-81.
7. Chennavasin P, Seiwell R, Brater DC, et al. Pharmacodynamic analysis of the furosemide-probenecid interaction in man. Kidney Int. 1979;16(2):187-95.
8. Cook JA, Smith DE, Cornish LA, et al. Kinetics, dynamics, and bioavailability of bumetanide in healthy subjects and patients with congestive heart failure. Clin Pharmacol Ther. 1988;44(5):487-500.
9. Brater DC. Diuretic therapy. N Engl J Med. 1998;339(6):387-95.
10. Huang CM, Atkinson AJ, Levin M, et al. Pharmacokinetics of furosemide in advanced renal failure. Clin Pharmacol Ther. 1974;16(4):659-66.
11. Hou W, Sanyal AJ. Ascites: diagnosis and management. Med Clin North Am. 2009;93(4): 801-17.
12. Fuller R, Hoppel C, Ingalls ST. Furosemide kinetics in patients with hepatic cirrhosis with ascites. Clin Pharmacol Ther. 1981;30(4):461-7.
13. Villeneuve JP, Verbeeck RK, Wilkinson GR, et al. Furosemide kinetics and dynamics in patients with cirrhosis. Clin Pharmacol Ther. 1986;40(1):14-20.
14. Mielniczuk LM, Tsang SW, Desai AS, et al. The association between high-dose diuretics and clinical stability in ambulatory chronic heart failure patients. J Card Fail. 2008;14(5):388-93.
15. Thomson MR, Nappi JM, Dunn SP, et al. Continuous versus intermittent infusion of furosemide in acute decompensated heart failure. J Card Fail. 2010;16(3):188-93.
16. Dormans TP, van Meyel JJ, Gerlag PG, et al. Diuretic efficacy of high dose furosemide in severe heart failure: bolus injection versus continuous infusion. J Am Coll Cardiol. 1996;28(2):376-82.
17. Allen LA, Turer AT, Dewald T, et al. Continuous versus bolus dosing of furosemide for patients hospitalized for heart failure. Am J Cardiol. 2010;105(12):1794-7.
18. Felker GM, Lee KL, Bull DA, et al. Diuretic strategies in patients with acute decompensated heart failure. N Engl J Med. 2011;364(9):797-805.
19. Sica DA. Metolazone and its role in edema management. Congest Heart Fail. 2003;9(2): 100-5.
20. Ghose RR, Gupta SK. Synergistic action of metolazone with "loop" diuretics. Br Med J (Clin Res Ed). 1981;282(6274):1432-3.
21. Brater DC, Pressley RH, Anderson SA. Mechanisms of the synergistic combination of metolazone and bumetanide. J Pharmacol Exp Ther. 1985;233(1):70-4.
22. Jentzer JC, DeWald TA, Hernandez AF. Combination of loop diuretics with thiazide-type diuretics in heart failure. J Am Coll Cardiol. 2010;56(19):1527-34.
23. Cooper HA, Dries DL, Davis CE, et al. Diuretics and risk of arrhythmic death in patients with left ventricular dysfunction. Circulation. 1999;100(12):1311-5.
24. Greenberg A. Diuretic complications. Am J Med Sci. 2000;319(1):10-24.
25. Tannen RL. Diuretic-induced hypokalemia. Kidney Int. 1985;28(6):988-1000.
26. Helgeland A, Hjermann I, Holme I, et al. Serum triglycerides and serum uric acid in untreated and thiazide-treated patients with mild hypertension. The Oslo study. Am J Med. 1978;64(1):34-8.
27. Johnson MW, Mitch WE. The risks of asymptomatic hyperuricaemia and the use of uricosuric diuretics. Drugs. 1981;21(3):220-5.
28. Klein L, O'Connor CM, Leimberger JD, et al. Lower serum sodium is associated with increased short-term mortality in hospitalized patients with worsening heart failure: results from the Outcomes of a Prospective Trial of Intravenous Milrinone for Exacerbations of Chronic Heart Failure (OPTIME-CHF) study. Circulation. 2005;111(19):2454-60.

29. Stanton BA, Kaissling B. Adaptation of distal tubule and collecting duct to increased Na delivery. II. Na^+ and K^+ transport. Am J Physiol. 1988;255(6 Pt 2):F1269-75.
30. Kobayashi S, Clemmons DR, Nogami H, et al. Tubular hypertrophy due to work load induced by furosemide is associated with increases of IGF-1 and IGFBP-1. Kidney Int. 1995;47(3):818-28.
31. Bock JS, Gottlieb SS. Cardiorenal syndrome: new perspectives. Circulation. 2010;121(23): 2592-600.
32. Brilla CG, Pick R, Tan LB, et al. Remodeling of the rat right and left ventricles in experimental hypertension. Cir Res. 1990;67(6):1355-64.
33. Vesey DA, Cheung C, Pat B, et al. Erythropoietin protects against ischaemic acute renal injury. Nephrol Dial Transplant. 2004;19(2):348-55.
34. Tojo A, Onozato ML, Kobayashi N, et al. Angiotensin II and oxidative stress in Dahl Salt-sensitive rat with heart failure. Hypertension. 2002;40(6):834-9.
35. Decaux G, Soupart A, Vassart G. Non-peptide arginine-vasopressin antagonists: the vaptans. Lancet. 2008;371(9624):1624-32.
36. Cotter G, Dittrich HC, Weatherley BD, et al. The PROTECT pilot study: a randomized, placebo-controlled, dose-finding study of the adenosine A1 receptor antagonist rolofylline in patients with acute heart failure and renal impairment. J Card Fail. 2008; 14(8):631-40.
37. Ring RH. The central vasopressinergic system: examining the opportunities for psychiatric drug development. Curr Pharm Des. 2005;11(2):205-25.
38. Bankir L. Antidiuretic action of vasopressin: quantitative aspects and interaction between V1a and V2 receptor-mediated effects. Cardiovasc Res. 2001;51(3):372-90.
39. Pouzet B, Serradeil-Le Gal C, Bouby N, et al. Selective blockade of vasopressin V2 receptors reveals significant V2-mediated water reabsorption in Brattleboro rats with diabetes insipidus. Nephrol Dial Transplant. 2001;16(4):725-34.
40. Gheorghiade M, Abraham WT, Albert NM, et al. Relationship between admission serum sodium concentration and clinical outcomes in patients hospitalized for heart failure: an analysis from the OPTIMIZE-HF registry. Eur Heart J. 2007;28(8):980-8.
41. Bettari L, Fiuzat M, Felker GM, et al. Significance of hyponatremia in heart failure. Heart Fail Rev. 2012;17(1):17-26.
42. Schrier RW, Gross P, Gheorghiade M, et al. Tolvaptan, a selective oral vasopressin V2-receptor antagonist, for hyponatremia. N Engl J Med. 2006;355(20):2099-112.
43. Gheorghiade M, Niazi I, Ouyang J, et al. Vasopressin V2-receptor blockade with tolvaptan in patients with chronic heart failure: results from a double-blind, randomized trial. Circulation. 2003;107(21):2690-6.
44. Gheorghiade M, Gattis WA, O'Connor CM, et al. Effects of tolvaptan, a vasopressin antagonist, in patients hospitalized with worsening heart failure: a randomized controlled trial. JAMA. 2004;291(16):1963-71.
45. Gheorghiade M, Orlandi C, Burnett JC, et al. Rationale and design of the multicenter, randomized, double-blind, placebo-controlled study to evaluate the Efficacy of Vasopressin antagonism in Heart Failure: Outcome Study with Tolvaptan (EVEREST). J Card Fail. 2005;11(4):260-9.
46. Gheorghiade M, Konstam MA, Burnett JC, et al. Short-term clinical effects of tolvaptan, an oral vasopressin antagonist, in patients hospitalized for heart failure: the EVEREST Clinical Status Trials. JAMA. 2007;297(12):1332-43.
47. Konstam MA, Gheorghiade M, Burnett JC, et al. Effects of oral tolvaptan in patients hospitalized for worsening heart failure: the EVEREST Outcome Trial. JAMA. 2007;297(12):1319-31.

48. Udelson JE, McGrew FA, Flores E, et al. Multicenter, randomized, double-blind, placebo-controlled study on the effect of oral tolvaptan on left ventricular dilation and function in patients with heart failure and systolic dysfunction. J Am Coll Cardiol. 2007;49(22):2151-9.
49. Ghali JK, Koren MJ, Taylor JR, et al. Efficacy and safety of oral conivaptan: a V1A/V2 vasopressin receptor antagonist, assessed in a randomized, placebo-controlled trial in patients with euvolemic or hypervolemic hyponatremia. J Clin Endocrinol Metab. 2006;91(6):2145-52.
50. Udelson JE, Smith WB, Hendrix GH, et al. Acute hemodynamic effects of conivaptan, a dual V(1A) and V(2) vasopressin receptor antagonist, in patients with advanced heart failure. Circulation. 2001;104(20):2417-23.
51. Goldsmith SR, Elkayam U, Haught WH, et al. Efficacy and safety of the vasopressin V1A/V2-receptor antagonist conivaptan in acute decompensated heart failure: a dose-ranging pilot study. J Card Fail. 2008;14(8):641-7.
52. Abraham WT, Shamshirsaz AA, McFann K, et al. Aquaretic effect of lixivaptan, an oral, non-peptide, selective V2 receptor vasopressin antagonist, in New York Heart Association functional class II and III chronic heart failure patients. J Am Coll Cardiol. 2006;47(8):1615-21.
53. Soupart A, Gross P, Legros JJ, et al. Successful long-term treatment of hyponatremia in syndrome of inappropriate antidiuretic hormone secretion with satavaptan (SR121463B), an orally active nonpeptide vasopressin V2-receptor antagonist. Clin J Am Soc Nephrol. 2006;1(6):1154-60.
54. King JD, Rosner MH. Osmotic demyelination syndrome. Am J Med Sci. 2010;339(6):561-7.
55. Lampl C, Yazdi K. Central pontine myelinolysis. Eur Neurol. 2002;47(1):3-10.
56. Verbalis JG, Goldsmith SR, Greenberg A, et al. Hyponatremia treatment guidelines 2007: expert panel recommendations. Am J Med. 2007;120(11 Suppl 1):S1-21.
57. Vallon V, Mühlbauer B, Osswald H. Adenosine and kidney function. Physiol Rev. 2006;86(3):901-40.
58. Yao K, Ina Y, Nagashima K, et al. Effect of the selective adenosine A1-receptor antagonist KW-3902 on lipopolysaccharide-induced reductions in urine volume and renal blood flow in anesthetized dogs. Jpn J Pharmacol. 2000;84(3):310-5.
59. Dittrich HC, Gupta DK, Hack TC, et al. The effect of KW-3902, an adenosine A1 receptor antagonist, on renal function and renal plasma flow in ambulatory patients with heart failure and renal impairment. J Card Fail. 2007;13(8):609-17.
60. Ponikowski P, Mitrovic V, O'Connor CM, et al. Haemodynamic effects of rolofylline in the treatment of patients with heart failure and impaired renal function. Eur J Heart Fail. 2010;12(11):1238-46.
61. Massie BM, O'Connor CM, Metra M, et al. Rolofylline, an adenosine A1-receptor antagonist, in acute heart failure. N Engl J Med. 2010;363(15):1419-28.

CHAPTER

3

Guideline Based Standard Therapy for Heart Failure: The Role of RAAS Blockers and Beta Blockers

Prakash C Deedwania, Enrique Carbajal

INTRODUCTION

Heart failure (HF) is associated with increased morbidity and mortality. With the improved survival of patients with myocardial infarction (MI), those with long-standing hypertension as well as increased life expectancy, it is likely that prevalence of HF will escalate further in the coming years. In general, the prognosis of patients with HF can be worse than many cancers, however, with the increasing use of guideline recommended therapies, such as neurohormonal blockade, there has been considerable improvement in the prognosis of patients with HF. During the last several decades, many studies have demonstrated the benefits of treatment with angiotensin converting enzyme inhibitors (ACEIs) or angiotensin receptor blockers (ARBs) and beta-blocking (BB) drugs.[1,2] Based on the evidence available from well-designed randomized controlled trials (RCT), various national and international guidelines have now established specific recommendations for the use of renin angiotensin aldosterone system (RAAS) blockers and beta blocking agents in HF.[1,2]

In the following section, we will review the evidence supporting the use of RAAS blockers and BB agents in patients with HF secondary to left ventricular (LV) systolic dysfunction.

GUIDELINE-BASED THERAPY FOR HEART FAILURE

Because HF is a progressive disorder early identification of those at risk of developing signs and symptoms of HF is of critical importance. The most recent ACC/AHA guidelines (Fig. 1) have emphasized identification of individuals in stages A/B of HF with the goal of early intervention to prevent progressive deterioration in cardiac dysfunction and subsequent prevention of symptomatic HF. Stage A patients are those who have risk factors [e.g., those with hypertension (HTN), diabetes mellitus (DM), obesity, coronary artery disease (CAD), etc.] that can subsequently lead to cardiac dysfunction and development of HF. Treatment of these underlying risk factors should attenuate/prevent the subsequent development of cardiac dysfunction.

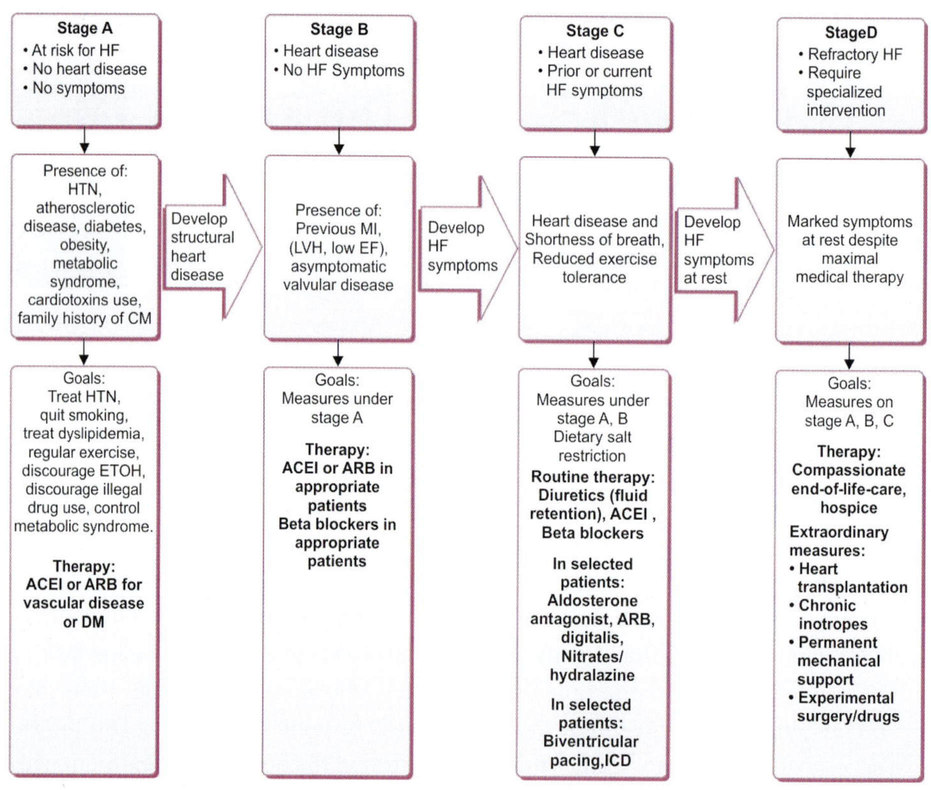

Figure 1: Staging of heart failure and recommended therapy at various stages. HF, heart failure; HTN, hypertension; CM, cardiomyopathy; LVH, left ventricular hypertrophy; EF, ejection fraction; MI, myocardial infarction; ETOH, alcohol; ACEI, angiotensin converting enzyme inhibitor; ARB, angiotensin receptor blocker; DM, diabetes mellitus; ICD, implantable cardioverter-defibrillator.

Source: *Adapted from* Hunt SA, et al. 2009 Focused update incorporated into the ACC/AHA 2005 guidelines for the diagnosis and management of heart failure in adults. Circulation. 2009;119:e391-479.

Stage B patients are those who have LV hypertrophy and/or impaired LV function but who are still asymptomatic. Early intervention with neurohormonal blockers with RAAS blockers and BB as appropriate should prevent the process of cardiac remodeling and further progression of LV dysfunction. The stage C denotes patients who have developed symptoms of HF due to the underlying cardiac dysfunction and require treatment for both symptoms of HF as well as improvement of the related adverse prognosis. Stage D patients are those who have significantly advanced and/or refractory HF who are generally candidates for specialized advanced treatment strategies including mechanical support devices, inotropic drugs, and consideration for cardiac transplantation and/or other surgical procedures.

The drugs that have proved to be unequivocally beneficial in prolonging survival and improving symptoms in patients with LV systolic dysfunction and HF are primarily those that block the heightened neuroendocrine activity and include RAAS, blocking drugs (ACEIs, ARBs, and ARB agents), and beta blocking agents. Although diuretics are frequently used and necessary in patients with congestive symptoms with fluid accumulation, there is no evidence that the chronic use of diuretic therapy improves survival. Furthermore, it is important to keep in mind that appropriate therapy for myocardial ischemia when present in the setting of HF is also associated with improved clinical outcome.

In this chapter, we will primarily focus on guideline-based therapy focused on neurohormonal blockade of the RAAS and sympatho-adrenergic systems. As shown in figure 2, both RAAS and sympathetic nervous system (SNS) are activated with the onset of myocardial dysfunction in response to decreased cardiac output. Initially, such a response is adaptive and helps to maintain adequate tissue perfusion of vital organs by causing peripheral vasoconstriction. However, continued chronic activation of RAAS and SNS has significant adverse consequences due to continued peripheral vasoconstriction, sodium retention and hemodynamic alterations (Fig. 3). In addition, activation of these systems, in particular the RAAS, has been shown to be associated with progressive myocardial remodeling which leads to worsening LV dysfunction. Because of the critical role of these neuroendocrine alterations in the pathophysiology of LV dysfunction and HF, there has been continued effort during the past several decades to use agents

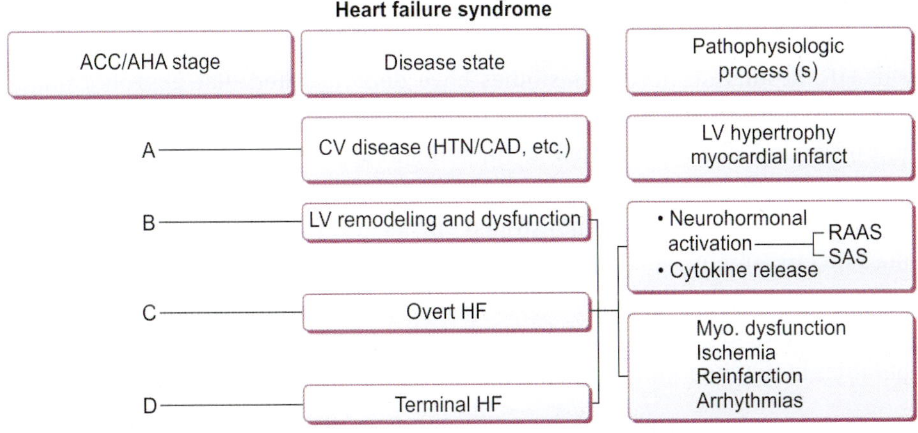

Figure 2: Various ACC/AHA stages of heart failure, the corresponding cardiovascular disease/ alterations and the underlying pathophysiology showing activation of RAAS and SAS with onset of LV dysfunction and related consequences. ACA, American College of Cardiology; AHA, American Heart Association; CV, cardiovascular; HTN, hypertension; CAD, coronary artery disease; LV, left ventricle; RAAS, renin angiotensin aldosterone system; SAS, sympathetic adrenergic system; HF, heart failure; Myo., myocardial.

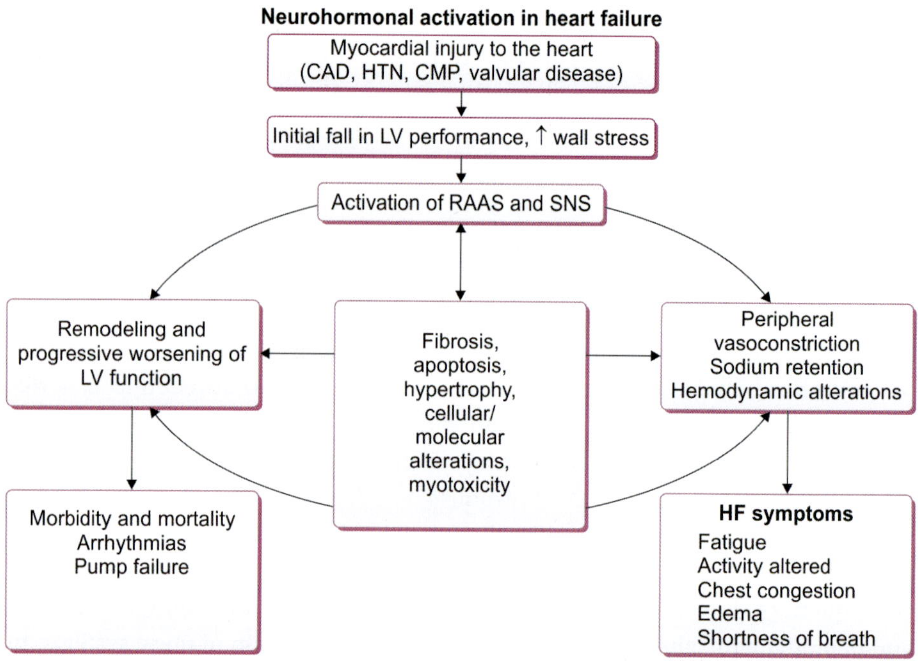

Figure 3: Importance of RAAS and SNS activation in pathophysiologic process of heart failure. RAAS, renin angiotensin aldosterone system; SNS, sympathetic nervous system; CAD, coronary artery disease; HTN, hypertension; CMP, cardiomyopathy; LV, left ventricle; ↑, increased; HF, heart failure.

effective in blocking the RAAS and SNS systems in an effort to not only improve the symptoms but also decrease associated morbidity and mortality in patients with HF. Results of numerous studies have demonstrated that neurohormonal blockade of RAAS and sympatho-adrenergic systems controls symptoms of HF, improves clinical status as well as functional capacity, enhances sense of well being, and reduces the associated morbidity and mortality in patients with HF.[3-10] It is because of these well-demonstrated effects of RAAS blocking drugs and beta blockers, treatment with these drugs is now recommended by all guidelines across the world for all patients with HF. In the following sections, we provide the pathophysiologic rationale and practical consideration for clinical use of these therapies in patients with HF.

RENIN ANGIOTENSIN ALDOSTERONE SYSTEM BLOCKING DRUGS

Angiotensin-Converting Enzyme Inhibitors

Angiotensin-converting enzyme inhibitors are the best studied class of drugs in patients with HF, with multiple beneficial effects. ACEI should be prescribed for all patients with LV dysfunction and HF unless there is a contraindication for their use or there is prior history of intolerance due to significant adverse experience with these agents. Because of the well-demonstrated survival benefit even in patients with asymptomatic LV dysfunction treatment with ACEI should not be delayed.

In patients with HF, inhibition of angiotensin-converting enzyme by ACEI produces a moderate increase in cardiac output with a concomitant significant decrease in right and left ventricular filling pressures, pulmonary and systemic vascular resistances, and mean arterial pressure without increasing the heart rate. It is not established whether these effects of ACEI are entirely due to the suppression of angiotensin-II production or increased bioavailability of bradykinin which augments kinin mediated prostaglandin production (Fig. 4). ACEIs have additional beneficial effects including reduction of ventricular arrhythmias, decreased end-systolic and end-diastolic dimensions, and improvements in symptoms, exercise duration, and quality of life.

Angiotensin-converting enzyme inhibitors have been evaluated in a number of RCTs in patients in various stages of HF.[3-9] These trials have consistently shown a significant reduction in mortality rates (Table 1).[3-9] Most trials enrolled patients

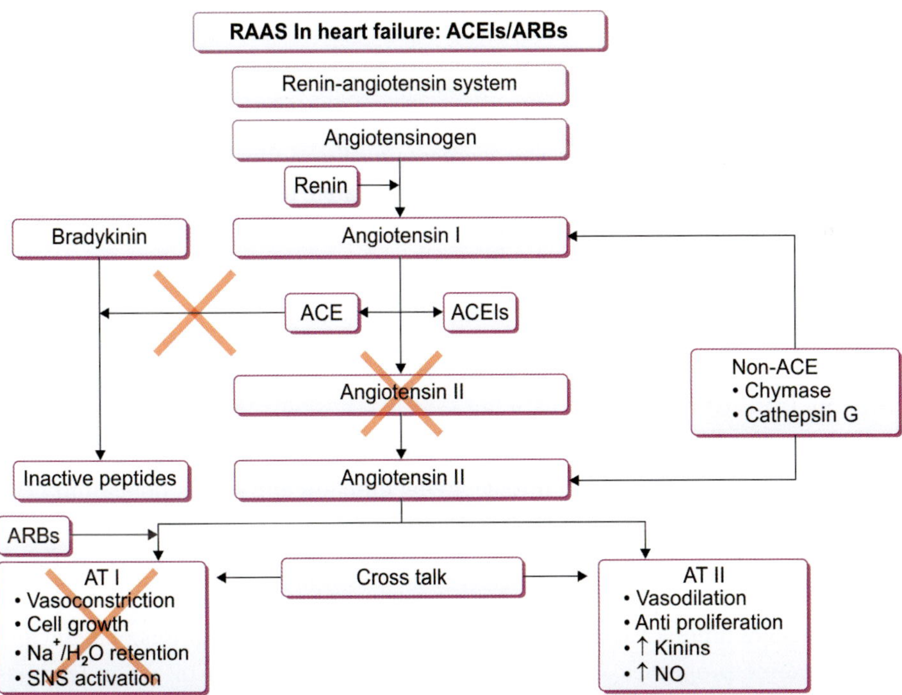

Figure 4: Mechanism of action of angiotensin converting enzyme inhibitors and angiotensin receptor blockers. RAAS, renin angiotensin aldosterone system; ACEIs, angiotensin converting enzyme inhibitors; ARBs, angiotensin receptor blockers; ATI-II, angiotensin II types I-II; Na^+, sodium; H_2O, water; SNS, sympathetic nervous system; ↑, increased; NO, nitric oxide.

Table 1 **Summary of results from various studies showing effects of angiotensin converting enzyme inhibitors on mortality**

Trial	*Mortality* *ACEI (%)*	*Controls*	*(%) RR (95% CI)*
Heart failure			
CONSENSUS I	39	54	0.56 (0.34–0.91)
SOLVD (Treatment)	35	40	0.82 (0.70–0.97)
SOLVD (Prevention)	15	16	0.92 (0.79–1.08)
Postmyocardial infarction			
SAVE (Captopril)	20	25	0.81 (0.68–0.97)
AIRE (Ramipril)	17	23	0.73 (0.60–0.89)
TRACE (Trandolapril)	35	42	0.78 (0.67–0.91)
SMILE (Zofenopril)	5	6.5	0.75 (0.40–1.11)

ACEI, angiotensin converting enzyme inhibitor; RR, relative risk; CI, confidence interval; CONSENSUS, Co-operative North Scandinavian Enalapril Survival Study; SOLVD, studies of left ventricular dysfunction; MI, myocardial infarction; SAVE, survival and ventricular enlargement; AIRE, acute infarction ramipril efficacy; TRACE, TRAndolapril Cardiac Evaluation; SMILE, survival of myocardial infarction long-term evaluation.

with reduced left ventricular ejection fraction (LVEF <35–40%) who were already being treated with diuretics with or without digitalis and in many trials patients were also getting vasodilating drugs. The aggregate results of these studies demonstrate a reduction in mortality of 20–25% in those treated with ACEI as compared to control groups. With consistent results seen in these RCTs, there is universal recommendation by all guideline committees to use ACEI in all patients with LV dysfunction and/or HF due to systolic dysfunction.

Practical Considerations Regarding Use of Angiotensin-Converting Enzyme Inhibitors

Treatment with ACEI should generally be initiated at low doses (Table 2) and followed by gradual increase in dosage. Renal function and serum potassium need to be assessed within 1–2 weeks of initiation of ACEIs and periodically thereafter, specifically in patients with preexisting hypotension, hyponatremia, diabetes, and chronic kidney disease [CKD; estimated glomerular filtration rate (eGFR) <60].

Differences among various ACE, are primarily related to pharmacokinetic and hemodynamic properties. Captopril has the shortest duration of action whereas enalapril, lisinopril, and other newer ACEIs have delayed onset of action and prolonged duration of hemodynamic effects. Because of its shorter duration of action, many clinicians prefer to start treatment with captopril specially in hospitalized patients who are ACEI naive and/or fluid depleted (due to excessive diuresis) to

Table 2 **List of evidence-based drugs and their dosage for heart failure**

Drug	*Initial daily dosage*	*Maximum dosage*
Angiotensin-converting enzyme inhibitors		
Captopril	6.25 mg 3 times	50 mg 3 times
Enalapril	2.5 mg twice	10–20 mg twice
Fosinopril	5–10 mg once	40 mg once
Lisinopril	2.5–5 mg once	20–40 mg once
Perindopril	2 mg once	8–16 mg once
Quinapril	5 mg twice	20 mg twice
Ramipril	1.25–2.5 mg once	10 mg once
Trandolapril	1 mg once	4 mg once
Angiotensin receptor blockers		
Candesartan	4–8 mg once	32 mg once
Losartan	25–50 mg once	50–100 mg once
Valsartan	20–40 mg twice	160 mg twice
Aldosterone antagonists		
Spironolactone	12.5–25 mg once	25 mg once or twice
Eplerenone	25 mg once	50 mg once
Beta blockers		
Bisoprolol	1.25 mg once	10 mg once
Carvedilol	3.125 mg twice	25 mg twice; 50 mg twice if >85 kg
Metoprolol succinate extended release (CR/XL)	12.5–25 mg once	200 mg once
Hydralazine/isosorbide dinitrate in combination		
With ACEI/ARB	Hydralazine 75 mg every 8 hours plus isosorbide dinitrate 40 mg every 8 hours	
Without ACEI/ARB	Hydralazine 50 mg every 6 hours plus isosorbide dinitrate 40 mg every 6 hours	

ACEI, angiotensin-converting enzyme inhibitor; mg, milligrams; kg, kilograms; ARB, angiotensin receptor blocker.

Source: *Adapted from* Hunt SA et al. 2009 Focused update incorporated into the ACC/AHA 2005 guidelines for the diagnosis and management of heart failure in adults: a report of the American College of Cardiology Foundation/American Heart Association Task Force on Practice Guidelines. Circulation. 2009;119:e391-479.

avoid the initial risk of hypotension particularly in those patients who have low blood pressure (SBP <80 mmHg). For most patients, stable treatment with longer acting agents starting at low doses should be initiated under careful monitoring. It is important to keep in mind that appropriate stable doses of diuretics need to be maintained in conjunction with the use of ACEI as fluid retention can blunt the therapeutic effects and fluid depletion can potentiate the adverse effects of ACEIs.

Angiotensin-converting enzyme inhibitors use is contraindicated if the patient has previously experienced life threatening adverse reactions (angioedema, anuric renal failure). ACEI should also be used with caution in patients who have low systemic blood pressure (SBP <80 mmHg), markedly increased serum creatinine (>3.0 mg/dL), bilateral renal artery stenosis, or elevated levels of serum potassium (>5.5 mEq/L).

Frequently, question is raised regarding the optimal dose of ACEI in patients with HF. RCTs conducted to evaluate the survival benefit of treatment with ACEI, the dose of ACEI was not determined by the patients' therapeutic response but was rather increased until the target dose or maximally tolerated dose was achieved. Despite this, ACEIs are frequently prescribed in clinical practice at much lower doses that are similar to those recommended for initiation of therapy rather than maintenance of therapy (Table 2). Clinician should generally attempt to use the doses that have been shown to reduce the risk of mortality and other cardiovascular events in RCTs. If the target doses of ACEI cannot be used or are poorly tolerated, intermediate doses should be used. It is also important to note that even though in some cases, symptoms may improve within a few days of starting treatment with ACEI, in general, the clinical response to ACEI is delayed and requires several weeks, months, or longer. Even if symptoms do not improve, long-term treatment with ACEI should be maintained to reduce risk of death or hospitalization.

Many patients with HF who have been previously receiving potassium supplementation in conjunction with diuretic therapy will not need such supplement once they are on adequate doses of ACEI. Therefore, it is important to monitor electrolytes and consider discontinuation of such supplementation at appropriate time. Because it is well known that use of nonsteroidal anti-inflammatory drugs (NSAIDs) can interfere with the favorable effects and enhance adverse effects of ACEI in patients with HF, their use should be avoided and/or minimized whenever possible. Concomitant use of aspirin has also been shown to be associated with decreased effects of ACEIs on cardiovascular morbidity and mortality. However, when all available data are considered the beneficial effects of ACEIs were still present, regardless of concomitant aspirin use, and most physicians now believe that when there is an appropriate indication for aspirin use, there is no harm in continuing it in conjunction with ACEI therapy.

Safety and Adverse Effects of Angiotensin-Converting Enzyme Inhibitors

Most of the adverse reactions of ACEIs are related to their principal pharmacological actions: those related to angiotensin suppression and kinin potentiation and general reactions (rash, taste disturbances). Important side effects are reviewed below.

Hypotension

The most common adverse effects of ACEI in patients with HF are hypotension and dizziness. Blood pressure generally declines without symptoms in almost every patient treated with an ACEI. Therefore, a decrease in blood pressure should be a concern only if it is associated with symptoms of cerebral hypoperfusion, postural symptoms, or worsening renal dysfunction. Significant hypotension when present is usually seen in the first few days of initiation of ACEI therapy or increase in the dosage. Patients who are ACEI naive and those who are dependent on the renin-angiotensin-aldosterone system for blood pressure maintenance are particularly at risk for hypotension. Similarly, patients with hyponatremia or hypovolemia, especially those receiving high-dose diuretic therapy are also at risk of hypotension. Hypotension usually resolves with continued therapy and can be avoided by reducing the diuretic dosage or stopping it for few days (often referred as diuretic holiday). Patients considered to be at risk for hypotension should be monitored closely for the first 2 weeks of treatment and with every dose escalation. In some patients (e.g., those with low blood pressure from the start) a period of brief hospitalization and close observation during the initiation of ACEI therapy might be necessary.

Cough

Cough is one of the most common reasons for withdrawal of ACEIs. In general, the frequency of cough is between 5 and 10% in Caucasians; however, it has been reported to be higher (up to 20%) in oriental and Asian patients. It is important to recognize that many patients with HF may have concomitant bronchitis, upper respiratory tract infection, etc., which might be the main reason for their cough. Therefore, it is very important to establish that the cough is indeed directly related to the use of ACEI before discontinuing their use. It is also important to realize that worsening HF leading to decompensation can itself lead to cough due to peribronchial edema. Therefore, it is crucial to establish the link between the use of ACEI and cough before considering discontinuation of this life saving therapy in patients with HF. ACEI induced cough generally occurs within the first few weeks to months of therapy and is usually nonproductive, generally persistent, and sometimes associated with an annoying "tickle" in the back of the throat. ACEI induced cough generally disappears within 1–2 weeks of discontinuation of treatment and re-appears with ACEI re-challenge. In a number of studies of ACEI, cough, it was demonstrated that cough did not recur with rechallenge and was probably a coincidental finding. Unless the cough is severe and quite bothersome to the patient, clinicians should encourage patients to continue taking these drugs because of the well-demonstrated benefit on cardiovascular morbidity and mortality.

Renal Dysfunction

Because of already reduced renal perfusion in many patients with HF, GFR is critically dependent on angiotensin mediated efferent arteriolar vasoconstriction. Therefore, ACEI might cause functional renal insufficiency by reducing the levels of angiotensin-II. The risk of renal dysfunction secondary to ACEI is greatest in patients who are dependent on renin angiotensin system (RAS) for support of renal homeostasis. It is, however, important to recognize that an increase in serum creatinine (e.g., > 0.3 mg/dL) is generally observed in 15–30% of patients with severe HF who are treated with ACEIs and in about 5–15% with mild to moderate HF. In most cases, this decline in renal function appears to be of little clinical significance. The risks are substantially greater if patient is taking NSAIDs or has baseline CKD and/or bilateral renal artery stenoses. In most cases, however, renal function usually returns to baseline or stabilizes at a new steady state despite continued treatment with the ACEI. Renal function usually improves after reduction in dosage of concomitantly administered diuretic, therefore, most patients can generally be managed without the need to withdraw treatment with ACEI. However, when clinically indicated discontinuing treatment or decreasing the dosage of the ACEI will rapidly resolve the renal dysfunction as well. In major clinical trials, the need for discontinuation of ACEI therapy because of renal impairment has been quite low (1–3%) and in some trials it was equivalent to that seen with placebo. The longer acting ACEIs, however, may be associated with a higher risk of renal dysfunction.

Hyperkalemia

Hyperkalemia can occur during ACEI therapy, and in some cases, it might be significant enough to cause cardiac conduction abnormalities. The risk of hyperkalemia is significantly higher in patients with baseline renal dysfunction and/or when renal dysfunction occurs as a result of ACEI use. Continued use of potassium sparing diuretics, potassium supplement, or salt substitute (which contains potassium) will obviously increase the risk of hyperkalemia and their use is generally prohibited. Concomitant use of aldosterone antagonists especially in presence of diabetes is also associated with increased risk of hyperkalemia and can be reduced by appropriate dose adjustments.

Angioedema

Angioedema is rare but a life threatening adverse effect that occurs only in less than 1% of patients taking ACEIs. It is now well established that angioedema occurs far more frequently in blacks. Because angioedema can be life threatening, any history or clinical suspicion of such reactions in the past should be considered a contraindication for ACEI therapy. Angiotensin receptor blockers can be considered as an alternative therapy as ARBs generally do not produce angioedema because they lack bradykinin potentiating effect. However, even therapy with ARBs be used with caution in patients with ACEI induced angioedema as there have been few reports of angioedema in patients treated with ARBs.

Angiotensin Receptor Blockers

Several RCTs have now shown that the renin angiotensin system can have partial escape during chronic therapy with ACEIs leading to increasing levels of angiotensin-II despite continued treatment with ACEIs. Such ACEI escape phenomenon occurs in part due to activation of alternative pathways for production of angiotensin-II in myocardial and vascular tissues (Fig. 4). These alternate pathways (especially chymase dependent) can be generally activated in the setting of myocardial injury secondary to infarction.

Because ARBs provide direct blockade of angiotensin II type-1 (AT1) receptors they have been utilized to counteract effects of angiotensin-II on tissues regardless of the site of origin of angiotensin II (Fig. 4). In addition, this effect is achieved without accumulation of bradykinin, which is primarily responsible for some adverse reactions associated with the use of ACEIs, such as persistent cough, angioedema, and significant hypotension.

Theoretically, the use of these drugs should be associated with beneficial effects on clinical outcomes similar to those observed with ACEI therapy and generally with fewer side effects. The ARBs have produced favorable hemodynamic effects during short- and long-term administration. Also, RCTs comparing ARBs with ACEIs have generally shown equivalent or enhanced benefits.

Several ARBs have been evaluated in the setting of HF and are available for clinical use (Table 2). Overall, placebo RCTs have demonstrated that long-term therapy with ARBs is associated with beneficial effects on hemodynamic, neurohormonal, and clinical parameters that are expected with RAS blockade. However, it is important to note that the overall experience with ARBs in large RCTs in HF is significantly less than that with ACEIs. Based on the clinical trials experience presently only 3 ARBs are approved for treatment of patients with HF (Table 2). Although these ARBs can be considered as an alternate RAS blocking therapy it is important to emphasize that treatment with ACEIs remain the first choice for inhibition of RAS in patients with HF. The use of ARBs should generally be reserved as an alternate therapy in patients who are intolerant to treatment with ACEI. The benefit of alternative therapy with an ARB was well demonstrated (Fig. 5) with candesartan in the candesartan in HF: assessment of reduction in mortality and morbidity (CHARM) alternative trial.[10]

Practical Considerations Regarding Use of ARBs

Similar to the use of ACEIs treatment with an ARB, when appropriate, should be started at the low doses (Table 2). In general, as discussed earlier, most considerations

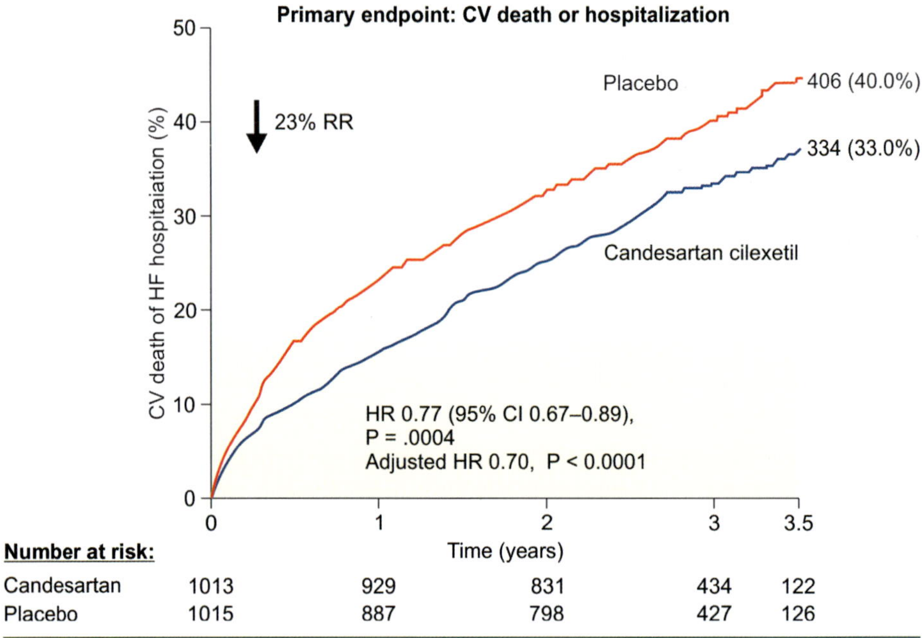

Figure 5: Results of CHARM alternative study showing efficacy of candesartan versus placebo in patients with systolic heart failure. CHARM, Candesartan in Heart failure Assessment of Reduction in Mortality and Morbidity; CV, cardiovascular; RR, relative risk; HF, heart failure; HR, hazard ratio; CI, confidence interval.

Source: *Adapted from* Granger CB, McMurray J, Yusuf S, et al. Effects of candesartan in patients with chronic heart failure and reduced left-ventricular systolic function intolerant to angiotensin-converting-enzyme inhibitors: the CHARM-Alternative trial. Lancet. 2003;362:7726.

regarding the use of ARBs are similar to those with ACEIs. Close monitoring of blood pressure, renal function, and serum K^+ is recommended starting at 1–2 weeks after initiation of ARB therapy and as needed subsequently. Titration of ARB doses is generally achieved by doubling doses every 2 weeks until the target dose is achieved or patient develops intolerance. The overall side effects related to the use of ARBs on renal function and serum potassium level are similar to those described above with ACEIs. However, angioedema (although reported in the literature) occurs rarely with ARBs.

BETA ADRENERGIC BLOCKERS

Activation of sympathetic adrenergic nervous system in response to cardiac dysfunction leads to higher levels of plasma catecholamines which are associated with deleterious effects on the heart (Fig. 3). Sympathetic activation causes profound vasoconstriction leading to increased afterload which subsequently increases ventricular pressures and volumes perpetuating the process of cardiac remodeling. In addition norepinephrine can itself induce cardiac hypertrophy and worsen myocardial ischemia in those with underlying CAD. Activation of SNS also impairs sodium excretion by kidney as well as it promotes release of aldosterone which also results in salt and water retention. Enhanced sympathetic activity can also provoke arrhythmias by increasing the automaticity of myocytes, increasing trigger activity in the heart, and promoting electrolyte imbalance. High levels of norepinephrine also potentiate the actions of the RAAS. Finally, norepinephrine can also trigger cardiac apoptosis by stimulating growth and increasing oxidative stress in terminally differentiated cells (Fig. 3). It is because of these deleterious effects of the SNS activation in patients with HF that treatment with beta blockers was considered useful in HF despite their well-known negative inotropic effects. Beta blockers work primarily by preventing the adverse consequences of enhanced SNS activity in patients with HF and these beneficial effects far outweigh their negative inotropic effects. As a matter of fact, long-term studies with beta blockers have shown that continued use of beta blockers is associated with positive cardiac remodeling which leads to significant improvement in LV performance associated with increased LVEF. There are several additional beneficial effects of beta blockers at the cellular level which are beyond the scope of this review.

It is important to note that so far only three beta blockers (carvedilol, bisoprolol, and sustained release metoprolol succinate) have been shown to be effective (Fig. 6) in patients with chronic HF.[11-14] It is important to realize that beneficial effects demonstrated with these three beta blockers are not indicative of a beta blocker class effect, as shown by the lack of effectiveness of bucindolol and lack of effectiveness of short acting metoprolol in clinical trials.[15-16]

Beta blockers have now been evaluated in numerous placebo controlled RCTs in HF patients with reduced LVEF (< 35–45%) who where already receiving treatment with diuretics and ACEIs, with or without digitalis. The aggregate experience from these trials indicates that long-term treatment with beta blockers reduced the symptoms of HF, improved the clinical status and reduced the risk of hospitalization for HF. More importantly, in all trials, treatment with beta blocker was associated a significant improvement (Fig. 6) in survival.[11-14] These benefits of beta blockers were seen in all subgroups of patients including those with milder or more severe HF, those with or without underlying CAD, those with or without DM, as well as in black and female patients.

Practical Considerations

Based on the consistent efficacy and significant survival benefit of the three beta blockers approved for treatment of HF, they are now recommended for all patients with chronic HF with reduced LVEF unless there is a contraindication or a history of intolerance. Because their significant favorable effect on cardiac remodeling, disease

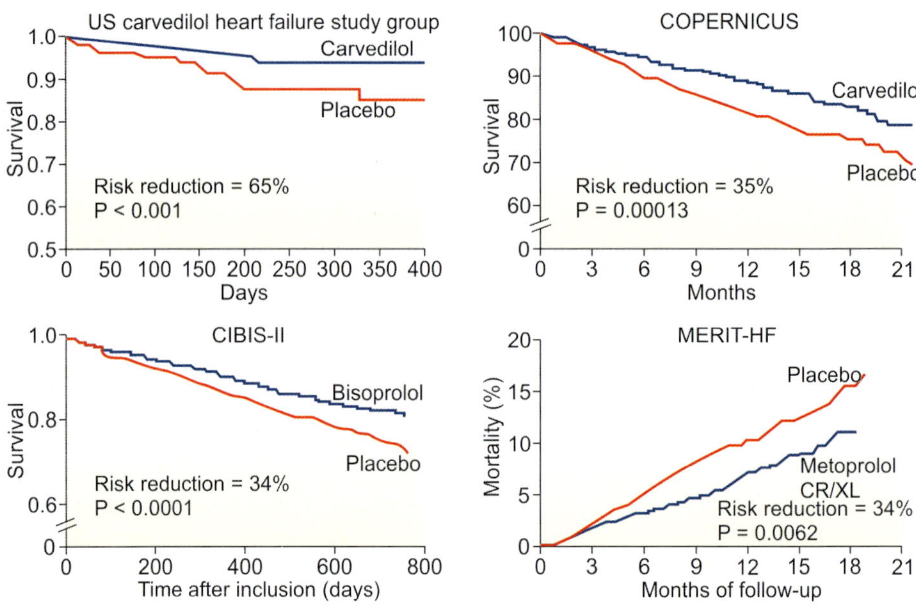

Figure 6: Results of RCTs demonstrating effects of selected beta blocker therapy in patients with HF secondary to LV systolic dysfunction. RCT, randomized controlled trials; HF, heart failure; LV, left ventricular; COPERNICUS, carvedilol prospective randomized cumulative survival study; CIBIS-II, cardiac insufficiency bisoprolol study II; MERIT-HF, metoprolol CR/XL randomized intervention trial in congestive heart failure.

Source: Based on data adapted from references 11-14.

progression, and survival, treatment with beta blockers should be initiated as soon as evidence of LV dysfunction is detected regardless of the lack and/or severity of symptoms. Treatment with beta blocker should be continued and optimized to reduce the risk of progressive LV dysfunction, further clinical deterioration, and prevent the risk of sudden cardiac death. The benefits of beta blocker therapy are evident even when the patient is not taking high doses of ACEIs. As a matter of fact when both drugs cannot be used in maximal doses the use of beta blocker has been shown to produce greater improvement in symptoms and reduction in risk of death in patients who are taking low dose ACEI. Therefore, it seems prudent to optimize the dosage of beta blockers rather than maximizing the dose of ACEIs especially in patients who develop symptomatic hypotension with higher doses of both classes of drugs.

Helpful Hints Regarding Use of Beta Blockers in Heart Failure

Beta blocker therapy should only be initiated when patient is stable and it is best to delay starting beta blockers during decompensated state. Recent data show that beta blocker therapy can be started safely before discharge even in patients hospitalized with HF who did not require intravenous therapy for HF. Treatment with a beta blocker should be initiated at very low dose (Table 2). If a lower dose has been well tolerated then dose should be increased gradually, usually doubling the dose at 2 weeks intervals. Careful monitoring of heart rate, blood pressure, and HF symptoms is needed during the initial period as well as during the entire up titration phase. All patients with current evidence or prior history of fluid retention should be on a diuretic before starting beta blocker therapy because diuretics are often needed to maintain sodium and fluid balance and prevent excessive fluid retention. Initiation of treatment with beta blocker can cause fluid retention, and lead to decompensated HF. Because of this, patients should be advised to weigh regularly on a daily basis and manage any weight increase by increasing the dose of diuretic to maintain the pretreatment weight. In presence of significant fluid retention, planned increment in the dose of beta blocker should be delayed until the patient's clinical condition has been stabilized. Utilizing such careful approach, most patients will tolerate the increase in dosing to the recommended target dosage.

The optimal dose of beta blocker is the target dose achieved in the clinical trial. The target dose in the RCTs was not based on the patients' therapeutic response but rather dependent on prespecified target dose. Lower doses were only used in these trials if the target dose could not be tolerated and most of these trials did not evaluate if lower dose would be as effective. Thus, clinician should make every effort to achieve the target dose of beta blocker shown to be effective in the clinical trials to ensure the maximal survival benefit. Once the target dose has been reached, most patients can continue long-term therapy without difficulty. It is important to educate the patient that the clinical response to beta blocker therapy is generally delayed and may require many months of treatment before improvement is noted. Even when symptoms do not improve, long-term therapy with beta blocker should be maintained to reduce the risk of cardiac and sudden death. Abrupt withdrawal of beta blocker therapy is to be avoided because it can lead to clinical deterioration and beta blocker withdrawal syndrome. Because long-term treatment with beta blocker reduces the risk of worsening HF, discontinuation of treatment with these drugs after an episode of decompensated HF will not diminish, and in fact might increase the subsequent risk of clinical decompensation. Therefore, even when patients develop fluid retention with or without worsening symptoms, it is advisable to continue beta blocker therapy and adjust the dose of diuretics. Only when the clinical deterioration is accompanied by hypoperfusion and/or requires use of intravenous inotropic agents, it may be necessary to decrease the dose or in rare cases hold beta blocker therapy temporarily until the clinical status is stabilized. Beta blocker should be reintroduced once patient is stable to reduce the risk of worsening HF and adverse clinical outcome.

Safety and Adverse Experience

As discussed earlier, initial therapy with beta blocker can cause fluid retention in some patients. Such fluid retention is generally asymptomatic but can occasionally lead to worsening of HF symptoms. Patients with fluid retention prior to treatment are at higher risk of retaining fluid during treatment with beta blockers and thus the clinician should be certain that patients are euvolemic before initiating beta blocker therapy. As described above, any increase in weight or worsening signs and symptoms of HF should be quickly managed with increased dosage of diuretic. However, the occurrence of fluid retention or decompensation of HF is generally not a reason for permanent withdrawal of beta blocker treatment.

Treatment with beta blocker can be associated with general fatigue and tiredness, therefore, it is important to educate the patients about such side effects in advance and ask them not to discontinue beta blocker therapy. Patient should be reassured that fatigue is generally short lasting and resolves within a few weeks of initiation of beta blocker therapy. In some cases, the fatigue may be significant enough to limit further increase in dose and rarely may require a reduction if symptoms are severe. But treatment should not be discontinued unless there is evidence of hypoperfusion.

Bradycardia and slowing of AV nodal conduction is an expected effect of beta blockers. In most patients, bradycardia is asymptomatic and requires no treatments. However, if high grade (2nd or 3rd degree) AV block develops, the dose of beta blocker should be reduced and careful evaluation should be made regarding other conditions or agents that can cause bradycardia or heart block. In some cases where bradycardia or AV block persists and when significant, pacemaker placement should be considered to permit continued use of beta blocker therapy.

Although hypotension can occur with beta blocker therapy (especially with carvedilol due to its alpha blocking action), it is usually asymptomatic. When hypotension is associated with dizziness, lightheadedness, or blurred vision, it might be necessary to reduce the dose and/or change the beta blocker to a non-alpha blocking agent. The risk of hypotension can also be minimized by administering beta blockers and ACEIs/ARBs at different times of the day. If hypotension still persists, a decrease in the dose of ACEI/ARB might be necessary, and in some cases, the dose of diuretic might need to be reduced in patients who are volume depleted.

CLINICAL APPLICATION OF GUIDELINE-BASED THERAPY

Despite the overwhelming evidence of benefits with evidence-based therapy utilizing RAAS blocking drugs and beta blocking agents in patients with HF and LV systolic dysfunction, their application in clinical practice is less than ideal. The burden of HF is enormous and increasing across the world. Heart failure remains a leading cause of hospitalization in the United States. In addition, the patients with HF suffer from significant morbidity and mortality. All of these consequences of

Table 3 Relative benefits of various evidence-based drug therapies for heart failure

Guideline-suggested therapy	*RRR (%) (RCT)*	*RRR (%) (meta-analyses)*
ACEI/ARB	17	20
Beta-Blocker	34	31
Aldosteone antagonist	30	25
Hydralazine/nitrate	43	NA

RRR, relative risk reduction; RCT, randomized clinical trials; ACEi, angiotensin converting enzyme inhibitor; ARB, angiotensin receptor blockers; NA, not applicable.

Source: *Adapted from* Fonarow GC, Yancy CW, Hernandez AF, et al. Potential impact of optimal implementation of evidence-based heart failure therapies on mortality. Am Heart J. 2011;161:1024-30.e3.

HF can be substantially reduced by adequate implementation of evidence-based guideline recommended therapy.[17] A recent analysis emphasized the degree of benefit in reducing mortality that can be achieved with the use of evidence-based therapy in patients with HF (Table 3).[18] This analysis emphasized that optimal implementation of evidence-based therapies with ACEIs/ARBs, beta blockers, aldosterone antagonists, and hydralazine-nitrate combination could potentially prevent as many as 47,500 deaths per year in the United States. These data clearly emphasize that considerable opportunity exists for implementation of evidence-based guideline recommended therapy in patient with HF due to LV systolic dysfunction to improve the associated adverse prognosis.

REFERENCES

1. Hunt SA, Abraham WT, Chin MH, et al. 2009 Focused update incorporated into the ACC/AHA 2005 guidelines for the diagnosis and management of heart failure in adults: a report of the American College of Cardiology Foundation/American Heart Association Task Force on Practice Guidelines: developed in collaboration with the International Society of Heart and Lung Transplantation. Circulation. 2009;119:e391-479.
2. Lindenfeld J, Albert NM, Boehmer JP, et al. HFSA 2010 Comprehensive Heart Failure Practice Guideline. J Card Fail. 2010;16:e1-194.
3. The CONSENSUS Trial Study Group. Effects of enalapril on mortality in severe congestive heart failure. Results of the Cooperative North Scandinavian Enalapril Survival Study (CONSENSUS). N Engl J Med. 1987;316:1429-35.
4. The SOLVD investigators. Effect of enalapril on survival in patients with reduced left ventricular ejection fractions and congestive heart failure. N Engl J Med. 1991;325:293-302.
5. The SOLVD Investigators: Effect of enalapril on mortality and the development of heart failure in asymptomatic patients with reduced left ventricular ejection fractions. N Engl J Med. 1992;327:685-91.
6. Pfeffer MA, Braunwald E, Moyé L, et al. Effect of captopril on mortality and morbidity in patients with left ventricular dysfunction after myocardial infarction. Results of the survival and ventricular enlargement trial. The SAVE Investigators. N Engl J Med. 1992;327:669-77.

7. The Acute Infarction Ramipril Efficacy (AIRE) Study Investigators. Effect of ramipril on mortality and morbidity of survivors of acute myocardial infarction with clinical evidence of heart failure. Lancet. 1993;342:821-8.
8. Køber L, Torp-Pedersen C, Carlsen JE, et al. A clinical trial of the angiotensin-converting-enzyme inhibitor trandolapril in patients with left ventricular dysfunction after myocardial infarction. Trandolapril Cardiac Evaluation (TRACE) Study Group. N Engl J Med. 1995;333(25):1670-6.
9. Ambrosioni E, Borghi C, Magnani B. The effect of the angiotensin-converting-enzyme inhibitor zofenopril on mortality and morbidity after anterior myocardial infarction. The Survival of Myocardial Infarction Long-Term Evaluation (SMILE) Study Investigators. N Engl J Med. 1995;332(2):80-5.
10. Granger C, McMurray J, Yusuf S, et al. Effects of candesartan in patients with chronic heart failure and reduced left-ventricular systolic function intolerant to angiotensin-converting-enzyme inhibitors: the CHARM-Alternative trial. Lancet. 2003;362:772-6.
11. Packer M, Bristow MR, Cohn JN, et al. The effect of carvedilol on morbidity and mortality in patients with chronic heart failure. U.S. Carvedilol Heart Failure Study Group. N Engl J Med. 1996;334:1349-55.
12. Packer M, Coats AJ, Fowler MB, et al. Carvedilol Prospective Randomized Cumulative Survival Study Group (COPERNICUS). Effect of carvedilol on survival in severe chronic heart failure. N Engl J Med. 2001;344:1651-8.
13. CIBIS-II investigators and committees: The cardiac insufficiency bisoprolol study II (CIBIS-II): A randomized trial. Lancet. 1999;353:9-13.
14. Effect of metoprolol CR/XL in chronic heart failure: Metoprolol CR/XL Randomised Intervention Trial in Congestive Heart Failure (MERIT-HF). Lancet. 1999;353:2001-7.
15. Beta-Blocker Evaluation of Survival Trial Investigators. A trial of the beta-blocker bucindolol in patients with advanced chronic heart failure. N Engl J Med. 2001;344: 1659-67.
16. Poole-Wilson P, Swedberg K, Cleland J, et al. Comparison of carvedilol and metoprolol on clinical outcomes in patients with chronic heart failure in the Carvedilol Or Metoprolol European Trial (COMET): randomised controlled trial. Lancet. 2003;362:7-13.
17. Deedwania PC, Carbajal E. Evidence-Based Therapy for Heart Failure. Med Clin North Am. 2012;96:915-31.
18. Fonarow GC, Yancy CW, Hernandez AF, et al. Potential impact of optimal implementation of evidence-based heart failure therapies on mortality. Am Heart J. 2011;161:1024-30.e3.

CHAPTER

4

Emerging Role of Aldosterone Receptor Blockers in Heart Failure

Manjunath C Harlapur, Prakash C Deedwania

INTRODUCTION

Aldosterone is an integral part of renin-angiotensin-aldosterone system (RAAS) and it has diverse pathophysiological role in congestive heart failure (CHF). Based on the current understanding about aldosterone antagonists from the preclinical research to several clinical trials, aldosterone blockade has an established role in the management of heart failure (HF). This section highlights the importance of the RAAS pathway, current understanding including the guidelines from the major organizations and future direction in the management of HF.

BASIC CONCEPT OF RENIN-ANGIOTENSIN-ALDOSTERONE SYSTEM AND CARDIOVASCULAR HEMODYNAMICS

The homeostasis of the fluid balance in the body is very closely regulated by complex mechanism called RAAS. This system involves several hormones and multiple organs in the body. Renin, a polypeptide hormone with 340 amino acids, is produced by the specialized juxtaglomerular cells adjacent to macula densa cells of distal tubules in the kidney. Renin, also known as "angiotensinogenase", is mainly produced in response to decreased blood flow to the kidney and also by the decrease in sodium concentration in the proximal tubules in the nephrons of the kidney. Angiotensinogen is a polypeptide hormone, formed in the hepatocytes of the liver. It is cleaved by renin to another peptide called angiotensin I. Angiotensin I is further broken into angiotensin II by angiotensin-converting enzyme (ACE) which is produced by the endothelium of lung and vascular system. Angiotensin II serves several important functions including promotion of systemic arteriolar vasoconstriction in kidneys as well as systemic vasculatures, leading to increased blood pressure. In kidneys, angiotensin II promotes the sodium reabsorption from the proximal convoluted tubules of the kidneys, while exchanging for the potassium and hydrogen, which are excreted in the urine. Angiotensin II also promotes the sodium absorption from the mucosa of colon, salivary glands, and sweat glands. Other important function of angiotensin II in the blood is to increase the release of aldosterone, a mineralocorticoid synthesized in the zona glomerulosa of adrenal glands. Thus, formed aldosterone further activates the distal tubular and collecting duct cells of the kidney to reabsorb more sodium and water, leading to increase in intravascular volume and raise in the systemic blood pressure, while potassium is excreted from the body. The activity of aldosterone is not only controlled by the angiotensin II, but also by the potassium concentration, adrenocorticotropic hormone (ACTH), and serum sodium levels.[1,2] Initially, aldosterone was thought to be produced only from the adrenal glands; however, it is very well known that aldosterone is also synthesized in other organs including myocardium and blood vessels, especially when there is evidence of injury, which have been discussed in subsequent segments.

ROLE OF ALDOSTERONE IN CARDIOVASCULAR DISEASE AND HEART FAILURE

Aldosterone has been attributed to several deleterious effects and negative cardiac remodeling (Fig. 1). It promotes synthesis of collagen and progression to myocardial fibrosis, which has harmful effects such as impaired relaxation leading to diastolic HF. The important role of aldosterone antagonists has been studied in detail from the preclinical disease process to advanced HF and the importance of this class of medications warrants systematic clinical research studies and in-depth

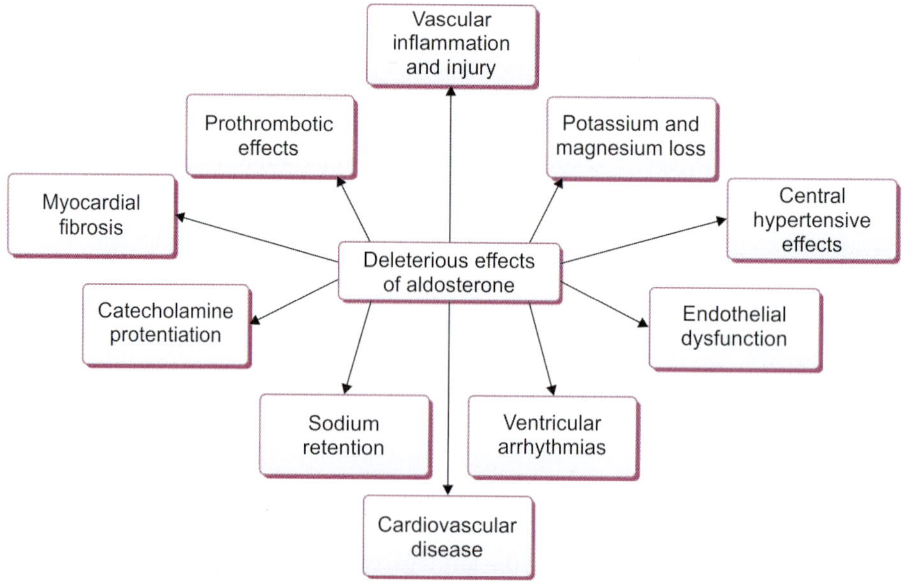

Figure 1: Effects of aldosterone on various components that contribute in heart failure.

understanding. The role of RAAS system blockade is an established therapeutic regimen in the management of HF.

There are two important facts in understanding why it is important to use the aldosterone antagonists, over and above the conventional use of angiotensin-converting enzyme inhibitor (ACEI)/angiotensin receptor blockers (ARBs) therapy. ACEIs decrease the level of angiotensin II which is an important trigger for the production of aldosterone. It is reasonable to think that by blocking the production of angiotensin II, the release of aldosterone can be decreased and subsequent deleterious effects of elevated levels of aldosterone. However, studies have shown that when ACEI is used alone, the production of aldosterone is not completely inhibited and overtime, residual levels of aldosterone are still detected, this phenomenon is called "aldosterone escape".[3] It is because of aldosterone escape phenomenon, aldosterone receptor antagonist therapy has been considered in addition to ACEI to further block the deleterious effects of aldosterone and pleiotropic actions of aldosterone.

With the discovery of extra-adrenal source for aldosterone synthesis in the recent past, RAAS pathway has regained significance in the management of HF. Extra-adrenal sources of aldosterone are currently described in myocardium, systemic blood vessels, and also in the brain.[4,5] Apart from the systemic effects as described before, the production of aldosterone has also been shown to have deleterious paracrine effects like endothelial dysfunction, where aldosterone is produced locally. This is another reason to use the aldosterone antagonists in HF. There are several mechanisms that have been well described in etiopathogenesis of systemic cardiovascular (CV) dysfunction, which eventually manifests as HF. These mechanisms include free radical-induced cellular injury, endothelial dysfunction, coronary artery dysfunction, atherosclerosis, arrhythmia, and hypertension. Any of these factors alone or in combination can occur concurrently resulting in additive consequences. Aldosterone has been shown not only to have the association with these mechanisms, but also the treatment with aldosterone antagonists has been shown to ameliorate some of these pathological changes.

In the animal models, selective blockade of aldosterone with eplerenone has been shown to decrease the production of free radical production with potential antiatherosclerotic properties.[6] Eplerenone has been shown to inhibit the formation of superoxide, which is known to damage the cells during the oxidative stress and also it has been shown to impair the nitric oxide (NO)-dependent relaxation of smooth muscle of the vasculature in experimental model.[7] Endothelial dysfunction and increased inflammation have been described to cause cellular damage.[8] Aldosterone can cause endothelial dysfunction by blocking the production of NO.[9] Spironolactone, an aldosterone antagonist, has been shown to increase NO levels in vasculature,[10] which has favorable antiatherosclerotic properties. Atherosclerosis is a gradual pathological process leading to ischemic CV disease, which eventually progresses to HF. In the transgenic mice, cardiac-specific increase in aldosterone has been reported to be associated with coronary artery dysfunction, which underscores the importance of aldosterone blocking at the local myocardial level apart from systemic blockade.[11] Hypertension is a very important risk factor in etiopathogenesis of CV diseases and is associated with increased risk of myocardial infarction, stroke, HF, and nephropathy. The combined action of aldosterone with angiotensin II (RAAS pathway) has been described to have additive harmful effect on these organs in multiple ways. One mechanism is that elevated aldosterone and angiotensin II further increase arterial blood pressure as well as have direct toxic effect on the vessel wall and myocardium. In the animal models, eplerenone, a selective ARB has been shown to decrease the injury to brain with prolonged survival.[12] Aldosterone also creates the substrate for arrhythmogenesis in heart due to autonomic system dysfunction by diminishing parasympathetic activity while escalating sympathetic activity. The mechanisms of these harmful effects on the electrical activity in heart have been well described. In brief, aldosterone reduces the afferent nerve signals from the carotid sinus baroreceptors by direct effect as well as by blunting of heart rate response to blood pressure variation.[13] In the United Kingdom (UK) heart study, the autonomic dysfunction, measured by heart rate variability, was an independent risk predictor of mortality in HF.[14] Aldosterone increases sympathetic system activity presumably due to lower NO production. Administration of spironolactone in CHF patients has been shown to restore heart rate variability supporting the concept of parasympatholytic effect of aldosterone.[15] Aldosterone is also shown to be produced by endothelial cells and smooth muscle of vasculature and heart. Extra-adrenal production of the aldosterone is known to be associated with inflammation and vascular injury. Apart from HF, high level of aldosterone has been shown to be associated with myocardial infarction, hypertrophy of the left ventricle, and it is associated with poor clinical outcomes in these settings.

Elevated levels of aldosterone have been shown to be associated with myocardial fibrosis which is a critical pathway in the pathogenesis of HF.[16] In the rat model of postinfarction-induced HF, Cittadini et al. have shown that aldosterone blockade has positive left ventricular (LV) remodeling effects by both improvement in systolic and diastolic function and decreased fibrosis.[17] There was also decrease in the level of norepinephrine and decreased incidence of ventricular fibrillation due to increase in the fibrillation threshold in the experimental model of the HF.[17]

ROLE OF ALDOSTERONE ANTAGONISTS IN HEART FAILURE

As discussed earlier, activation of RAAS plays a pivotal role in the initiation as well as progression of HF. It has been shown that despite adequate blockade of RAAS with ACEI/ARB, there could be aldosterone escape. As discussed earlier, the higher levels of aldosterone are deleterious in patients with HF due to variety of actions. Aldosterone blockade has been evaluated and found to be highly effective in reducing morbidity and mortality in HF.

There are presently two ARBs that are available for clinical use. Spironolactone is the classic drug and eplerenone, the newer medication. Spironolactone has been used over half a century, mainly as antihypertensive drug. It is a weak antihypertensive agent that is labeled as diuretic and has potassium-sparing properties. In the last decade, it has regained the importance due to emerging knowledge about the pathophysiology of HF related to RAAS pathway. In the kidneys, spironolactone blocks the absorption of sodium and water, while promoting the reabsorption of potassium in the collecting tubules of kidneys. It is important to note that in the setting of moderate chronic kidney disease and coadministration of other medications (like ACEI/ARB), the use of spironolactone has been associated with the risk of hyperkalemia. Spironolactone has several other hormonal effects, such as estrogenic, antiandrogenic, and progestogenic effects. Gynecomastia seen with treatment of spironolactone is related to imbalance between increased estrogen levels and decrease in testosterone levels. Spironolactone causes displacement of androgen from the androgen receptors, increased metabolic clearance of testosterone, and increased conversion of testosterone to estrogen in the peripheral tissue.[18,19] Low testosterone state mainly leads to hirsutism, androgenic alopecia, acne, and seborrhea which may not be well tolerated by the female patient population. Spironolactone also has antiprogestogenic activity leading to menstrual irregularities in women and dyslipidemia.[20]

The newer drug, eplerenone is a selective aldosterone blocker and, therefore, it is gaining the recognition because of the lack of gynecomastia and other side effects due to absence of activation of glucocorticoid, progesterone, or androgen receptors as compared to spironolactone. Due to lower protein-binding property of eplerenone, it is about 20-fold less potent at the mineralocorticoid receptor level, even though it is as efficacious as spironolactone. However, eplerenone has similar side-effect profile related to electrolyte imbalance, primarily hyperkalemia due to potassium reabsorption in the setting of chronic kidney disease and in patients who are already on medications (like ACEI/ARB) that cause hyperkalemia. The clinical use of these two medications has been discussed in the following sections.

CLINICAL TRIALS WITH ALDOSTERONE RECEPTORS ANTAGONISTS IN HEART FAILURE

There are three major clinical studies that support the use of aldosterone receptor antagonists in systolic HF and one study in patients with isolated diastolic dysfunction with preserved LV function. First, the randomized aldactone evaluation

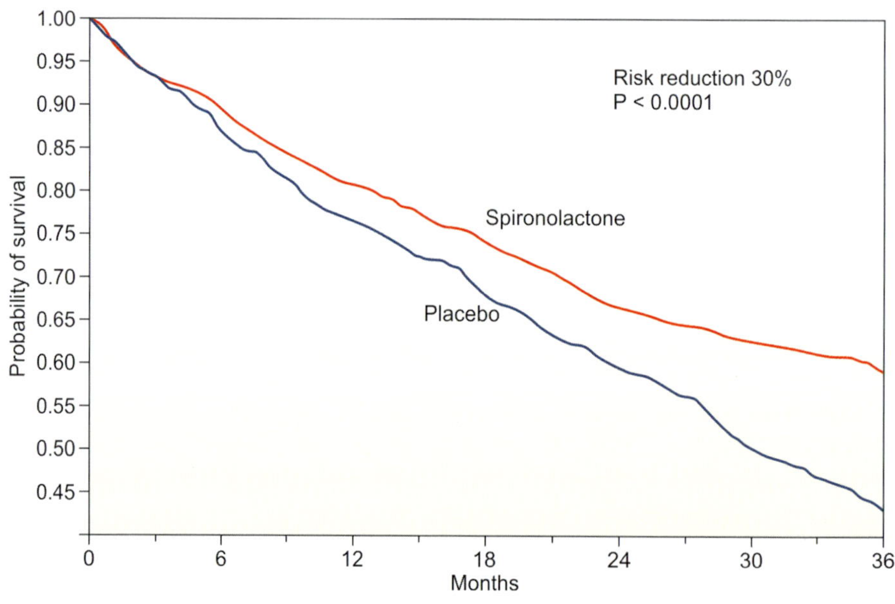

Figure 2: The results showing Kaplan-Meier curves for survival in the randomized aldactone evaluation study (RALES).[21]

Source: *From* Pitt B, Zannad F, Remme WJ, et al. The effect of spironolactone on morbidity and mortality in patients with severe heart failure. Randomized Aldactone Evaluation Study Investigators. N Engl J Med. 1999;341(10):709-17. Copyright© Massachusetts Medical Society, *with permission*.

study (RALES)[21] was a double-blind, randomized controlled study which enrolled over 1,650 patients with chronic to severe HF and a left ventricular ejection fraction (LVEF) less than 35% with New York Heart Association (NYHA) Class III and IV. The patients in RALES were already treated with an ACEI, a loop diuretic, and digoxin. Spironolactone was used for the therapy in one arm of the study and the placebo was used for other group of patients. The interim analysis demonstrated that spironolactone was effective in reducing the mortality and the study was discontinued after 24 months. The spironolactone group showed a decrease in the number for primary outcomes; 35% mortality as compared to 46% in placebo arm [relative risk (RR) of death = 0.70; 95% confidence interval (CI), 0.60–0.82; P < 0.001] (Fig. 2). There was also significantly lower incidence of hospitalization and also significant improvement in the symptoms in the cohort treated with spironolactone as compared to placebo group. However, there were two main concerns noted in the RALES study. The incidence of enlargement of breast (gynecomastia) or breast pain (mastalgia) was reported in 10% of men in the spironolactone arm as compared to 1% in placebo arm. There was also minimal elevation of serum potassium levels

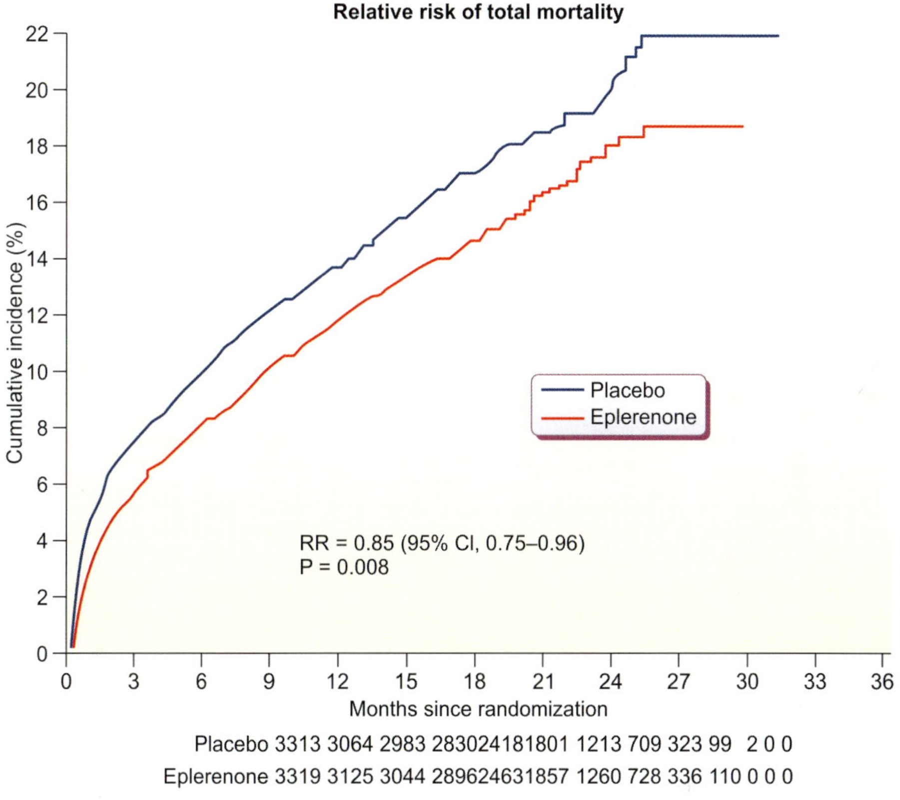

Figure 3: Primary endpoint of total mortality in the eplerenone post-acute myocardial infarction heart failure efficacy and survival study (EPHESUS).[22]

Source: *From* Pitt B, Remme W, Zannad F, et al. Eplerenone, a selective aldosterone blocker, in patients with left ventricular dysfunction after myocardial infarction. N Engl J Med. 2003;348(14):1309-21. Copyright© Massachusetts Medical Society, *with permission*.

in the cohort treated with spironolactone in the study, although risk of serious hyperkalemia was minimal in both groups of patients.

Second study, the eplerenone post-acute myocardial infarction heart failure efficacy and survival study (EPHESUS)[22] was done to evaluate the effect of eplerenone, a selective aldosterone blocker on morbidity and mortality among patients with acute myocardial infarction complicated by LV dysfunction and HF. This was a double-blind, randomized clinical trial and one group was treated with titrating dose of eplerenone (3,319 patients) and other group received placebo group (3,313 patients) in addition to optimal medical therapy. With mean follow-up of 16 months, there were 407 CV deaths in the eplerenone group versus 483 in the placebo group (RR = 0.83; 95% CI, 0.72–0.94; P = 0.005) (Fig. 3). The rate of other primary end-point, death from CV causes, or hospitalization for CV events

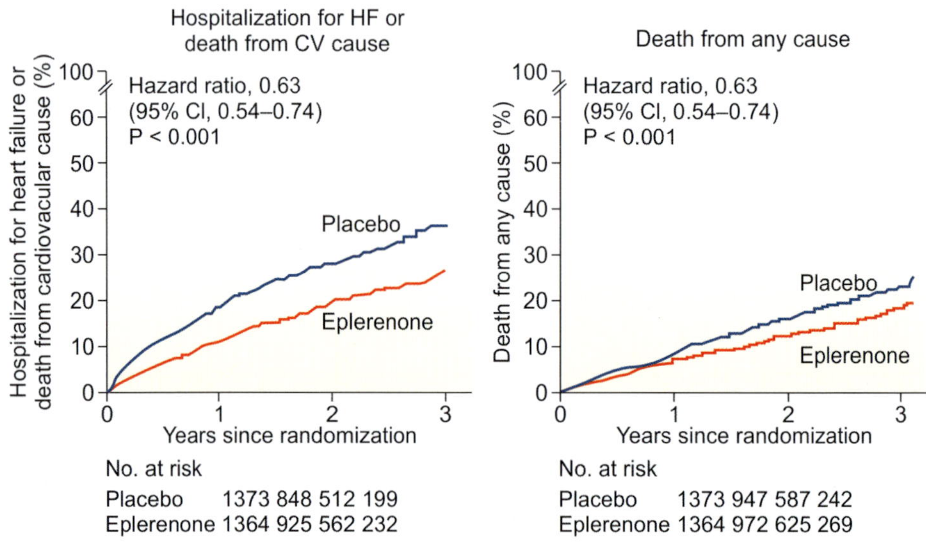

Figure 4A and B: (A) Hospitalization for heart failure (HF) or death from cardiovascular (CV) cause; and (B) death from any cause in the Eplerenone in Mild Patients Hospitalization and Survival in Heart Failure Study (EMPHASIS-HF).[23]

Source: *From* Zannad F, McMurray JJ, Krum H, et al. Eplerenone in patients with systolic heart failure and mild symptoms. N Engl J Med. 2011;364(1):11-21. Copyright© Massachusetts Medical Society, *with permission.*

was also significantly lower in patient group treated with eplerenone (RR = 0.87; 95% CI, 0.79–0.95; P = 0.002). The secondary end-point, incidence of death from any cause, or hospitalization was lower in the eplerenone group (RR = 0.92; 95% CI, 0.86–0.98; P = 0.02). There was also a reduction in the rate of sudden death from cardiac causes (RR = 0.79; 95% CI, 0.64–0.97; P = 0.03). The rate of serious hyperkalemia was 5.5% in the eplerenone group and 3.9% in the placebo group (P = 0.002) whereas the rate of hypokalemia was 8.4% in the eplerenone group and 13.1% in the placebo group (P ≤ 0.001).

Third study, the eplerenone in mild patients hospitalization and survival in heart failure study (EMPHASIS-HF), was a randomized, double-blind trial to study the effects of eplerenone in patients with chronic systolic HF with mild HF symptoms. In this study, 2,737 patients with the NYHA Class II HF and an ejection fraction (EF) of 35% or less were randomly assigned to receive eplerenone or placebo in addition to standard medical therapy. The study was stopped prematurely due to definite benefit in eplerenone group with a median follow-up period of 21 months. There was survival benefit; 10.8% mortality in eplerenone group as compared to 13.5% in placebo group (P = 0.01) in addition to decrease in hospitalizations related to HF (Figs. 4A and B). However, there was an increased incidence of hyperkalemia in eplerenone group as compared to placebo group; 11.8% of patients in the eplerenone group and 7.2% of those in the placebo group ($P \leq 0.001$).[23]

Apart from these large trials to study the effect of aldosterone antagonists in systolic HF, the Aldosterone Receptor Blockade in Diastolic Heart Failure (Aldo-DHF) study was done to evaluate the effect of aldosterone blockers in the patients with diastolic HF with preserved LVEF (LVEF >50%). In this study, 422 patients were randomized to receive the spironolactone in the active treatment arm and placebo in other arm. There were two primary endpoints in this study. First, the exercise capacity [measured by peak oxygen consumption (peak VO_2)] on bicycle ergometry that was not different in patients treated with spironolactone. However, the second primary endpoint showed significant benefit in decreasing the filling pressures in the heart (measured by echocardiographic parameters E/E′) in the group treated with spironolactone as compared to placebo group in 1-year follow-up. Other secondary endpoints, left ventricular mass index (LVMI) and N-terminal pro-brain natriuretic peptide (NT-proBNP) were also favorably decreased in patients treated with spironolactone. Furthermore in this study, there was no severe hyperkalemia [serum potassium (K) level >5.5 mmol/L] in patients who were treated with spironolactone suggesting the tolerable side-effect profile in this patient population.

Apart from these major studies, there are several other smaller trials that have shown other benefits with use of aldosterone blocking agents. The study by Chan AK et al. showed that addition of spironolactone in addition to ARB therapy was associated with improvement in the LV systolic function and also decreased the LV hypertrophy.[24] Fletcher et al. have shown that intravenous administration of spironolactone has additional benefits due to improving cardiac vagal control mechanism as evaluated by heart rate variability and improved sensitivity to baroreceptor reflex sensitivity.[25]

CURRENT EVIDENCE-BASED GUIDELINES FOR ALDOSTERONE BLOCKING DRUGS

The earlier guidelines published by the American College of Cardiology (ACC)/ American Heart Association (AHA) recommend the use of aldosterone receptor antagonist spironolactone with decreased LV function and Class III/IV HF as long as the kidney function is normal and serum potassium levels are normal.[26] After these guidelines were published, the EPHESUS study[22] results became available demonstrating the benefits of eplerenone in the patients with EF of less than 40%, after acute myocardial infarction. Subsequently in 2009, the guidelines[27] were updated based on the results of this study. More recently, the EMPHASIS-HF study[23] highlighted the role of eplerenone in patients with mild HF with the NYHA Class II who are on standard medical therapy. Future guidelines may likely incorporate these important beneficial data and recommend using the aldosterone antagonists, specifically eplerenone in patients with milder forms of HF.

Currently, all the national guidelines recommend aldosterone receptors antagonists in patients with moderately severe to severe symptoms of HF and reduced LVEF. Specifically, spironolactone is recommended for patients with the NYHA functional Class III, IV HF symptoms, and recent hospitalization. Eplerenone is recommended for the patients with LVEF less than or equal to 40% and clinical evidence of HF or diabetes within 14 days of myocardial infarction. The importance of kidney function is to be stressed again and it is recommended to restrict the use of these medications for the patients with creatinine value of equal to or less than 2.5 mg/dL in men and 2.0 mg/dL for women and potassium levels should be less than 5.0 mEq/L. It is very important to recognize that this group of patients is also on other medications that seem to alter the potassium homeostasis. ACEI and ARBs are known to cause the elevation in the potassium levels, while diuretic medications (thiazide and loop diuretics) are known to decrease the potassium by excreting more potassium in the kidneys and some patients with HF are also on oral potassium supplementation for hypokalemia. The drugs like digoxin and other antiarrhythmic medications have favorable profile when the potassium levels are in the optimal range. Therefore, extreme caution is advised while starting the aldosterone blockade medications in these circumstances. Hypokalemia and hyperkalemia should be avoided to prevent the conduction and arrhythmogenic abnormalities leading to increase the risk of sudden cardiac death. It is recommended to keep the potassium level in the range of 4.0–5.0 mEq/L. The importance of the dietary and medication compliance is also equally important to optimally manage the HF patients and also to avoid inadvertent dangers related to electrolyte imbalance. To avoid the potential side effects, it is recommended to start the aldosterone antagonists at lower dose and then, titrate to the higher dose while closely monitoring the potassium levels and kidney function. Spironolactone is started with initial dose of 12.5 mg or 25 mg daily and titrated to maximum daily dose of 50 mg daily. Initial dose for eplerenone is 25 mg and then titrated to maximum dose of 50 mg daily. The risk of hyperkalemia is high when the baseline creatinine is more than 1.6 mg/dL. Elderly patients and those patients with thin body mass index are more prone to develop hyperkalemia. Nonsteroidal anti-inflammatory medications and cyclooxygenase-2 inhibitors should be avoided whenever possible. ARBs are contraindicated in patients with creatinine clearance less than 30 mL/min. Periodic monitoring of potassium level should be done and further changes in terms of potassium intake and medication usage need to be carefully evaluated based on the potassium levels. If the patient is on combination of medications that tend to increase the potassium levels like ACEI or ARB simultaneously, careful attention is needed. The safety of combination with ACEI plus ARB and aldosterone antagonists has not been adequately studied and triple combination with these medications is not recommended.

CLINICAL UTILIZATION OF ALDOSTERONE RECEPTOR ANTAGONIST IN HEART FAILURE

Aldosterone receptor antagonists are less commonly prescribed in spite of clinical trial evidence and recommendations by the guidelines. One of the major concerns to the practicing physicians is side-effect profile of ARBs, especially for the patients with renal dysfunction and hyperkalemia. Congestive HF patients are usually on ACEI/ARBs and often have chronic kidney disease, which makes it even more complicated. There is potential higher risk of hyperkalemia, hypotension, and worsening renal function. The RALES study[21] also showed that chronic use of spironolactone was associated with about 8% incidence of painful gynecomastia. Other hormonal side effects related to spironolactone include sexual dysfunction, hirsutism, and menstrual dysregulation in female.

FUTURE PERSPECTIVES ABOUT ALDOSTERONE ANTAGONISTS IN HEART FAILURE MANAGEMENT

The current guidelines recommend the use of aldosterone antagonists in patients with reduced LV systolic dysfunction with moderate-to-severe HF symptoms based on the larger clinical trials. However, the complex mechanism of activation of RAAS occurs early in the process of HF. Future studies should be considered to evaluate the role of aldosterone receptor antagonists in patients with milder LV systolic function who have no symptoms or mild symptoms may be considered. Overall, aldosterone antagonist therapy is cheaper and it can be cost-effective in the management of HF and has acceptable side-effect profile when used carefully.

Another area for future consideration regulating the use of aldosterone antagonists is in the management of diastolic HF. Sato et al. have shown that use of aldosterone antagonists could improve diastolic function by attenuating the LV hypertrophy, depicted by decreased LVMI after treating the patients with spironolactone over 1 year period.[28] This regression was still significant after controlling for the baseline antihypertensive medications. This was smaller study in 20 patients and results were analyzed after 60 weeks of therapy. Even though, the preliminary unpublished results of the Aldo-DHF study[29] in patients with preserved EF and HF with spironolactone did not show any significant improvement in the maximum peak VO_2 at 1 year. However, there was improvement in the diastolic parameters evaluated by echocardiographic measurements (E/E′). It is known that the process of cardiac remodeling leading to HF takes long time for the cellular and tissue changes. Therefore, it is essential to conduct a study of sufficient length and earlier in the course of LV systolic dysfunction to evaluate the effects of appropriate intervention designed to reverse the cardiac remodeling process and resultant clinical benefit from such therapy. The long-term benefit regarding the role of aldosterone antagonist, spironolactone in diastolic HF is being prospectively examined in the trial of aldosterone antagonist therapy in adults with preserved systolic function,[30] conducted by the National Heart, Lung and Blood Institute. The results of the TOPCAT study should provide the valuable insight regarding the role of aldosterone antagonism in the management of patients with diastolic HF.

REFERENCES

1. Biglieri EG, Arteaga E, Kater CE. Effect of ACTH on aldosterone and other mineralocorticoid hormones. Ann N Y Acad Sci. 1987;512:426-37.
2. Aguilera G, Fujita K, Catt KJ. Mechanisms of inhibition of aldosterone secretion by adrenocorticotropin. Endocrinology. 1981;108(2):522-8.
3. Borghi C, Boschi S, Ambrosioni E, et al. Evidence of a partial escape of renin-angiotensin-aldosterone blockade in patients with acute myocardial infarction treated with ACE inhibitors. J Clin Pharmacol. 1993;33(1):40-5.
4. Silvestre JS, Robert V, Heymes C, et al. Myocardial production of aldosterone and corticosterone in the rat. Physiological regulation. J Biol Chem. 1998;273(9):4883-91.
5. Takeda Y, Miyamori I, Yoneda T, et al. Regulation of aldosterone synthase in human vascular endothelial cells by angiotensin II and adrenocorticotropin. J Clin Endocrinol Metab. 1996;81(8):2797-800.
6. Rajagopalan S, Duquaine D, King S, et al. Mineralocorticoid receptor antagonism in experimental atherosclerosis. Circulation. 2002;105(18):2212-6.
7. Schäfer A, Fraccarollo D, Hildemann SK, et al. Addition of the selective aldosterone receptor antagonist eplerenone to ACE inhibition in heart failure: effect on endothelial dysfunction. Cardiovasc Res. 2003;58(3):655-62.
8. Funder JW. Aldosterone, mineralocorticoid receptors and vascular inflammation. Mol Cell Endocrinol. 2004;217(1-2):263-9.
9. Ikeda U, Kanbe T, Nakayama I, et al. Aldosterone inhibits nitric oxide synthesis in rat vascular smooth muscle cells induced by interleukin-1 beta. Eur J Pharmacol. 1995;290(2):69-73.
10. Farquharson CA, Struthers AD. Spironolactone increases nitric oxide bioactivity, improves endothelial vasodilator dysfunction, and suppresses vascular angiotensin I/angiotensin II conversion in patients with chronic heart failure. Circulation. 2000;101(6):594-7.
11. Garnier A, Bendall JK, Fuchs S, et al. Cardiac specific increase in aldosterone production induces coronary dysfunction in aldosterone synthase-transgenic mice. Circulation. 2004;110(13):1819-25.
12. Rocha R, Stier CT. Pathophysiological effects of aldosterone in cardiovascular tissues. Trends Endocrinol Metab. 2001;12(7):308-14.
13. Wang W, McClain JM, Zucker IH. Aldosterone reduces baroreceptor discharge in the dog. Hypertension. 1992;19(3):270-7.
14. Nolan J, Batin PD, Andrews R, et al. Prospective study of heart rate variability and mortality in chronic heart failure: results of the United Kingdom heart failure evaluation and assessment of risk trial (UK-heart). Circulation. 1998;98(15):1510-6.
15. Yee KM, Struthers AD. Aldosterone blunts the baroreflex response in man. Clin Sci (Lond). 1998;95(6):687-92.

16. Brilla CG. Aldosterone and myocardial fibrosis in heart failure. Herz. 2000;25(3):299-306.
17. Cittadini A, Monti MG, Isgaard J, et al. Aldosterone receptor blockade improves left ventricular remodeling and increases ventricular fibrillation threshold in experimental heart failure. Cardiovasc Res. 2003;58(3):555-64.
18. Prisant LM, Chin E. Gynecomastia and hypertension. J Clin Hypertens (Greenwich). 2005;7(4):245-8.
19. Rose LI, Underwood RH, Newmark SR, et al. Pathophysiology of spironolactone-induced gynecomastia. Ann Intern Med. 1977;87(4):398-403.
20. Nakhjavani M, Hamidi S, Esteghamati A, et al. Short term effects of spironolactone on blood lipid profile: A 3-month study on a cohort of young women with hirsutism. Br J Clin Pharmacol. 2009;68(4):634-7.
21. Pitt B, Zannad F, Remme WJ, et al. The effect of spironolactone on morbidity and mortality in patients with severe heart failure. Randomized Aldactone Evaluation Study Investigators. N Engl J Med. 1999;341(10):709-17.
22. Pitt B, Remme W, Zannad F, et al. Eplerenone, a selective aldosterone blocker, in patients with left ventricular dysfunction after myocardial infarction. N Engl J Med. 2003;348(14):1309-21.
23. Zannad F, McMurray JJ, Krum H, et al. Eplerenone in patients with systolic heart failure and mild symptoms. N Engl J Med. 2011;364(1):11-21.
24. Chan AK, Sanderson JE, Wang T, et al. Aldosterone receptor antagonism induces reverse remodeling when added to angiotensin receptor blockade in chronic heart failure. J Am Coll Cardiol. 2007;50(7):591-6.
25. Hunt SA, American College of Cardiology, American Heart Association Task Force on Practice Guidelines, et al. ACC/AHA 2005 guideline update for the diagnosis and management of chronic heart failure in the adult: a report of the American College of Cardiology/American Heart Association Task Force on Practice Guidelines (Writing Committee to Update the 2001 Guidelines for the Evaluation and Management of Heart Failure). J Am Coll Cardiol. 2005;46(6):e1-82.
26. Hunt SA, Abraham WT, Chin MH, et al. 2009 focused update incorporated into the ACC/AHA 2005 Guidelines for the Diagnosis and Management of Heart Failure in Adults: a report of the American College of Cardiology Foundation/American Heart Association Task Force on Practice Guidelines developed in collaboration with the International Society for Heart and Lung Transplantation. J Am Coll Cardiol. 2009;53(15):e1-90.
27. Sato A, Hayashi M, Saruta T. Relative long-term effects of spironolactone in conjunction with an angiotensin-converting enzyme inhibitor on left ventricular mass and diastolic function in patients with essential hypertension. Hypertens Res. 2002;25(6):837-42.
28. Edelmann F, Schmidt AG, Gelbrich G, et al. Rationale and design of the 'aldosterone receptor blockade in diastolic heart failure' trial: a double-blind, randomized, placebo-controlled, parallel group study to determine the effects of spironolactone on exercise capacity and diastolic function in patients with symptomatic diastolic heart failure (Aldo-DHF). Eur J Heart Fail. 2010;12(8):874-82.
29. Desai AS, Lewis EF, Li R, et al. Rationale and design of the treatment of preserved cardiac function heart failure with an aldosterone antagonist trial: a randomized, controlled study of spironolactone in patients with symptomatic heart failure and preserved ejection fraction. Am Heart J. 2011;162(6):966-72.e10.
30. Fletcher J, Buch AN, Routledge HC et al. Acute aldosterone antagonism improves cardiac vagal control in humans. J Am Coll Cardiol. 2004;43(7):1270-5.

CHAPTER

5

Inotropic Therapy for Heart Failure: Past, Present, and Future

Paul J Hauptman, Patrick McCann

"However beautiful the strategy, you should occasionally look at the results."

Sir Winston Churchill

INTRODUCTION

Few scientific stories are more complicated in the annals of cardiovascular (CV) therapeutics than the trials and tribulations associated with the inotrope class of medications. Beginning in the 1970s, an intensive effort in drug development was initiated and expanded over a period of a quarter of a century in the areas of both acute decompensated heart failure (ADHF) and chronic symptomatic heart failure.[1,2] Despite remarkably favorable findings in short-term phase II studies, the promise of inotropic drugs has not been fulfilled and the reasons are complex and varied. The failures are particularly stark in chronic HF since positive short-term hemodynamic data led investigators and industry sponsors to launch of multiple large long-term randomized multicenter studies. Almost simultaneously, the increasing appreciation for the neurohormonal model of HF progression served to successfully redirect the focus of drug development to antagonists of the renin-angiotensin-aldosterone and sympathetic nervous systems.

In this chapter, we review the potential mechanistic benefits and risks associated with inotropic agents; account for the extensive failures; outline current evidence-based practice in a variety of clinical settings; and discuss newer approaches in drug development. Ultimately, the muted interest in and general pessimism about new inotropic drugs may provide an opportunity, as long as the lessons of the past are recognized. Future regulatory requirements will undoubtedly include both short- and long-term safety end-points plus conservative efficacy margins constructed to justify use in limited and clearly defined cohorts of patients with heart failure. Conversely, use of a uniform 'one size fits all' approach pursued in earlier clinical trials will almost certainly limit the chances of future success. Indeed, while the key to new drug development in this area will still be based on finding a mechanistic approach that improves cardiac performance without increasing oxygen consumption and energy expenditure, identification, and subsequent study inclusion of patients most likely to benefit based on responder analyses from pilot studies will be of paramount importance.

POTENTIAL MECHANISTIC BENEFITS AND RISKS

Early interest focused on increasing intracellular cyclic adenosine monophosphate (cAMP) either through enhanced generation by direct beta adrenergic receptor stimulation or decreased degradation via the effects of phosphodiesterase type III inhibition. As a secondary messenger, cAMP leads to activation of protein kinase A, which allows phosphorylation of calcium channels promoting increased calcium influx and hence increased contractile force generation (Figs. 1A and B). Although acute effects can be useful to achieve short-term hemodynamic goals, a chronic increase in cAMP has proved detrimental[3] partly mediated through increased tachyarrhythmias and oxygen consumption.

Subsequently, knowledge about the essential mechanisms of myocardial contraction and the interplay between contractile proteins, metabolic pathways, ion channels, and calcium transients progressed, leading to a number of novel approaches, several of which are emphasized in this chapter. The list of agents subjected to clinical evaluation includes calcium sensitizers, myosin activators, and fatty acid oxidation inhibitors (Table 1); all but the last can be categorized as belonging to the inotrope class. In addition, gene delivery of SERCA2a represents a nonpharmacologic approach that, if successful, would shift focus of therapeutic targeting to the repletion of the structural components of the calcium handling apparatus that are depleted or impaired in the setting of heart failure.[4]

The oldest known inotropic treatment for heart failure, digitalis, exerts its effects in a manner that depends on its serum concentation. At serum blood levels that do not exceed 0.9 ng/mL,[5] effects are predominantly manifested at the level of the baroreceptor, increasing its sensitivity and thereby decreasing central sympathetic discharge and increasing parasympathetic tone. At higher serum levels, inotropic effects will predominate, mediated through inhibition of membrane bound alpha subunits of the sodium potassium ATPase which indirectly promotes sodium-calcium exchange. This suggests that the neurohormonal rather than the direct inotropic effects may be responsible for the observation of clinical benefit, however, limited. In that context, it is noteworthy that in the Digitalis Investigation Group Study,[6] digoxin had no impact on overall mortality but favorable trends were seen at the low serum dose range.

Another class of agent directly enhances the response of myofilaments to calcium, a process known as "calcium sensitization". Some calcium sensitizers have additional mechanisms of action, such as the opening of adenosine triphosphate

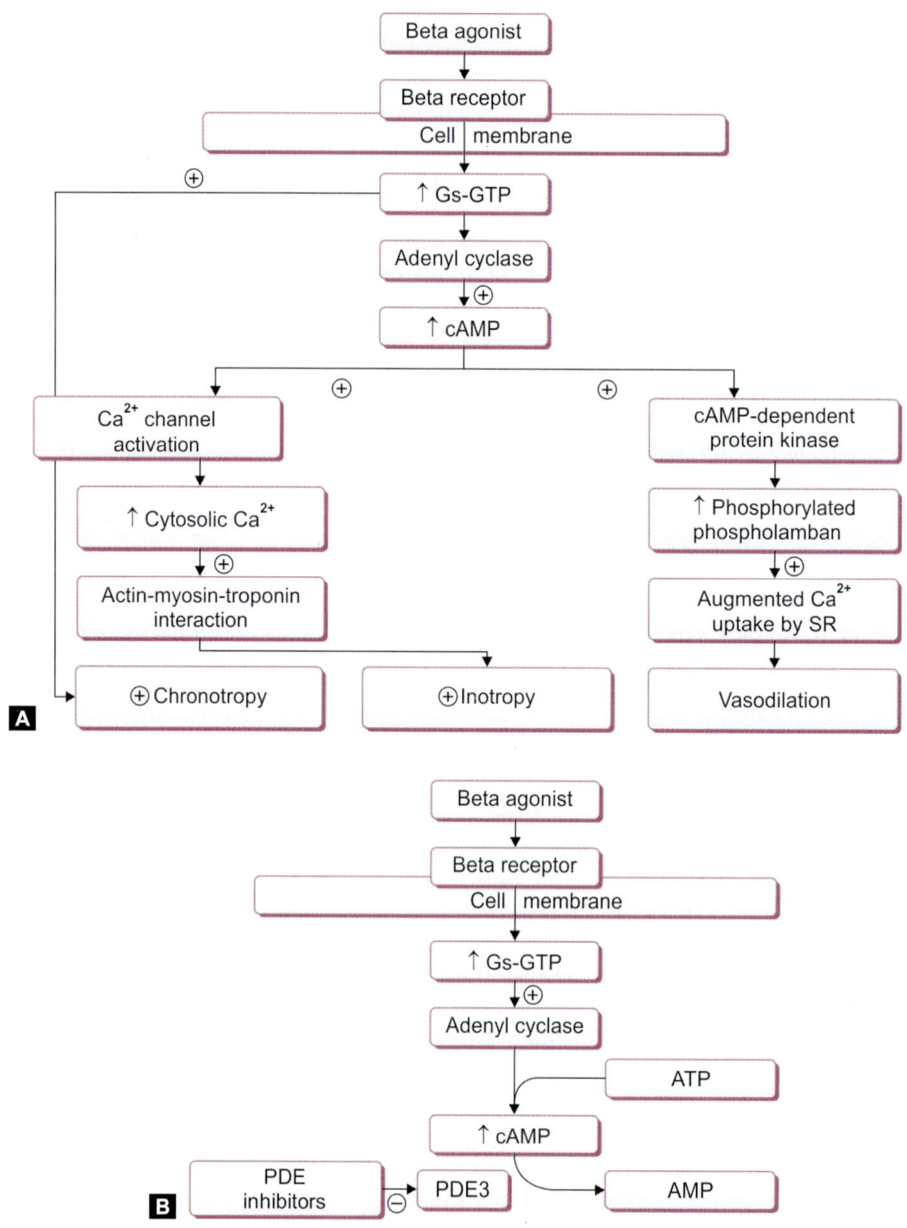

Figure 1A and B: Schema of mechanism of action of beta sympathomimetic agents and phosphodiesterase III inhibitors. Gs-STP, gamma s guanosine triphosphate; cAMP, cyclic adenosine monophosphate; SR, sarcoplasmic recticulum; ATP, adenosine triphosphate; PDE, phosphodiesterase.

Source: *Modified from* Overgaard CB, Dzavik V. Inotropes and vasopressors: review of physiology and clinical use in cardiovascular disease. Circulation. 2008;118:1047-56, *with permission*.

Table 1 **Potential targets for inotropic drugs**

Mechanism	*Examples*
Na^+-K^+-ATPase inhibition	Digoxin, istaroxime
Activation of cAMP-PKA pathway	Dopamine, dobutamine, milrinone, enoximone
Calcium sensitization	Levosimendan
SERCA2a activation	Istaroxime
Cardiac myosin activators	Omecamtiv mecarbil
Ryanodine receptor-stabilization	Ivabradine

(ATP)-dependent potassium channels or phosphodiesterase inhibition. In general, diastolic relaxation and myocardial energetics are not adversely impacted, unlike with most agents that increase cAMP. In addition, at least theoretically, catecholamine-induced and chronotropic dependent changes in calcium release that occur with increased demand will increase the inotropic effect of the sensitizer. Furthermore, arteriolar and venous vasodilation in pulmonary, cardiac, and systemic circuits may occur with the opening of potassium channels in vascular smooth muscle cells lining the vasculature. Nevertheless, the promise of these agents has not been fully realized.

It may also be seen as a central tenet that any intrope that increases heart rate or prolongs systolic ejection time without decreasing heart rate will likely have detrimental effects on diastolic filling. Moreover, increased chronotropy often contributes to arrhythmias and/or sudden cardiac death. Even with improved acute hemodynamics, increased neurohormonal activation and increased intracellular calcium influx can lead to maladaptive remodeling, increased ischemia, and other effects that can accelerate rather than retard HF progression.

THE PAST: THE RISE AND FALL OF ORAL INOTROPES

The Drugs

Multiple oral inotropes have failed in clinical trials including vesnarinone, milrinone, ibopamine, pimobendan, enoximone, and flosequinan.[7-14] Historically, the oral doses selected for the randomized clinical trials were based on interpretation of dose response in short-term invasive hemodynamic studies that demonstrated reductions in pulmonary capillary wedge pressure and increases in cardiac index. Documentation of these acute responses was deemed necessary and appropriate prior to the evaluation of long-term drug effects on mortality end points. While elevated filling pressures have been associated with poorer outcomes, it is not clear if acute reduction can be sustained or serve as a reasonable therapeutic target during chronic management. In addition, the Evaluation Study of Congestive Heart Failure and Pulmonary Artery Catheterization Effectiveness (ESCAPE) study demonstrated that invasively derived hemodynamics do not add value in the routine management of patients with decompensated heart failure.[15] Nevertheless, the lack of translation of the favorable acute response to longer-term benefit was unexpected. In this section, we further highlight several of the drugs and results from phase 2 and 3 clinical trials.

Pimobendan

One of the early generation calcium sensitizers with phosphodiesterase (PDE)-III activity, pimobendan was assessed in the Pimobendan In COngestive heart failure (PICO) trial in which 317 patients with New York Heart Association (NYHA) Class II or III symptoms were randomized to one of two doses of active study drug versus placebo.[10] Although the trial showed a borderline improvement in exercise duration on bicycle ergometry after 24 weeks of therapy, the treatment groups had an increased risk of mortality and no improvement in quality of life compared to the placebo arm. Subsequently, the Effects of Pimobendon On Chronic Heart failure (EPOCH) study in Japan[11] did not demonstrate a reduction in death or cardiovascular hospitalizations in patients with advanced heart failure symptoms. Both studies may have been underpowered and in EPOCH less than one quarter of patients were on a beta blocker at baseline.

Vesnarinone

A drug with pluripotent effects on multiple ion channels and weak PDE inhibition, vesnarinone appeared promising in a small placebo-controlled study of patients with ejection fraction less than 30% and ongoing symptoms. There was a 62% reduction in mortality at 6 months and a 50% reduction in a combined end-point of death or worsening HF[16] compared with placebo. However, these results were only evident in patients receiving the 60 mg dose. At 120 mg, there was an increase in mortality that resulted in early termination of that study arm. With such a narrow therapeutic window, additional study was required. In fact, the drug at 30 and 60 mg was subsequently found to be detrimental with a 26% increased risk of sudden cardiac death and a 16% increase in all-cause mortality.[7]

Enoximone

Another PDE inhibitor, enoximone, has been evaluated in multiple trials including several carried out in a contemporaneous setting when beta blocker therapy was viewed as standard of care. The drug was studied in several interesting patient cohorts. For example, EnoxiMone in intravenous inOTropE-dependent subjects (EMOTE) was a novel investigation designed to determine whether low dose oral enoximone could help safely wean patients with advanced HF from intravenous

(IV) inotrope therapy.[12] In this double blind, placebo-controlled trial, 201 patients with NYHA Class III or IV symptoms, requiring either intermittent or continuous IV inotropic therapy, were randomized to enoximone or placebo. Subjects receiving intermittent IV inotropes were administered study medication at 25 or 50 mg three times a day. Subjects receiving continuous IV inotropes were administered 50 or 75 mg three times a day for 1 week and then the dose was reduced to 25 or 50 mg three times a day. The primary end-point of the trial was constructed in order to evaluate whether low-dose oral enoximone could alleviate the need for IV inotrope therapy at 30 days to a greater extent than placebo. This end-point was not reached.

The Studies of Oral Enoximone Therapy in Advanced Heart Failure (ESSENTIAL) trial was a more standard examination of the effects of enoximone on symptoms, exercise capacity, and major clinical outcomes in patient with advanced HF who were also treated with beta-blockers and other guideline recommended background therapy.[13] The study consisted of two identical randomized, double blind, placebo-controlled trials. ESSENTIAL-I recruited patients in North and South America while ESSENTIAL-II recruited patients from Europe. The trials had three co-primary end-points: (i) the composite of time to all-cause mortality or cardiovascular hospitalization, analyzed in the two ESSENTIAL trials combined; (ii) the 6-month change from baseline in the 6-minute walk test distance (6MWTD); and (iii) patient global assessment (PGA) at 6 months, both analyzed in each trial separately.[13] The trials enrolled 1,854 subjects with an ejection fraction of less than or equal to 30%, left ventricular (LV) end-diastolic diameter greater than 3.2 cm/m^2, symptoms of dyspnea or fatigue at rest or at minimal exertion [New York Heart Association Class III-IV] for more than 2 months, and at least one hospitalization or two outpatient visits requiring IV diuretic or vasodilator therapy within 12 months before screening. Results were mostly negative: the first and third endpoints did not differ between the treatment groups; the 6-MWTD increased with enoximone compared to placebo in ESSENTIAL-I but not in ESSENTIAL-II. Further clinical evaluation has not been pursued in the United States.

Levosimendan

Intravenous levosimendan, a calcium sensitizer, is the inotropic agent most recently subjected to an extensive clinical development program. Levosimendan produces greater contractility by enhancing the binding of calcium to cardiac troponin C. Specifically, calcium binding to troponin C causes structural changes that expose the myosin-binding sites on actin, thereby allowing crossbridge formation; levosimendan enhances the binding of calcium by reversibly eliciting a conformational change in troponin C.[17]

Despite structural similarity with molecules belonging to the PDE-inhibitor family, levosimendan does not increase intracellular levels of cAMP or intracellular calcium to levels high enough to explain its positive inotropic effect at therapeutic concentrations.[18] Levosimendan also stimulates ATP-sensitive K^+ channels that are suppressed by intracellular ATP and opens cardiac mitochondrial ATP-sensitive K^+ channels, a potentially cardioprotective mechanism linked to preconditioning in response to oxidative stress.[19]

Regardless of these insights into the mechanism of action and very intriguing early data from studies, such as Levosimendan Infusion versus Dobutamine in severe low-Output heart failure (LIDO) study and CAlcium Sensitizer or Inotrope or None in low-Output Heart Failure Study (CASINO),[20,21] the drug failed in larger more definitive studies due to safety issues[22] or lack of efficacy.[23] In the randomized multicenter evaluation of intravenous levosimendan efficacy (REVIVE) study, the primary composite end-point which included reduction in pulmonary capillary wedge pressure, patient reported dyspnea relief, and need for rescue therapy was met but increases in atrial fibrillation and other arrhythmias were observed.[22] In the Survival of patients with Acute Heart Failure in need of Intravenous Inotropic Support (SURVIVE) study, the measurement of the primary outcome of all-cause mortality following infusion of levosimendan versus dobutamine extended out to 180 days, an unrealistic time frame for a therapeutic effect given limited exposure to the drug (despite its long half-life due to a pharmacologically active metabolite).[23] The drug is approved for use in some European countries but not in the United States and there is little indication that it or any other related drug will be able to meet the high regulatory bar set by the Food and Drug Administration (FDA).

Istaroxime

This novel drug enhances cardiac contractility through inhibition of the sodium-potassium ATPase and increased activation of the Sarcoplasmic/Endoplasmic Reticulum Calcium ATPase [(SERCA) Fig. 2]. Augmented SERCA activity results in calcium accumulation within the myocyte during systole and rapid removal of calcium during diastole. This augmentation results in improved inotropy and lusitropy. Studies with istaroxime have demonstrated an improvement in systolic and diastolic function with little change in myocardial oxygen consumption.[24] The Hemodynamic Effects of Istaroxime in Patients with HF and Reduced LV Systolic Function (HORIZON-HF) study was a phase II trial in which 120 patients hospitalized for HF exacerbation were randomly assigned to a 6-hour infusion of one of three doses of istaroxime or placebo.[25] The trial demonstrated a reduction in pulmonary capillary wedge pressure in all treatment arms compared to placebo, lower heart rate and increased systolic blood pressure.

Furthermore, subjects treated with the highest dose demonstrated an increase in cardiac index, decrease in LV end-diastolic volume, and improvement in diastolic function. No major adverse events were noted.

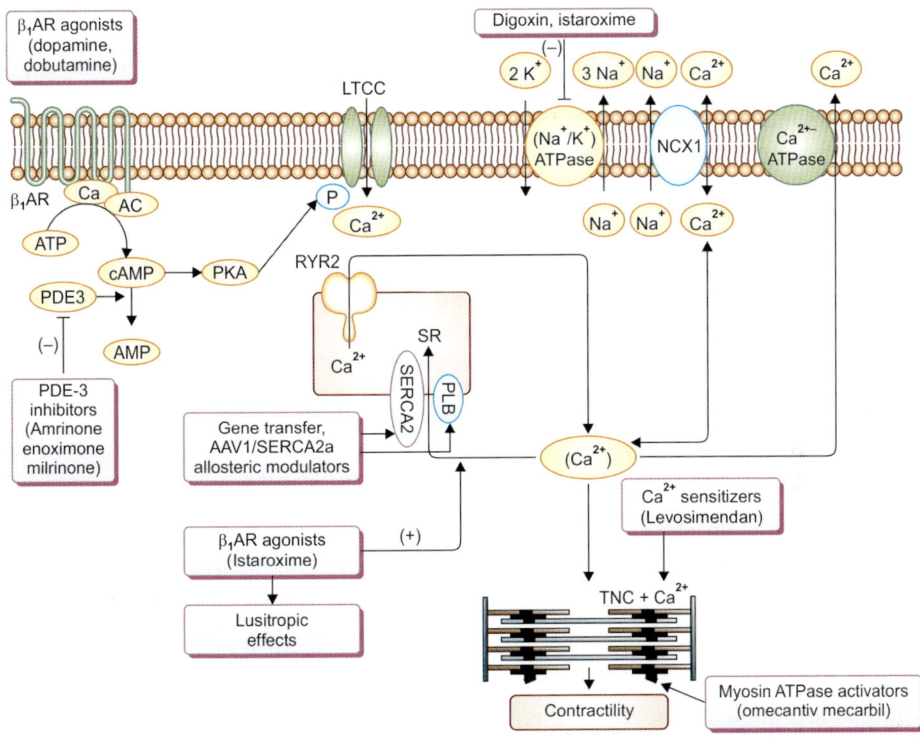

Figure 2: Schema of mechanism of action of several novel inotropic drugs. Calcium entry via L-type Ca^{2+} channels (LTCCs) activates Ca^{2+} release from the sarcoplasmic reticulum (SR) via ryanodine receptor 2 (RYR2) which results in an increase in intracellular Ca^{2+} concentration and induces cardiac contraction. Ca^{2+} uptake into the sarcoplasmic reticulum via sarcoplasmic reticulum Ca^{2+}-ATPase 2 (SERCA2) and its extrusion via the Na^+/Ca^{2+} exchanger 1 (NCX1) and sarcolemmal Ca^{2+}-ATPase allows relaxation. β_1AR, β_1-adrenergic receptor; AAVI/SERCA2, adeno-associated viral-vector (AAV1) carrying the SERCA2 gene; AC, adenylcyclase; PDE3, phosphodiesterase 3; PDE3I, PDE3 inhibitor; PKA, protein kinase A; PLB, phospholamban; TNC, troponin C.

Source: *From* Tamargo J, Lopez-Sendon J. Novel therapeutic targets for the treatment of heart failure. Nat Rev Drug Discov. 2011;10:536-55, *with permission.*

However, while the initial results appeared promising, clinical efficacy, and safety have not yet been determined and there are no additional studies underway to clarify this drug's potential benefit.

Possible Explanations for the Failure of Oral Inotropic Agents

The reasons for the difference between effects on short-term surrogate end-points with IV formulations and meaningful long-term clinical end-points following chronic oral administration are not definitively known. The list of possible explanations for the failure of the oral formulations includes inappropriate dosing, incorrect dosing interval, deleterious effects of large peak-to-trough differences in serum concentrations, chronically increased metabolic demand and oxygen consumption, and proarrhythmia. Variables to consider include long-term impact on myocardial energetics, impact on heart rate, changes in diastolic filling, drug-drug interactions and presence, and/or adequate dosing of concomitant therapy with neurohormonal antagonists. Indeed, the lack of concomitant treatment with aldosterone or beta adrenergic antagonists in many of these early studies is particularly noteworthy as is the absence of implantable cardioverter defibrillators that might have prevented premature sudden deaths precipitated by pro-arrhythmic effects of some oral inotropes.

THE PRESENT: CURRENT PRACTICE

Acute Decompensated Heart Failure

Despite the setbacks that plagued drug development in chronic HF, IV inotropes (in particular dobutamine and milrinone) have been used for treatment of acute decompensated heart failure for many years. While these agents might not be approved if data generated in studies from 20 years ago were presented to contemporary regulatory agencies, such as the FDA, the drugs serve an important role for patients who have low cardiac output syndrome unresponsive to standard approaches. Their use spans a range of clinical scenarios when short-term goals, such as symptom relief and improved end-organ perfusion, are of vital clinical importance.

Clinical Setting

Inotropic therapy is a viable option in select patients when heart failure exacerbations are punctuated by low-cardiac output, end-organ hypoperfusion, and borderline blood pressure. Multiple mechanisms that regulate the basal contractile force of the myocardium, including length dependent activation of cross bridges, contraction frequency-dependent activation of contractile force, and catecholamine induced inotropy, influence the force and velocity of contraction as well as relaxation and energy consumption of the myocardium. We refer the reader to a chapter that helps to define the elements involved in myocyte contraction and the abnormalities that occur in the setting of heart failure.[26]

The major inotropic agents are dopamine, dobutamine, and milrinone. The first two are beta adrenergic agonists, and mediate their cardiac effect largely through β-1 receptors. The third bypasses the beta receptor but like the other agents utilizes cAMP as a secondary messenger. The relative value of these agents is debated but if the patient is on a concomitant β-blocker, milrinone is the most likely to lead to a hemodynamic response at conventional doses.[27] The fact that milrinone is also more appropriately characterized as an inodilator, due to its vasodilatory effects on the pulmonary vasculature, adds to the strength of the argument in favor of its use. However, it is important to emphasize that patients who require inotropic therapy have a high short-term mortality and there are no well-designed placebo-controlled trials of IV inotropes versus placebo for chronic infusions. In the Randomized Evaluation of Mechanical Assistance for the Treatment of Congestive Heart Failure (REMATCH) study, medically treated patients of whom 72% were on IV inotrope experienced a mortality rate of 100% at just over 2 years of follow-up.[28] In a Medicare cohort requiring chronic continuous IV inotrope, mortality was 42.6% at 6 months.[29] Therefore, it is advisable to set realistic goals for inotropic therapy, with a focus on symptom relief.

Dopamine

For decades, dopamine has been known to have significant hemodynamic effects, through dose dependent stimulation of beta (β-), alpha (α-), and dopaminergic receptors and release of norepinephrine from sympathetic nerve terminals. At low dose (1–3 μg/kg/min), dopamine can cause renal and peripheral vasodilation; doses achieved through intermediate infusion rates of 4–8 μg/kg/min also stimulate α- and β-adrenergic receptors in the vasculature and myocardium. The β-adrenergic stimulation results in positive inotropic and chronotropic actions causing increased heart rate, stroke volume, and cardiac output. Alpha-adrenergic stimulation results in peripheral and venous constriction which causes increased arterial pressure and increased cardiac filling pressure as a result of increased venous return to the heart. At higher infusion rates (greater than 8 μg/kg/min), the α-adrenergic effect becomes predominant resulting in more vasoconstriction.

The use of "renal dose dopamine" (dose of 1–3 μg/kg/min) has long been debated as an intervention to induce renal vasodilation and enhance renal function. A meta-analysis of low doses of dopamine given to reduce the incidence and severity of renal failure in critically ill patients revealed no improvement in rates of death or renal failure and the overall clinical effect on diuresis was similar to dobutamine.[30] The clinician must be aware of the risk of tachyarrhythmias and ischemia which can be observed even with low doses.

Dobutamine

A frequent choice for low-output syndrome, dobutamine is a sympathomimetic drug that exerts its effect through direct stimulation of β1-receptors with little α-adrenergic effect leading to increased cardiac contractility and peripheral vasodilation. Stroke volume, stroke work, and cardiac output are all increased. The major dose limiting side effects are tachycardia and increased atrial and ventricular ectopy. These issues were highlighted in the Prospective Randomized Evaluation of Cardiac Ectopy with Dobutamine or Natrector Therapy (PRECEDENT) study in which the safety and clinical effectiveness of dobutamine was examined compared with the vasodilator nesiritide. The patients were randomized to receive either agent and assessment was made by 24-hour Holter recordings before and during study drug therapy. Dobutamine was associated with substantial proarrhythmic and chronotropic effects, whereas nesiritide reduced ventricular ectopy or had a neutral effect.[31] The investigators concluded that nesiritide may be a safer short-term treatment than dobutamine for patients with decompensated heart failure; however, nesiritide is unlikely to improve cardiac index to the same degree in dobutamine-naïve patients not on beta blocker.

When dobutamine therapy is initiated, the lowest possible dose should be utilized to produce the desired effect. Increasing severity of hypoperfusion usually requires higher doses. There may be little benefit from increasing the dose above 10 μg/kg/min and other therapies should be considered. Tachyphylaxis is known to occur with prolonged infusions, and eosinophilic hypersensitivity including myocarditis has been reported,[32] although the clinical relevance of the latter finding is unclear.

Milrinone

As a PDE-III inhibitor, milrinone prevents degradation of cAMP, thus increasing protein kinase A (PKA) activity. In general, administration does not require invasive hemodynamic monitoring. Initiation with a bolus is also discouraged to avoid an early hypotensive effect; by 30 minutes, the hemodynamic effects are not distinguishable between administrations by bolus followed by continuous infusion versus continuous infusion alone.[33] The formal recommendation for a starting dose is 0.25–0.75 μg/kg/min with dose adjustment in the presence of renal failure; the authors frequently use doses as low as 0.125 μg/kg/min with good effect.

Colucci and colleagues, in a study performed before the use of β-blockers for heart failure, demonstrated that patients in the lowest baseline quartile of contractility responded better to milrinone than dobutamine.[26] The reason for this finding likely relates to the down regulation of β-receptors due to increased levels of circulating norepinephrine in the patients with the most advanced HF. In a subsequent study by Lowes et al., dobutamine produced an increase in cardiac index in patients maintained on β-blockers but only at doses that are not typically used to treat HF (15–20 μg/kg/min) compared to conventional dosing with milrinone, as the effect of the latter is not mediated through β-receptors.[34] Milrinone as a vasodilator can reduce right ventricular afterload, an important consideration if significant elevations of pulmonary arterial pressure or pulmonary vascular resistance are present. Another advantage over dobutamine is that tachyphylaxis is generally not observed.

However, the routine use of milrinone in the setting of decompensated HF is not considered standard of care. In the Outcomes of a Prospective Trial of Intravenous Milrinone for Exacerbations (OPTIME) study, no benefit from milrinone treatment versus placebo was observed in hospital days, other measurements of chronic heart failure improvement, or the ability to institute oral drugs that improve long-term prognosis. In contrast, milrinone caused an increase in early adverse events related to hypotension and atrial arrhythmias.[35] Further, intermittent scheduled infusions of IV inotropic agents for the chronic management of HF are not appropriate due to lack of convincing placebo-controlled data about both safety and efficacy.

Guidelines

Current guidelines from the major professional societies [European Society of Cardiology (ESC), American College of Cardiology (ACC)/American Heart Association (AHA), and Heart Failure Society of America (HFSA)] are reviewed in table 2.[36-38] Thematically, it is clear that use of IV inotropes is limited to patients with advanced symptoms and hemodynamic compromise. The evidence is not based

Table 2 Guidelines

ESC Guidelines	*Strength of recommendation*	*Level*
Inotropic agents are not recommended unless the patient is hypotensive (systolic blood pressure <85 mmHg), hypoperfused, or shocked because of safety concerns (atrial and ventricular arrhythmias, myocardial ischemia, and death)	III	C
An intravenous infusion of an inotrope (e.g. dobutamine) should be considered in patients with hypotension (systolic blood pressure <85 mmHg) and/or hypoperfusion to increase cardiac output, increase blood pressure and improve peripheral perfusion. The ECG should be monitored continuously because inotropic agents can cause arrhythmias and myocardial ischemia	IIa	C
Heart Failure Society of America Guidelines		
Intravenous inotropic therapy, such as dobutamine may be considered to relieve symptoms and improve end-organ function in patients with advanced HF characterized by LV dilation, reduced LVEF, and diminished peripheral perfusion or end-organ dysfunction (low-output syndrome), particularly if these patients have marginal systolic blood pressure (<90 mmHg), have symptomatic hypotension despite adequate filling pressure, or are unresponsive to, or intolerant of intravenous vasodilators	May be considered	C
These agents may be considered in similar patients with evidence of fluid overload if they respond poorly to intravenous diuretics or manifest diminished or worsening renal function	May be considered	C
Intravenous inotropes (milrinone or dobutamine) are not recommended unless left heart filling pressures are known to be elevated or cardiac index is severely impaired based on direct measurement or clear clinical signs	Is not recommended	C

Contd...

Contd...

It is recommended that administration of intravenous inotropes in the setting of ADHF is accompanied by continuous or frequent blood pressure monitoring of cardiac rhythm	Is recommended	C
If symptomatic hypotension or worsening tachyarrhythmias develop during administration of these agents, discontinuation or dose reduction should be considered	Should be considered	C
ACC/AHA Guidelines		
Intravenous inotropic therapy, such as dopamine, dobutamine, or milrinone might be reasonable for those patients presenting with documented severe systolic dysfunction, low-blood pressure, and evidence of low-cardiac output, with or without congestion, to maintain systemic perfusion and preserve end-organ performance	IIb	C
Continuous intravenous infusion of a positive inotropic agent for palliation of symptoms	IIb	C
Use of parenteral inotropic drugs in normotensive patients with acute decompensated HF without evidence of decreased organ perfusion is not recommended	III	B
Long-term use of an infusion of a positive inotropic drug may be harmful and is not recommended for patients with current or prior symptoms of HF and reduced LVEF, except as palliation for patients with end-stage disease who cannot be stabilized with standard medical treatment	III	C
Routine intermittent infusions of vasoactive and positive inotropic agents are not recommended for patients with refractory end-stage HF	III	A

ESC, European Society of Cardiology; ECG, electrocardiogram; HF, heart failure; LV, left ventricular; LVEF, left ventricular ejection fraction; ADHF, acute decompensated heart failure; ACC, American College of Cardiology; AHA, American Heart Association.

on multiple large placebo-controlled clinical trials; nevertheless, the European guidelines do provide an impressive algorithmic approach[36] that facilitates decision-making when use of these agents is under consideration.

Chronic Symptomatic Heart Failure

There are currently no oral inotropes (excluding digoxin) currently on the United States market and/or approved by the FDA for any indication including use in patients with HF. Indeed, drugs that are approved for other indications but have some potential for inotropic effects (e.g., cilostazol which has PDE-III inhibitory effects) are contraindicated in patients with HF.

Other Settings

Bridge to Beta blockade

In a small minority of patients with decompensated heart failure, the use of milrinone can be considered as a bridge to β-blockade.[39,40] However, in most cases, as demonstrated in the COPERNICUS study, patients with advanced heart failure tolerate initiation of β-blockers without the need for inotropic support as long as clinical euvolemia is present and low doses are used.[41] Indeed, the benefit of carvedilol in this cohort was pronounced.

Bridge to Transplant or Ventricular Assist Device

Continuous infusions of IV inotrope are frequently used in patients awaiting heart transplantation; the need for such agents elevates the patient on the transplant waiting list in the United States.[42] These patients are also often evaluated for placement of a left ventricular assist device as a bridge-to-transplant or destination therapy; in some cases, IV inotropes are continued after device placement to support the right ventricle. A similar approach is often taken in other HF surgery, especially if right ventricular failure and/or pulmonary hypertension are present, which can in turn limit left ventricular filling and reduce blood pressure. Given the absence of tachyphylaxis and pulmonary vasodilatory effects, our group has used milrinone in this setting.

Postcardiotomy Syndrome

Pharmacological support is often necessary during and after weaning from cardiopulmonary bypass in patients who have developed low-cardiac output syndrome, arbitrarily defined as a cardiac index less than 2.4 L/min/m^2 with evidence of end-organ dysfunction.[43] Causes of low-cardiac ouput include effects of cardioplegia, precipitation of cardiac ischemia during aortic cross-clamping, reperfusion injury, inflammatory and coagulation cascade activation, and the presence of unrepaired preexisting cardiac disease. In addition to potential measures such as optimization of volume status, reduction of systemic vascular resistance, temporary pacing and temporary mechanical circulatory support, therapy with inotropes should be instituted promptly. Although no single agent is universally superior in this setting, dobutamine has the most desirable side-effect profile of the β-agonists, whereas PDE inhibitors may increase flow through arterial grafts, reduce mean arterial pressure, and improve right-sided heart performance in pulmonary hypertension.[43] Concomitant vasopressor therapy may be necessary but can compromise renal blood flow.

Several studies have tested the role of prophylactic inotropic or vasopressor therapy in weaning from cardiopulmonary bypass. In one study, preemptive milrinone administration before separation from cardiopulmonary bypass was found to attenuate postoperative deterioration in cardiac function and reduce the need for additional inotropes.[44] In off-pump bypass, the use of preemptive milrinone may ameliorate increases in mitral regurgitation and improve hemodynamic indices.[45] Milrinone and dobutamine were both found to be effective in improving general hemodynamic parameters compared with placebo in a European multicenter, randomized, open-label trial.[46]

Right Ventricular Support

Significant right ventricular free-wall ischemia results in dilation of the right ventricle. As a consequence, a rapid increase in intrapericardial pressures and intraventricular septal shift can alter LV geometry, impairing LV filling and contractile performance.[47,48] These changes in hemodynamics may precipitate shock. Administration of excess IV fluid to improve a preload in the right ventricle can result in deterioration of LV performance. Dobutamine improves myocardial performance in this setting[49] but milrinone is an excellent choice if pulmonary artery pressure is elevated or extended right ventricular support is anticipated. Cardiac monitoring is necessary for hypotension and arrhythmias, which can profoundly worsen hemodynamics.

Palliation with Intravenous Inotropic Agents

The ACC/AHA guidelines state "continuous IV infusion of a positive inotropic agent may be considered for palliation of symptoms in patients with refractory end-stage HF" and categorize infusions as a Class IIb (level of evidence C) recommendation.[37] Additional consensus opinion supports this option as well with the additional proviso that deactivation of the shock function of implantable cardioverter defibrillators should be considered when inotropic therapy is selected.[50,51] The mortality rate in this patient cohort is high but IV inotropes may also contribute to a reduction in hospital days, possibly mediated through improved symptoms.[29]

If chronic continuous inotropic therapy is under consideration for palliative management, right heart catheterization may be necessary to document a hemodynamic response. According to regulations of the Centers for Medicare and Medicaid Services, demonstration of a 20% increase in cardiac index or a 20% decrease in pulmonary capillary wedge pressure is required for reimbursement.[52,53]

A clinical conundrum arises when a patient does not have baseline hemodynamic data available but has already been started on inotropic therapy and HF symptoms have abated. In these cases, despite the risk of deterioration, it is often necessary to completely stop the drug and obtain baseline hemodynamic measurements in order to document a subsequent improvement with re-initiation of inotrope if indefinite continuous therapy is anticipated.

Patients who receive this therapy are often candidates for hospice but from a practical standpoint, two barriers exist. First, some hospice medical directors have limited experience with HF and may view the use of IV inotropes as a "life prolonging" treatment.[54] Second, the costs associated with infusions may exceed the per diem for hospice care.[55]

FUTURE DEVELOPMENT OF INOTROPIC DRUGS

Although the focus of drug development in the last decade has been on neurohormonal antagonists and anticytokine agents, recent failures in this area[56-60] may have revitalized a modest degree of interest in inotropic therapy. At present, most of the focus has been in omecamtiv mecarbil, a drug with a novel mechanism of action. However, while we await the definitive studies, caution is prudent given the history of the inotrope class.

Omecamtiv Mecarbil: A Novel Drug

Omecamtiv mecarbil (formerly CK-1827452) is a cardiac specific myosin activator in active clinical trials. Specifically, myosin binds and hydrolyzes ATP, weakly binds to actin via a calcium-sensitive mechanism, and then releases phosphate, forming a strong bond with actin, which results in a powerful force generating stroke.[61-63] The rate-limiting step in this process is the transition from the weakly bound actin-myosin-ADP-Pi complex, to the strongly bound actin-myosin-ADP complex configuration. Omecamtiv is an allosteric activator of the myosin S1 domain (which allows the medication to modulate both enzymatic and mechanical properties of cardiac myosin[64]). It accelerates the rate limiting step in actin-myosin crossbridging through enhanced removal of phosphate, causing rapid transition of actin-myosin to its strongly bound state. It also reduces ATP hydrolysis by inhibiting nonproductive phosphate release.[65] These cellular alterations result in recruitment of additional myosin heads and the generation of a stronger contractile force leading to increased left ventricular systolic ejection time, sarcomere shortening, and stroke volume without altering blood pressure or velocity of contraction.[64]

Several reports suggest that the drug does not alter myocardial oxygen consumption, myocyte calcium levels, or the rate of left ventricular pressure development (dP/dt).[65,66] In contrast, cAMP-mediated inotropic agents, such as dobutamine, affect cardiac function by increasing the rate of LV dP/dt and decreasing the systolic ejection time.[67] Thus, omecamtiv mecarbil may induce beneficial effects on cardiac function by means of a novel mechanism that seems to avoid the undesired effects of other inotropic agents.

In an early clinical study with escalating doses of the IV formulation, Cleland et al.[68] assessed drug tolerability and cardiac function in 45 patients with chronic stable systolic heart failure (ejection fraction <40%). Similar to its effect in healthy patients,[64] omecamtiv mecarbil showed dose- and concentration-dependent increases in cardiac function with increases in systolic ejection time, stroke volume, and fractional shortening at concentrations more than 500 ng/mL. There was a small decrease in heart rate noted as well, which was thought to be a reflexive response to an increased stroke volume. Thus, only a small reduction in diastolic duration was noted.

Currently, the drug is being studied in the ATOMIC-AHF trial,[69] a phase II study in which patients are randomized to a 48-hour infusion of study drug or placebo within 24 hours of initiation of IV diuretic therapy, during a hospitalization for decompensated heart failure. The primary end-point is dyspnea relief with a range of secondary outcomes including patient global assessment and surrogate markers, such as change in level of NT-proBNP.

However, unless the drug consistently lowers heart rate (preferably through a non-reflex mediated mechanism), a prolongation of systole may not be advantageous unless it somehow also improves myocardial energetics. This is particularly relevant if acute IV therapy is considered a bridging approach to chronic oral administration of the drug.

New Indications: Palliation with Oral Inotropic Drugs

An intriguing alternative to IV inotropic therapy for patients with terminal heart failure who are not candidates for transplant, advanced surgical interventions, or experimental approaches, is the use of oral agents in the inotrope class. Since survival is not the goal, the potentially negative effect on mortality may be a reasonable trade-off in some patients in order to achieve improved symptoms. However, there is a paucity of data in this area, limited to small-scale studies as with oral levosimendan[70] and enoximone.[71] To date, there has been no significant interest in a formal drug development program, in part, because regulatory requirements would need to be altered to allow the primary end-point to be defined by improvement in quality of life or symptom control.

Looking Forward

Is there an ideal inotrope? The challenge of regulatory requirements in an imperfect world: The attributes of the ideal inotrope include a range of salutary effects (Table 3)

Table 3 Attributes of the ideal inotrope

• Offers early and sustained symptom relief
• Promotes diuresis and vasodilation (venous/arterial)
• Improves end-organ function
• Does not exacerbate ischemia
• Does not exacerbate arrhythmias
• Does not have significant drug-drug interactions
• Decreases LOS, readmissions, and mortality
• Easy to administer and inexpensive

LOS, length of stay.

that provide an unrealistic target for drug development. Indeed, given the record of failure in this therapeutic area and the enhanced regulatory focus on safety, the pathway for approval for a novel inotrope is not straightforward. Even the definition and utility of acute end-points remain uncertain.[72] The use of composite or combined end-points is useful but consensus has not been reached about the time points for efficacy and safety measurements. Given the high event rates of hospitalization, adverse events, such as symptomatic arrhythmia and mortality, these studies require fewer patients than those designed to evaluate the impact of interventions in chronic HF. The need for rescue with additional IV vasoactive therapy and/or mechanical support is a particularly appealing way to define worsening of heart failure but these decisions are likely based on physician global assessment and subject to variation by physician and site. Further, there remains significant heterogeneity in the severity of illness among patients with decompensated HF. Nevertheless, an inotrope that does not increase heart rate, oxygen demand, or frequency and severity of arrhythmia could have a meaningful impact on both acute and chronic heart failure management. Without question, given the epidemiology of heart failure and its increasing prevalence, there is an ongoing and unmet need in this therapeutic area.[73]

REFERENCES

1. Colucci WS, Wright RF, Braunwald E. New positive inotropic agents in the treatment of congestive heart failure. Mechanisms of action and recent clinical developments. 1. N Engl J Med. 1986;314:290-9.
2. Colucci WS, Wright RF, Braunwald E. New positive inotropic agents in the treatment of congestive heart failure. Mechanisms of action and recent clinical developments. 2. N Engl J Med. 1986;314:349-58.
3. Overgaard CB, Dzavik V. Inotropes and vasopressors: review of physiology and clinical use in cardiovascular disease. Circulation. 2008;118:1047-56.
4. Kawase Y, Ly HQ, Prunier F, et al. Reversal of cardiac dysfunction after long-term expression of SERCA2a by gene transfer in a pre-clinical model of heart failure. J Am Coll Cardiol. 2008;51:1112-19.
5. Adams KF, Gheorghiade M, Uretsky BF, et al. Clinical benefits of low serum digoxin concentrations in heart failure. J Am Coll Cardiol. 2002;39:946-53.
6. The Digitalis Investigation Group. The effect of digoxin on mortality and morbidity in patients with heart failure. N Engl J Med. 1997;336:525-33.
7. Cohn JN, Goldstein SO, Greenberg BH, et al. A dose-dependent increase in mortality with vesnarinone among patients with severe heart failure. Vesnarinone trial investigators. N Engl J Med. 1998;339:1810-6.
8. Packer M, Carver JR, Rodeheffer RJ, et al. Effect of oral milrinone on mortality in severe chronic heart failure. The PROMISE Study Research Group. N Engl J Med. 1991;325:1468-75.
9. Morimoto Y, Kasai A, Nagano K, et al. Acute and chronic effects of a new oral inotropic agent, ibopamine hydrochloride, on hemodynamic and metabolic response to ergometer exercise in patients with severe congestive heart failure. Kokyu To Junkan 1989;37:773-8.
10. Lubsen J, Just H, Hjalmarsson AC, et al. Effect of pimobendan on exercise capacity in patients with heart failure: main results from the Pimobendan in Congestive Heart Failure (PICO) trial. Heart. 1996;76:223-31.

11. The EPOCH Study Group. Effects of pimobendan on adverse cardiac events and physical activities in patients with mild to moderate chronic heart failure-the effects of pimobendan on chronic heart failure study (EPOCH). Circ J. 2002;66: 149-57.
12. Feldman AM, Oren RM, Abraham WT, et al. Low dose oral enoximone enhances the ability to wean patients with ultra-advanced heart failure from intravenous inotropic support: results of the oral enoximone in intravenous inotrope-dependent subjects trial. Am Heart J. 2007;154:861-9.
13. Metra M, Eichhorn E, Abraham WT, et al. Effects of low-dose oral enoximone administration on mortality, morbidity, and exercise capacity in patients with advanced heart failure: the randomized, double-blind, placebo-controlled, parallel group ESSENTIAL trials. Eur Heart J. 2009;30:3015-26.
14. Packer M, Rouleau J, Swedberg K, et al. Effect of flosequinan on survival in chronic heart failure: preliminary results of the PROFILE study [abstract]. Circulation. 1993;88 (Suppl I):301.
15. Binanay C, Califf RM, Hasselblad V, et al. Evaluation study of congestive heart failure and pulmonary artery catheterization effectiveness: the ESCAPE trial. JAMA. 2005;294:1625-33.
16. Feldman AM, Bristow MR, Parmley WW, et al. Effects of vesnarinone on morbidity and mortality in patients with heart failure. N Engl J Med. 1993;329:149-55.
17. Ng TM. Levosimendan, a new calcium-sensitizing inotrope for heart failure. Pharmacotherapy. 2004;24:1366-84.
18. Szilágyi S, Pollesello P, Levijoki J, et al. Two inotropes with different mechanism of action: contractile, PDE-inhibitory and direct myofibrillar effects of levosimendan and enoximone. J Cardiovasc Pharmacol. 2005;46:369-76.
19. Hassenfuss G, Pieske B, Castell M, et al. Influence of the novel inotropic agent levosimendan on isometric tension and calcium cycling in failing human myocardium. Circulation. 1998;98:2141-7.
20. Follath F, Cleland JG, Just H, et al. Efficacy and safety of intravenous levosimendan compared with dobutamine in severe low-output heart failure (the LIDO study): a randomised double-blind trial. Lancet. 2002;360:196-202.
21. Cleland JG, Ghosha J, Freemantle N, et al. Clinical trials update and cumulative meta-analyses from the American College of Cardiology: WATCH, SCD-HeFT, DINAMIT, CASINO, INSPIRE, STRATUS-US, RIO-Lipids and cardiac resynchronization therapy in heart failure. Eur J Heart Fail. 2004;6:501-8.
22. Packer M, Colucci W, Fisher L, et al. Effect of levosimendan on the short-term clinical course of patients with acutely decompensated heart failure. JACC Heart Failure. 2013;1:103-11.
23. Mebazaa A, Nieminen MS, Packer M, et al. Levosimendan vs dobutamine for patients with acute decompensated heart failure. JAMA. 2007;297:1883-91.
24. Sabbah HN, Imai M, Cowart D, et al. Hemodynamic properties of a new generation positive luso-inotropic agent for the acute treatment of advanced heart failure. Am J Cardiol. 2007;99:41A-6A.
25. Gheorghiade M, Blair JE, Filippatos GS, et al. Hemodynamic, echocardiographic and neurohormonal effects of istaroxime, a novel intravenous inotropic and lusitropic agent: a randomized controlled trial in patients hospitalized with heart failure. J Am Coll Cardiol. 2008;51:2276-85.
26. Colucci WS, Wright RF, Jaski BE, et al. Milrinone and dobutamine in severe heart failure: differing hemodynamic effects and individual patient responsiveness. Circulation. 1986;73:III175-83.

27. Lowes BD, Tsvetkova T, Eichhorn EJ, et al. Milrinone versus dobutamine in heart failure subjects treated chronically with carvedilol. Int J Cardiol. 2001;81:141-9.
28. Rose EA, Gelijns AC, Moskowitz AJ, et al. Randomized evaluation of mechanical assistance for the treatment of congestive heart failure (REMATCH) study group. N Engl J Med. 2001;345:1435-43.
29. Hauptman PJ, Mikolajcak P, George A, et al. Chronic inotropic therapy in end-stage heart failure. Am Heart J. 2006;152:1096.e1-8.
30. Friedrich JO, Adhikari N, Herridge MS, et al. Meta-analysis: low-dose dopamine increases urine output but does not prevent renal dysfunction or death. Ann Intern Med. 2005;142:510-24.
31. Burger AJ, Horton DP, Lejemtel R, et al. Effect of nesiritide (B-type natriuretic peptide) and dobutamine on ventricular arrhythmias in the treatment of patients with acutely decompensated congestive heart failure: The PRECEDENT study. Am Heart J 2002;144:1102-8.
32. Takkenberg JJ, Czer LS, Fishbein MC, et al. Eosinophilic myocarditis in patients awaiting heart transplantation. Crit Care Med. 2004;32:714-21.
33. Baruch L, Patacsil P, Hameed A, et al. Pharmacodynamic effects of milrinone with and without a bolus loading infusion. Am Heart J. 2001;141:266-73.
34. Lowes BD, Simon MA, Tsvetkova TO, et al. Inotropes in the beta-blocker era. Clin Cardiol. 2000;23(Suppl III):11-16.
35. Cuffe MS, Califf RM, Adams KF, et al. Short-term intravenous milrinone for acute exacerbation of chronic heart failure. JAMA. 2002;287:1541-7.
36. Dickstein K, Cohen-Solal A, Filippatos G, et al. ESC guidelines for the diagnosis and treatment of acute and chronic heart failure 2008: the Task Force for the Diagnosis and Treatment of Acute and Chronic Heart Failure 2008 of the European Society of Cardiology. Developed in collaboration with the Heart Failure Association of the ESC (HFA) and endorsed by the European Society of Intensive Care Medicine (ESICM). Eur Heart J. 2008;29:2388-442.
37. 2009 Focused Update: ACCF/AHA Guidelines for the Diagnosis and Management of Heart Failure in Adults. Circulation. 2009;119:1977-2016.
38. Heart Failure Society of America, Lindenfeld J, Albert NM, et al. HFSA 2010 Comprehensive heart failure practice guideline. J Card Fail. 2010;16:e1-194.
39. Hauptman PJ, Woods D, Pritzker MR, et al. Novel use of a short-acting intravenous beta blocker in combination with inotropic therapy as a bridge to chronic oral beta blockade in patients with advanced heart failure. Clin Cardiol. 2002;25:247-9.
40. Shakar SF, Abraham WT, Gilbert EM, et al. Combined oral positive inotropic and beta-blocker therapy for treatment of refractory class IV heart failure. J Am Coll Cardiol. 1998;31:1336-40.
41. Packer M, Coats AJ, Fowler MD, et al. Effect of carvedilol on survival in severe chronic heart failure. N Engl J Med. 2001;344:1651-8.
42. Allocation of thoracic organs. Available at: http://optn.transplant.hrsa.gov/policiesandbylaws2/policies/pdfs/policy_9.pdf. Accessed October 29, 2012.
43. Gillies M, Bellomo R, Doolan L, et al. Bench-to-bedside review: inotropic drug therapy after adult cardiac surgery: a systematic literature review. Crit Care. 2005;9:266-79.
44. Kikura M, Sato S. The efficacy of preemptive milrinone or amrinone therapy in patients undergoing coronary artery bypass grafting. Anesth Analg. 2002;94:22-30.
45. Omae T, Kakihana Y, Mastunaga A, et al. Hemodynamic changes during off-pump coronary artery bypass anastomosis in patients with coexisting mitral regurgitation: improvement with milrinone. Anesth Analg. 2005;101:2-8.

46. Feneck RO, Sherry KM, Withington PS, et al. Comparison of the hemodynamic effects of milrinone with dobutamine in patients after cardiac surgery. J Cardiothorac Vasc Anesth. 2001;15:306-15.
47. Dell'Italia LJ. Reperfusion for right ventricular infarction. N Engl J Med. 1998;338:978-80.
48. Calvin JE. Acute right heart failure: pathophysiology, recognition, and pharmacological management. J Cardiothorac Vasc Anesth. 1991;5:507-13.
49. Ferrario M, Poli A, Previtali M, et al. Hemodynamics of volume loading compared with dobutamine in severe right ventricular infarction. Am J Cardiol. 1994;74:329-33.
50. Goodlin SJ, Hauptman PJ, Arnold R, et al. Consensus statement: Palliative and supportive care in advanced heart failure. J Card Fail. 2004;10:200-9.
51. Allen LA, Stevenson LW, Grady KL, et al. Decision making in advanced heart failure: a scientific statement from the American Heart Association. Circulation. 2012;125:1928-52.
52. Home Parenteral Inotropic Therapy: Data Collection Form. https://coverage.cms.fu.com/lcd_area/lcd_uploads/5044_15/HomeParenteralInotropicTherapyDataCollectionForm.pdf. Accessed 10/29/2012.
53. Available from: http://www.cgsmedicare.com/jc/pubs/adv/pdf/1995/December%201995.pdf. Accessed 10/29/2012.
54. Kutner J, Goodlin SJ, Connor SR, et al. Hospice care for heart failure patients. J Pain Symptom Manage. 2005;29:525-8.
55. Rich MW, Shore BL, et al. Dobutamine for patients with end-stage heart failure in a hospice program? J Pall Med. 2003;6:93-7.
56. O'Connor CM, Gattis WA, Adams KF, et al. Tezosentan in patients with acute heart failure and acute coronary syndromes: results of the randomized intravenous tezosentan study (RITZ-4). J Am Coll Cardiol. 2003;41:1452-7.
57. Packer M, Califf RM, Konstam MA, et al. Comparison of omapatrilat and enalapril in patients with chronic heart failure: the Omapatrilat Versus Enalapril Randomized Trial of Utility in Reducing Events (OVERTURE). Circulation. 2002;106:920-6.
58. Cohn JN, Pfeffer MA, Rouleau J, et al. Adverse mortality effect of central sympathetic inhibition with sustained release moxonidine in patient with heart failure (MOXCON). Eur J Heart Fail. 2003;5:659-67.
59. Chung ES, Packer M, Lo KF, et al. Randomized, double-blind, placebo-controlled, pilot trial of infliximab, a chimeric monoclonal antibody to tumor necrosis factor-alpha, in patients with moderate-to-severe heart failure: results of the anti-TNF Therapy Against Congestive Heart Failure (ATTACH) trial. Circulation. 2003;107:3133-40.
60. Mann DL, McMurray JJ, Packer M, et al. Targeted anticytokine therapy in patients with chronic heart failure: results of the Randomized Etanercept Worldwide Evaluation (RENEWAL). Circulation. 2004;109:1594-602.
61. Teerlink JR. A novel approach to improve cardiac performance: cardiac myosin activators. Heart Fail Rev. 2009;14:289-98.
62. Malik FI, Morgan BP. Cardiac myosin activation part 1: from concept to clinic. J Mol Cell Cardiol. 2011;51:454-61.
63. Holmes KC, Angert I, Kull FJ, et al. Electron cryo-microscopy shows how strong binding of myosin to actin releases nucleotide. Nature. 2003;425:423-27.
64. Teerlink JR, Clarke CP, Saikali KG, et al. Dose-dependent augmentation of cardiac systolic function with the selective cardiac myosin activator, omecamtiv mecarbil: a first-in-man study. Lancet. 2011;378:667-75.
65. Malik FI, Hartman JJ, Elias KA, et al. Cardiac myosin activation: a potential therapeutic approach for systolic heart failure. Science. 2011;331:1439-43.
66. Shen YT, Malik FI, Zhao X, et al. Improvement of cardiac function by a cardiac myosin activator in conscious dogs with systolic heart failure. Circ Heart Fail. 2010;3:522-7.

67. Banfor PN, Preusser LC, Campbell TJ, et al. Comparative effects of levosimendan, OR-1896, OR-1855, dobutamine, and milrinone on vascular resistance, indexes of cardiac function, and O2 consumption in dogs. Am J Physiol Heart Circ Physiol. 2008;294:H238-48.
68. Cleland JG, Teerlink JR, Senior R, et al. The effects of the cardiac myosin activator, omecamtiv mecarbil, on cardiac function in systolic heart failure: a double-blind, placebo-controlled, crossover, dose-ranging phase 2 trial. Lancet. 2011;378:676-83.
69. ClinicalTrials.gov: A service of the U.S. National Institutes of Health www.clinicaltrials.gov identifier: NCT01300013 accessed October 29, 2012.
70. Nieminen MS, Cleland JG, Eha J, et al. Oral levosimendan in patients with severe chronic heart failure—the PERSIST study. Eur J Heart Fail. 2008;10:1246-54.
71. Dec GW, Fifer MA, Herrmann HC, et al. Long-term outcome of enoximone therapy in patients with refractory heart failure. Am Heart J. 1993;125:423-9.
72. Packer M. Proposal for a new clinical end point to evaluate the efficacy of drugs and devices in the treatment of chronic heart failure. J Card Fail. 2001;7:176-82.
73. Tamargo J, Lopez-Sendon J. Novel therapeutic targets for the treatment of heart failure. Nat Rev Drug Discov. 2011;10:536-55.

CHAPTER

6

Hospitalization for Heart Failure: Pathophysiology, Classification, and Management Considerations

Muthiah Vaduganathan, Mihai Gheorghiade

INTRODUCTION

Heart failure (HF) accounts for over 1 million admissions annually in the United States. Despite relatively low in-hospital mortality [~3–5%, comparable to that of acute myocardial infarction (MI)], this clinical entity carries a mortality rate of up to 15% and a rehospitalization rate up to 30% within 60–90 days of hospital discharge.[1] The unique characteristics, common predictors, prognostic markers, and clinical profiles have only recently been defined by a number of international registries.[1-5] Limited data exist regarding the postdischarge course of this patient population, although recent large phase III clinical trials have begun to shift to more definite clinical end-points.[6]

Hospitalization for heart failure (HHF) is a complex clinical syndrome that does not represent a single clinical entity, but rather is the final common pathway of a number of diverging processes.[7] Furthermore, the optimal treatment of HHF patients remains unclear with numerous unmet clinical needs. A "one-size-fits-all" approach is likely not plausible based on the heterogenous cardiac substrate and diverse set of inciting and amplifying factors. A number of contributing mechanisms have been proposed that may play a role in the pathogenesis of HHF including hemodynamic perturbations, myocardial injury, renal dysfunction, neurohormonal activation, and inflammation. The individual contributions of these processes are yet to be defined. This review provides an overview of the major pathophysiological pathways contributing to HHF and also provides a therapy-oriented classification scheme that may assist clinicians with early and late management. Tailored therapy to focus on cardiac and noncardiac abnormalities contributing to HHF may improve postdischarge prognosis.

PATHOPHYSIOLOGY

Clinical Course and Definition of Congestion

Hospitalization for HF is formally defined as the rapid onset or change in the signs and symptoms of HF, resulting in the need for urgent therapy, often necessitating admission.[8] Congestion remains the main reason for admissions and readmissions in HF (as opposed to low cardiac output).[9] Ultimately, the combination of an abnormal cardiac substrate, a precipitating cause, and the amplifying circumstances leads to worsening cardiac function and relative volume overload.[9] These varied potential mechanisms converge into a shared outcome of elevated left ventricular (LV) filling pressures leading to pulmonary and systemic congestion. Different congestive etiologies have varying timing of onset and duration ranging from acute events (e.g., hypertensive crisis, ischemia, and arrhythmias) to more long-term gradual processes (e.g., worsening HF). "Clinical congestion" manifests as a constellation of presenting signs and symptoms including dyspnea, jugular venous distension and edema. However, a small but significant subset of patients may be "flying under the radar" with elevated ventricular filling pressures, despite the lack of prominent signs and symptoms of HF. This phenomenon has been termed as "hemodynamic congestion".[9] Limited data have explored the relative time-course of clinical and hemodynamic congestion. However, it appears that hemodynamic congestion is present in the days or even weeks prior to initial presentation and may persist into the postdischarge period.[10] Indeed, elevation of natriuretic peptide levels that may represent hemodynamic congestion persists even after initial treatment of HHF and improvement of clinical congestion.[11]

Identifying Hemodynamic Congestion

Several supporting lines of evidence substantiate this as the possible underlying mechanism of HHF. Elevated pulmonary pressures appear to clearly precede the onset of clinical signs and symptoms of HF in basic science models.[12] Furthermore, direct and indirect correlates of LV filling pressures are known predictors of poor prognosis at time of discharge and into the early postdischarge period.[13,14] In *post-hoc* analyses of a large HHF clinical trial, body weight (as a surrogate of volume status) was shown to be predictive of subsequent readmissions (Figs. 1A–D).[15] Body weight may give rise to false negative measurements given that fluid redistribution to the lung (causing pulmonary edema and warranting admission) may not significantly alter body weight readings. Indeed, in the same retrospective analysis, Blair and colleagues found that body weight was not a predictor of postdischarge mortality.[15] Hemoconcentration (relative increase in hematocrit, albumin, and total protein levels during hospitalization) has been proposed as a potential target of in-hospital diuretic strategies, but this concept needs to be tested in a larger, more controlled setting.[16,17] Other means of identifying hemodynamic congestion at the time of discharge include natriuretic peptide measurement, testing for orthopnea, and assessment of exercise capacity (including six-minute walk test).[18]

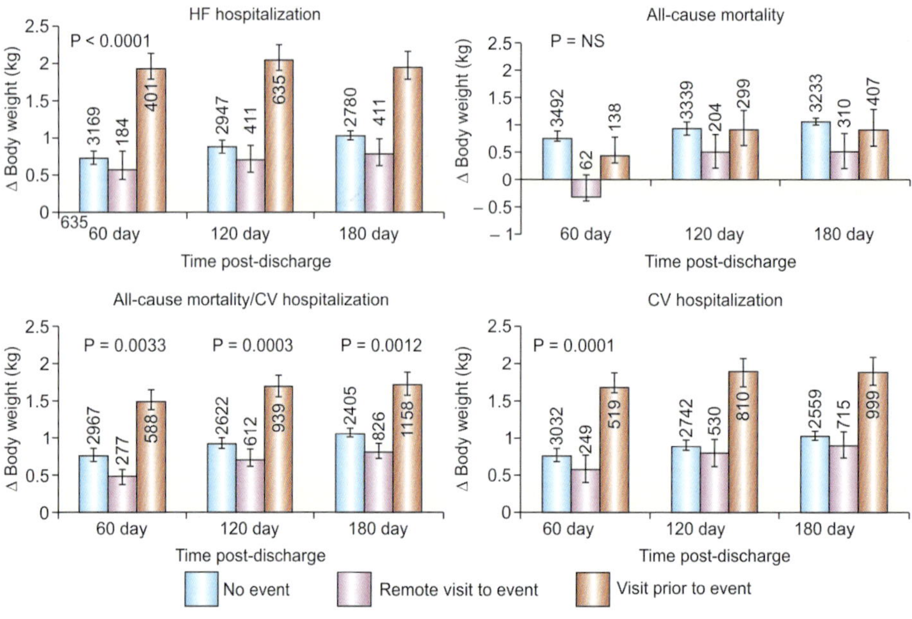

Figure 1A to D: Post-discharge changes in body width weight (BW) are plotted as the mean BW in patients without event, the mean BW at the clinic visit before an event, and at a remote clinic visit prior to the event in patients with events at 60, 120, and 180 days. (A) Represents hospitalization for heart failure (HF). (B) All-cause mortality. (C) All-cause mortality and cardiovascular hospitalization. (D) Cardiovascular hospitalization. Mean values are plotted with standard error from the mean. P-values are a comparison of changes in BW between patients with no event and the visit prior to the event.[15] CV, cardiovascular

Source: *From* Blair JE, Khan S, Konstam MA, et al. Weight changes after hospitalization for worsening heart failure and subsequent re-hospitalization and mortality in the EVEREST trial. Eur Heart J. 2009;30(13):1666-73, *with permission.*

Consequences of Congestion

Hemodynamic congestion or high LV filling pressures may contribute to progression of HF by increasing wall stress and subendocardial ischemia resulting in myocardial necrosis or apoptosis.[9] This process may also alter LV geometry (from ellipsoid to spherical shape) resulting in secondary mitral regurgitation (MR).[19,20] The increased LV filling pressures may contribute to diastolic dysfunction by delaying the drainage of venous blood from the coronary veins and right atrium.[21] Elevated right atrial pressure may reduce the perfusion gradient across the kidneys leading to worse renal function.[22,23] Finally, hemodynamic congestion may further activate the sympathetic axis, increase circulating neurohormonal factors, and upregulate inflammatory mediators.[24] This viscous cycle may be integrally involved in the progression of HF. Clinicians need to become aware of the potential for persistent hemodynamic congestion in a proportion of HHF patients at the time of discharge. In fact, patients are currently discharged with improved symptomatology, but persistently elevated LV filling pressures, as suggested by high B-type natriuretic peptide (BNP) levels.[25]

Neurohormonal Abnormalities

The available data suggests that in addition to hemodynamic abnormalities resulting in congestion, significant abnormalities in neurohormonal profile occur in patients with HHF before, during, and soon after discharge.[10] Although these abnormalities may be secondary to the overall congestive process, they may contribute to the progression of HF and represent a major target for therapy. Circulating catecholamines, vasopressin, and other neurohormonal mediators may have cardiac-specific and systemic effects that contribute to acute and chronic worsening HF.

PHENOTYPICAL CLASSIFICATION OF HEART FAILURE

Contemporary classification schemes[8] focus on presenting clinical scenarios at the time of admission. The relative prevalence of each of these scenarios, estimated by the EuroHeart Failure Survey II (EHFS II) is as follows (in order of decreasing incidence): decompensated HF (65.4%), pulmonary edema (16.2%), high systolic blood pressure (SBP) (11.4%), cardiogenic shock (3.9%), and isolated right-sided HHF (3.2%).[3] Although, this stratification allows for rapid triage, it must be recognized that this clinical definition does not provide any insight into the potential etiology or subsequent course of therapeutic action. Thus, we propose to shift our paradigm to initially assess patients based on a phenotypical classification system that allows targeted therapies and specific interventions. HHF can be initially divided into patients with preserved versus reduced ejection fraction (EF), new-onset versus worsening preexisting HF, and with low- or high-blood pressure, with or without cardiac ischemia/necrosis, and with or without key cardiac/noncardiac comorbidities.

Preserved versus Reduced Ejection Fraction

HHF patients can be broadly divided into HF with reduced EF and HF with preserved EF (HFpEF). The relative prevalence of HFpEF is approximately 50%.[26] In terms of overall clinical profiles, HFpEF patients tend to be older, more likely to be female, and have a history of hypertension (Table 1).[25,26] Beyond these basic demographic and comorbidity data, this unique subset of patients have been poorly characterized. In addition, the growing insight in HFpEF is mainly derived from ambulatory patients. Notwithstanding, the dominant role of hemodynamic congestion as a driver of hospitalization has also been shown for patients with HFpEF. These patients experience a more rapid rate of increase in pulmonary artery diastolic pressure measured by an implantable hemodynamic monitor before HF-related events.[27]

Table 1 **Preserved versus reduced systolic function patient characteristics**[7,26]

Characteristics at admission	*Patients with LVSD (n = 20, 118)*	*Patients with PSF (n = 21, 149)*
Demographics		
Age (years)	70.4 ± 14.3	75.1 ± 13.1
Male	62%	38%
Caucasian	71%	77%
African-American	21%	15%
Medical history		
Diabetes, insulin-treated	15%	17%
Diabetes, noninsulin-treated	24%	26%
Hypertension	66%	76%
Hyperlipidemia	34%	32%
Atrial arrhythmia	28%	33%
Vital signs on admission		
Body weight (kg)	78.5 (65.8, 94.0)	78.9 (64.0, 97.5)
Heart rate (beats/min)	89 ± 22	85 ± 21
SBP (mmHg)	135 ± 31	149 ± 33
DBP (mmHg)	77 ± 19	76 ± 19
Etiology		
Ischemic	54%	38%
Hypertensive	17%	28%
Idiopathic	18%	21%
Findings on admission		
Acute pulmonary edema	3%	2%
Chest pain	23%	24%
Uncontrolled hypertension	9%	12%
Dyspnea at rest	44%	44%
Dyspnea on exertion	63%	62%
Rales	63%	65%
Lower extremity edema	62%	68%
Jugular venous distention	33%	26%
Left ventricular EF (%)	24.3 ± 7.7	54.7 ± 10.2
Laboratory values		
Serum sodium (mEq/L)	137.7 ± 4.6	137.9 ± 4.8
Serum creatinine (mg/dL)	1.4 (1.1, 1.9)	1.3 (1.0, 1.8)
Serum hemoglobin (g/dL)	12.5 ± 2.0	11.9 ± 2.0

Contd...

Contd...

BNP (pg/mL)	1,170.0 (603.0, 2,280.0)	601.5 (320.0, 1,190.0)
Troponin I (ng/mL)	0.1 (0.1, 0.3)	0.1 (0.0, 0.3)
Medications on admission		
ACEI	45%	36%
ARB	11%	13%
Amlodipine	5%	10%
Aldosterone antagonist	10%	5%
β-blocker	56%	52%
Loop diuretic	63%	58%
Digoxin	30%	17%
Aspirin	42%	38%
Antiarrhythmic	13%	8%
Hydralazine	3%	3%
Nitrate	22%	21%
Statin*	40%	39%

LVSD, left ventricular systolic dysfunction; PSF, preserved systolic function; SBP, systolic blood pressure; DBP, diastolic blood pressure; EF, ejection fraction; BNP, B-type natriuretic peptide; ACEI, angiotensin-converting enzyme inhibitor; ARB, angiotensin receptor blocker.

Sources:

1. Reproduced with permission from Gheorghiade M, Pang PS. Acute heart failure syndromes. J Am Coll Cardiol. 2009;53(7):557-73.
2. Data presented as percent, mean ± SD, or median [25th, 75th percentiles]. Adapted and reproduced with permission from Fonarow GC, Stough WG, Abraham WT, et al. Characteristics, treatments, and outcomes of patients with preserved systolic function hospitalized for heart failure: a report from the OPTIMIZE-HF Registry. J Am Coll Cardiol. 2007;50(8):768-77.

*Statin is used among patients with coronary artery disease (CAD), cerebrovascular disease/transient ischemic attack, diabetes, hyperlipidemia, and peripheral vascular disease.

Left ventricular function is relatively maintained in this patient subset through various myocardial-driven compensatory mechanisms. However, these patients have shown to have substantial underlying systolic and diastolic dysfunction.[25,26] While the LVEF is considered normal at more than 50%,[8] patients with an LVEF of 35–50% and mild systolic dysfunction deserve attention as well, since the majority of prior HF trials defined reduced EF as less than 35%. HFpEF patients may be even more sensitive to blood pressure elevations and are more likely to present with a hypertensive etiology and baseline arrhythmias.[26] The postdischarge prognosis of patients with preserved and reduced EF are likely similar,[26] although this population requires further characterization with future studies. Interestingly, a number of hospital admissions and readmission in HFpEF are related to the patient's comorbidities rather than worsening HF itself. Nevertheless, in a 10-year follow-up of newly discharged patients with HF in the Enhanced Feedback for Effective Cardiac

Treatment (EFFECT) phase I study, LVEF did not predict repeated HF, coronary heart disease or cardiovascular readmissions. Furthermore, the lifetime risk for repeat rehospitalizations was similar between patients with reduced or preserved EF.[28] Similarly, mortality in HFpEF is in general unacceptably high.[29,30]

Thus, optimizing pharmacological and nonpharmacological therapies for cardiac and noncardiac comorbidities is particularly important in this HHF subset.[31] This has been addressed in detail in subsequent sections of this review. These interventions may be essential since evidence-based therapies targeting this subgroup are currently lacking. In order to successfully manage HFpEF, any exclusive focus on diastolic dysfunction as single most important target for new therapies may need to give way to the recognition of other mechanisms, such as an impaired ventricular-vascular coupling or abnormal exercise-induced and flow-mediated vasodilation.[32] Diastolic, systolic, vascular, and chronotropic capacities may individually contribute to the progressive loss of the ventricular-vascular reserve[33] that ultimately result in the requirement of hospitalization. Apart from the description of this population in the Organized Program to Initiate Lifesaving Treatment in Hospitalized Patients with Heart Failure (OPTIMIZE-HF),[26] more precise data are required on the clinical trajectories of this HHF subgroup prior to initiation of specific drug development for this indication.

De Novo versus Worsening Chronic Heart Failure

Hospitalization for HF is most commonly a result of worsening chronic HF (roughly 85%), while occurring as a new-onset process in the remainder (~15%). De novo HF presents more commonly with acute pulmonary edema, cardiogenic shock, and hypertensive crisis as the presenting clinical scenario.[3] Furthermore, this subset is more likely to experience a more abrupt change in fluid balance, generally incited by acute coronary syndrome (ACS). Patients with chronic HF likely experience a more gradual accumulation of fluid with high rates of prior ischemic disease and common clinical comorbidities (renal dysfunction, diabetes).[4] Interestingly, despite these variations in initial clinical presentation, the in-hospital mortality rates are fairly similar (if the cardiogenic shock subgroup is excluded).[3] On the other hand, postdischarge clinical course has been shown to be superior in patients with de novo HHF. These findings are perhaps due to the generally lower comorbid illness burden and the specific mechanisms underlying HHF in each subset. Fixable, reversible causes of HHF, such as ACS and hypertensive crisis appear to be more prevalent in the de novo HHF population, thus portending a better postdischarge prognosis.[4]

This postdischarge data emphasize the importance of early interventions to ameliorate reversible causes of congestion and acute decompensation. Thus, any patient with new-onset HHF should be thoroughly and systematically assessed for potentially reversible therapeutic targets.[34] These findings also emphasize the important disconnection between severity of presentation and postdischarge outcomes. Particular attention should be paid to the underlying cardiac substrate and comorbid illnesses, rather than the specific clinical scenario. For example, a patient presenting in hypertensive crisis with flash pulmonary edema may have uneventful postdischarge clinical course, while a patient with only mild symptoms but severely reduced myocardial function may have a poor prognosis. Thus, we choose to focus our classification scheme on factors that are known to influence postdischarge outcomes that have potential reversible or treatable causes.

Low Systolic Blood Pressure

The vast majority of patients admitted for HHF present with normal or high SBP. This vital sign represents a critical component of the "six-axis" model of HHF which is a quick tool to facilitate rapid assessment and initial management upon patient presentation.[35] This important hemodynamic variable has a strong, independent correlation with both in-hospital and postdischarge prognosis. Based on the data from the OPTIMIZE-HF registry, rates of postdischarge mortality ranged from 14.0% in patients with SBP less than 120 mm Hg to 5.4% in patients with SBP more than 160 mm Hg. These results have been consistently demonstrated across other large registries.[1,2,4] Systolic blood pressure represents one of the strongest prognostic markers in current risk stratification models.[36,37]

HHF patients with low SBP remains a clinical entity associated with extremely poor postdischarge prognosis and limited therapeutic options.[38] There is a critical unmet clinical need for "safer" novel inotropes that can safely improve cardiac output and blood pressure without adversely influencing other critical hemodynamic parameters (including myocardial oxygen demand, coronary perfusion, and heart rate). Therapies for this high-risk subset are particularly difficult in patients with concurrent coronary artery disease (CAD) given the high risk of ischemia/necrosis and reduced baseline myocardial flow reserve.[38]

Myocardial Ischemia and Coronary Artery Disease

Large registries have consistently demonstrated that approximately 40–50% of all patients admitted for HF have a history of CAD.[1-5] Indeed, in stable outpatients with chronic HF, ischemic etiology is an independent predictor of poor clinical outcomes.[39] However, the same results have not been observed in the HHF population, except in the subset presenting with cardiogenic shock.[40]

The interconnections between the ischemic disease and HHF range from a precipitant of admission (e.g., acute plaque rupture leading to de novo HF) to a contributor of worsening HF (e.g., due to underlying ischemic disease and progressive LV dysfunction). Recent standardized definitions have been proposed for acute MI in the setting of a HF hospitalization.[41] For practical purposes, a new ischemic event in HHF is defined as a troponin elevation over the 99th percentile above normal.[41] It has been estimated that approximately 20% of patients with HHF present initially with ACS (primarily new-onset HHF).[3] ST-elevation acute MI occurs in over 50% of patients presenting with cardiogenic shock.[3] Thus, the specific clinical scenario should shape the clinician's suspicion for acute plaque rupture.

"Demand ischemia" is on the other end of the spectrum and is extremely common in this patient population. Transient increases in myocardial demand (e.g., due to elevated LV filling pressures, neurohormonal, and sympathetic activation) and reductions in coronary blood flow (e.g., due to low blood pressure, increased heart rate, and endothelial dysfunction) may contribute to myocardial ischemia during hospitalization.[42] Troponin leak into systemic circulation can occur in patients with and without known CAD. In fact, plasma troponin levels were elevated in more than 50% of patients with known CAD and 40% with unknown CAD in prior experiences.[43]

The presence or absence of significant myocardial ischemia during hospitalization and a previous history of CAD greatly informs clinical decision-making. Certain vasoactive agents may be particularly harmful in this population and may contribute to increasing myocardial ischemia and LV dysfunction. Perhaps most dramatically, inotropes may induce myocardial ischemia/necrosis by increasing myocardial oxygen demand and causing significant subendocardial ischemia.[44] Indeed, ischemic etiology of HF may help risk-stratify patients and may predict adverse attendant effects of inotropic administration. Furthermore, these data may provide indirect evidence for the "step-wise" decline in cardiac function observed with each hospitalization in chronic worsening HF. Acute decompensation and subsequent inotropic support may create a vicious cycle of cardiac dysfunction and myocardial injury.[45] Similarly, vasodilators, such as nitroprusside and nesiritide may dilate superficial coronary vessels, thus inducing "coronary steal" from small penetrating vessels. In terms of therapeutic options for HHF patients with ischemia or at high risk for ischemia, nitrates may be safe and efficacious. However, the effectiveness of nitrate therapy in this high-risk subset on postdischarge outcomes has not been demonstrated.

Throughout hospitalization, myocardial preservation and minimization of troponin release should be a major goal of therapies, especially in patients with established CAD.[46-48] Recent data suggest that HF no longer represents a progressive, nonreversible condition.[49] An excellent example of this is hibernating myocardium. Optimal medical management or revascularization in selected cases may improve this viable, but dysfunctional myocardium.[50,51] Aggressive lipid-lowering strategies may help reduce overall ischemic event risk in well-selected HHF patients, despite recent equivocal results from the Controlled Rosuvastatin in Multinational Trial in Heart Failure (CORONA) trial.[52]

Renal Dysfunction and Worsening Renal Function

Baseline renal dysfunction at the time of presentation may play an integral role in the pathogenesis, in-hospital and postdischarge course of HHF.[53] The assessment of renal function is difficult since hemodynamics never reach steady-state during hospitalization. The vast majority of patients with HHF present with some degree of renal impairment, regardless of the presence of "true" kidney injury. This baseline dysfunction is likely a result of mild hemodynamic perturbations and resultant reductions in effective circulating volume. There is increasing appreciation for the central role of renal venous pressure (as opposed to kidney perfusion) in the pathogenesis of kidney injury in HHF.[19,20] Other modulating factors include systemic inflammation and neurohormonal activation during acute decompensation. In-hospital worsening of renal function is present in up to 30% of all HHF patients.[54] Both baseline renal dysfunction and worsening renal function during hospitalization have independent prognostic roles in this population.[53]

This comorbidity should be considered uniquely because of the direct impact of our therapies on renal function in the acute stabilization and postdischarge management of HHF patients. Renal dysfunction may significantly modulate the available therapies that can be utilized in this population, both in terms of safety and efficacy. However, the recent diuretic optimization strategies evaluation (DOSE) trial involving 308 HHF patients showed that there were no significant differences in renal function parameters with the use of different diuretic strategies (high versus low dose and bolus versus continuous infusion).[55] Furthermore, short-term transient changes in serum creatinine levels may not have prognostic significance when they occur after aggressive diuretic treatment with relief of signs of congestion.[17,55] A strategy of aggressive diuretic treatment with relief of congestion may be associated with short-term increase in serum creatinine levels in the absence of any relation with outcomes.[17,55-57] Despite these encouraging data, open questions remain regarding the optimal duration of diuretic therapy, potential end-points for therapeutic success during hospitalization and the reversibility of renal damage in the setting of HHF.

Overall, the optimal methods of fluid removal in this population continue to be investigated. It is likely that aggressive fluid management in the face of worsening renal function is appropriate to relieve renal venous pressures, unless renal dysfunction is persistent into the postdischarge period. From a clinical standpoint, the early identification, close monitoring of renal function, and periodic assessment of responsiveness to therapies remain major management principles.

Select Cardiac Comorbidities

"Deconstructing" the heart into its individual components and potential targets may help guide initial specific therapies.[58] Figure 2 summarizes the overall assessment and targeted management of five overlapping domains of

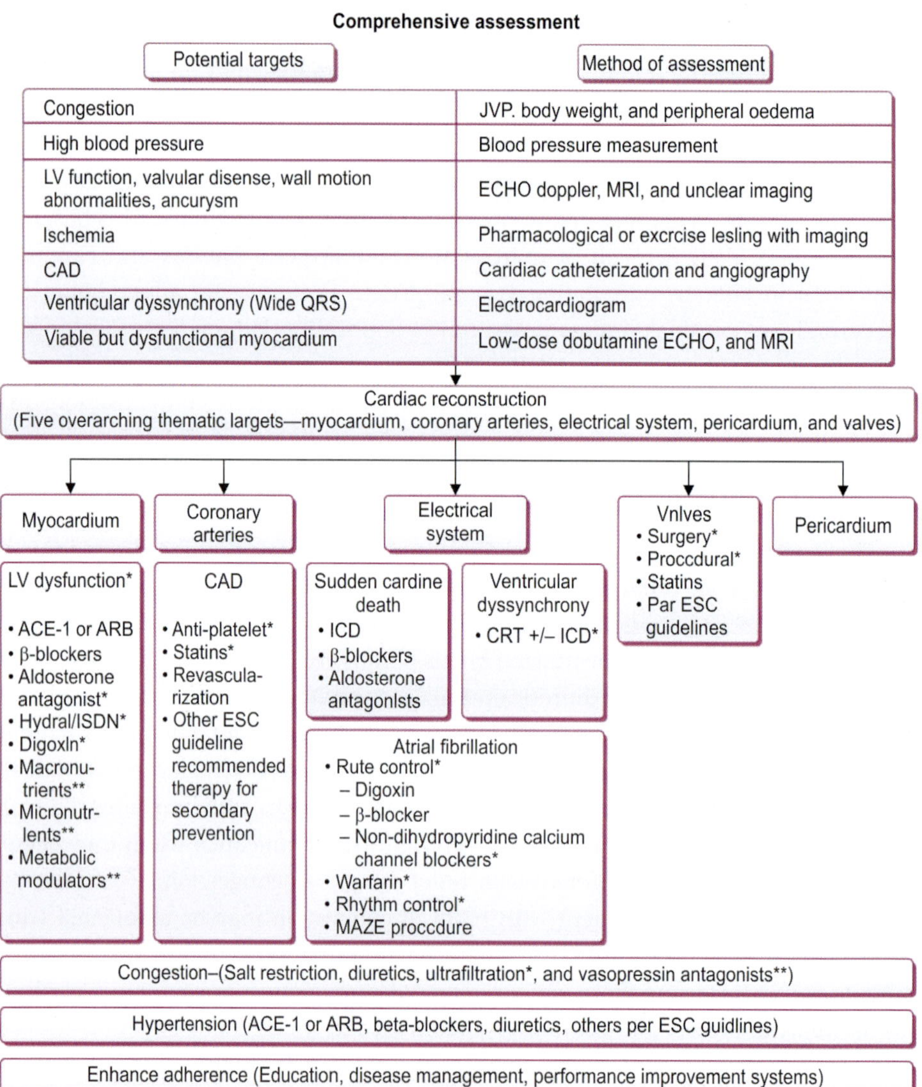

Figure 2: Comprehensive assessment and cardiac reconstruction.[58] ACEI, angiotensin converting enzyme inhibitor; AF, atrial fibrillation; AHFS, acute heart failure syndrome; ARB, angiotensin receptor blocker; CABG, coronary artery bypass grafting; CAD, coronary artery disease; CRT, chronic resynchronization therapy; ESC, European Society of Cardiology; Hydral, hydralazine; ICD, implantable cardioverter defibrillator; ISDN, isosorbide dinitrate; JVP, jugular venous pulse; LV, left ventricle.

Source: *From* Ambrosy A, Wilcox J, Nodari S, et al. Acute heart failure syndromes: assessment and reconstructing the heart. J Cardiovasc Med (Hagerstown). 2011;12(4):258-63, *with permission*.
*Select patients;
**Investigational agents;
#Viable but dysfunctional myocardium.

cardiovascular pathology (myocardium, coronary arteries, electrical system, valves, and pericardium).[58] We have briefly discussed current approaches to each of these potential targets.

Valves

Primary valvular pathologies may be operatively replaced or repaired. Secondary valve disease, especially MR from chronic LV dilatation that is common in patients with depressed LVEF, should be evaluated for surgery in select patients. Further data are required to define whether secondary MR represents a marker of severity of HF or a potential therapeutic target. Clinical attention should be paid to "silent" valvular disease, such as aortic stenosis in the elderly population who may not exhibit a prominent murmur on examination.

Electrical System

Patients with HHF often have atrial arrhythmias [most commonly atrial fibrillation (AF)], chronotropic incompetence, LV dyssynchrony and are at risk for ventricular fibrillation. Although heart rate is a major determinant of cardiac output in patients with HF, maintaining lower heart rates may also be beneficial to reduce cardiac workload. The "optimal" heart rate is likely a balance between hemodynamics and cardioprotection and remains an area of uncertainty. Atrial fibrillation can be managed similar to patients without HF with rate or rhythm control strategies. The combination of β-blocker therapy and lower-dose digoxin may be particularly effective in HHF patients with comorbid AF.[59] Furthermore, standard thrombotic prophylaxis should be initiated with warfarin or novel anticoagulants. Cardiac resynchronization therapy (CRT) in addition to standard therapy should be considered in patients with ventricular dyssynchrony, detected on electrocardiogram by widened QRS complex.[60] Although not very common, patients at risk for sudden cardiac death may benefit from postdischarge device implantation[61] and medical management with β-blockers and mineralocorticoid receptor antagonists.

Myocardium

Traditionally, the identification of viable, but dysfunctional myocardium was only performed in patients with CAD to evaluate for "stunned" or "hibernating" myocardium to assist in prediction of therapeutic response. However, recent data has suggested that multiple strategies beyond revascularization may improve myocardial viability[49] including stem cells, micro- and macronutrient supplementation, and LV assist devices. Contemporary treatment of LV dysfunction should extend beyond standard regimens of β-blockers and angiotensin-converting enzyme inhibitors (ACEIs)/angiotensin receptor blockers (ARBs) to include mineralocorticoid antagonists, digoxin, and hydralazine/nitrates.

Vascular

The importance of pulmonary hypertension (arterial or venous) as a major consequence of HF is well recognized, but specific treatment strategies are still experimental. Pulmonary hypertension at rest or at minimal excursion may be an especially important target for therapy for patients with HFpEF.[62] Normalization of blood pressure in patients who present with hypertension is also necessary.

Pericardium

Surgical or percutaneous pericardectomy is warranted if this pathology is hemodynamically significant.

Metabolic Needs

Despite its relatively small mass, the heart uses more energy than any other organ in the body. Every 30 days, the heart undergoes complete protein remodeling.[63] These incredible metabolic needs must be matched by adequate macro- and micronutrients, especially in settings of decreased cardiac reserve, such as HF. Micronutrients, such as coenzyme Q10 (co-Q10), L-carnitine, and thiamine are integral in helping the heart adapt to continuously changing environment and improve overall energy utilization. Interestingly, deficiencies in these compounds are present in various animal and human models of the failing myocardium.[64] Furthermore, our own therapies including statins (co-Q10)[65] and furosemide (thiamine)[66] can induce micronutrient deficiencies. Micronutrient supplementation may be a unique approach to correcting cellular level abnormalities present in HF that may translate to improved clinical symptomatology. Supplementation with n-3 polyunsaturated fatty acids (PUFAs), approved in Europe but not the United States, may augment cardiac performance. In rat models, n-3 PUFAs increase cardiac efficiency by reducing myocardial oxygen demand.[67] Initial clinical data suggest that n-3 PUFAs improve LV systolic function and may decrease hospitalization in patients with nonischemic cardiomyopathy.[68] Further investigations may be revealing of additional micronutrient strategies to optimize cardiac function.

Select Noncardiac Comorbidities

A systematic approach to the assessment and management of major cardiac and noncardiac comorbidities in HHF is required. Each individual patient should be considered in the context of his/her comorbid illnesses because this can significantly influence early and late management strategies. Chronic kidney disease and diabetes are present in 30–40% of patients at the time of presentation, while chronic obstructive pulmonary disease (COPD), sleep apnea, pulmonary hypertension,

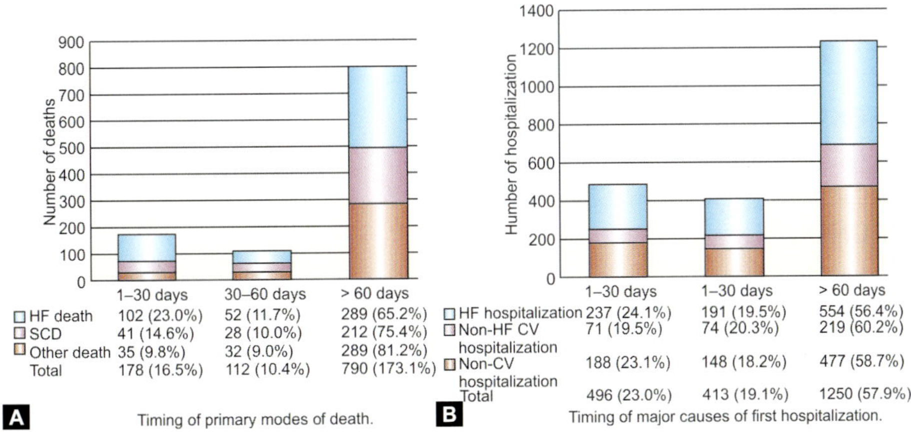

Figure 3A and B: Timing of primary modes of death and major causes of first hospitalization.[73] HF, heart failure; SCD, sudden cardiac death; CV, cardiovascular.

Source: *From* O'Connor CM, Miller AB, Blair JE, et al. Causes of death and rehospitalization in patients hospitalized with worsening heart failure and reduced left ventricular ejection fraction: results from Efficacy of Vasopressin Antagonism in Heart Failure Outcome Study with Tolvaptan (EVEREST) program. Am Heart J. 2010;159(5):841-9.e1, *with permission*.

anemia, and depression are present in smaller, but significant subgroups.[7] Large multivariate risk prediction models have identified each of these comorbid illnesses as independent prognosticators in this population.[69]

Briefly, based on current available data, targeted therapy should be offered for patients with comorbid COPD,[70,71] diabetes, and obstructive sleep apnea.[72] Since the majority of HF rehospitalizations are not directly HF-related (Figs. 3A and B),[73] a holistic, targeted approach against cardiac and noncardiac comorbidities is imperative to improve postdischarge outcomes.[74] Unfortunately, no prospective study has been conducted testing individualized targeted therapies in HHF subgroups with particular comorbidities. Thus, it is difficult to ascertain at this time whether the excess mortality risk in these high-risk groups is related to worsening HF or higher overall comorbid burden.

CONCLUSIONS

Hospitalization for HF is a common clinical entity associated with high postdischarge event rates, despite available therapies. The underlying pathophysiology of HHF is the presence of congestion that is final common pathway of a multitude of cardiac and noncardiac abnormalities. The classification of HHF patients must shift from a clinical scenario approach focused on symptoms to a phenotypical approach focused on correlation with postdischarge outcomes. Specific, tailored approaches must be targeted against known cardiac and noncardiac comorbidities. Future studies must rigorously test optimal medical and nonmedical therapies in specific HHF subgroups.

ACKNOWLEDGMENTS

None.

FUNDING

None.

REFERENCES

1. Gheorghiade M, Abraham WT, Albert NM, et al. Systolic blood pressure at admission, clinical characteristics, and outcomes in patients hospitalized with acute heart failure. JAMA. 2006;296(18):2217-26.
2. Adams KF, Fonarow GC, Emerman CL, et al. Characteristics and outcomes of patients hospitalized for heart failure in the United States: rationale, design, and preliminary observations from the first 100,000 cases in the Acute Decompensated Heart Failure National Registry (ADHERE). Am Heart J. 2005;149(2):209-16.
3. Nieminen MS, Brutsaert D, Dickstein K, et al. EuroHeart Failure Survey II (EHFS II): a survey on hospitalized acute heart failure patients: description of population. Eur Heart J. 2006;27(22):2725-36.
4. Tavazzi L, Maggioni AP, Lucci D, et al. Nationwide survey on acute heart failure in cardiology ward services in italy. Eur Heart J. 2006;27(10):1207-15.
5. Zannad F, Mebazaa A, Juillière Y, et al. Clinical profile, contemporary management and one-year mortality in patients with severe acute heart failure syndromes: The EFICA study. Eur J Heart Fail. 2006;8(7):697-705.
6. Konstam MA, Gheorghiade M, Burnett JC, et al. Effects of oral tolvaptan in patients hospitalized for worsening heart failure: the EVEREST Outcome Trial. JAMA. 2007;297(12):1319-31.
7. Gheorghiade M, Pang PS. Acute heart failure syndromes. J Am Coll Cardiol. 2009;53(7):557-73.
8. McMurray JJ, Adamopoulos S, Anker SD, et al. ESC Guidelines for the diagnosis and treatment of acute and chronic heart failure 2012: The Task Force for the Diagnosis and Treatment of Acute and Chronic Heart Failure 2012 of the European Society of Cardiology. Developed in collaboration with the Heart Failure Association (HFA) of the ESC. Eur Heart J. 2012;33(14):1787-847.
9. Gheorghiade M, Filippatos G, De Luca L, et al. Congestion in acute heart failure syndromes: an essential target of evaluation and treatment. Am J Med. 2006;119(12 Suppl 1):S3-S10.
10. Gheorghiade M, Pang PS, Ambrosy AP, et al. A comprehensive, longitudinal description of the in-hospital and post-discharge clinical, laboratory, and neurohormonal course of patients with heart failure who die or are re-hospitalized within 90 days: analysis from the EVEREST trial. Heart Fail Rev. 2012;17(3):485-509.
11. Metra M, Gheorghiade M, Bonow RO, et al. Postdischarge assessment after a heart failure hospitalization: the next step forward. Circulation. 2010;122(18):1782-5.
12. Adamson PB, Magalski A, Braunschweig F, et al. Ongoing right ventricular hemodynamics in heart failure: clinical value of measurements derived from an implantable monitoring system. J Am Coll Cardiol. 2003;41(4):565-71.

13. Drazner MH, Rame JE, Stevenson LW, et al. Prognostic importance of elevated jugular venous pressure and a third heart sound in patients with heart failure. N Engl J Med. 2001;345(8):574-81.
14. Lucas C, Johnson W, Hamilton MA, et al. Freedom from congestion predicts good survival despite previous class IV symptoms of heart failure. Am Heart J. 2000;140(6):840-7.
15. Blair JE, Khan S, Konstam MA, et al. Weight changes after hospitalization for worsening heart failure and subsequent re-hospitalization and mortality in the EVEREST trial. Eur Heart J. 2009;30(13):1666-73.
16. Davila C, Reyentovich A, Katz SD. Clinical correlates of hemoconcentration during hospitalization for acute decompensated heart failure. J Card Fail. 2011;17(12):1018-22.
17. Testani JM, Chen J, McCauley BD, et al. Potential effects of aggressive decongestion during the treatment of decompensated heart failure on renal function and survival. Circulation. 2010;122(3):265-72.
18. Gheorghiade M, Follath F, Ponikowski P, et al. Assessing and grading congestion in acute heart failure: a scientific statement from the acute heart failure committee of the heart failure association of the European Society of Cardiology and endorsed by the European Society of Intensive Care Medicine. Eur J Heart Fail. 2010;12(5):423-33.
19. Kono T, Sabbah HN, Rosman H, et al. Left ventricular shape is the primary determinant of functional mitral regurgitation in heart failure. J Am Coll Cardiol. 1992;20(7):1594-8.
20. Sabbah HN, Rosman H, Kono T, et al. On the mechanism of functional mitral regurgitation. Am J Cardiol. 1993;72(14):1074-6.
21. Grossman E, Oren S, Messerli FH. Left ventricular filling and stress response pattern in essential hypertension. Am J Med. 1991;91(5):502-6.
22. Damman K, Ng Kam Chuen MJ, MacFadyen RJ, et al. Volume status and diuretic therapy in systolic heart failure and the detection of early abnormalities in renal and tubular function. J Am Coll Cardiol. 2011;57(22):2233-41.
23. Mullens W, Abrahams Z, Francis GS, et al. Importance of venous congestion for worsening of renal function in advanced decompensated heart failure. J Am Coll Cardiol. 2009;53(7):589-96.
24. Colombo PC, Ganda A, Lin J, et al. Inflammatory activation: cardiac, renal, and cardio-renal interactions in patients with the cardiorenal syndrome. Heart Fail Rev. 2012;17(2):177-90.
25. Pang PS, Gheorghiade M, Dihu J, et al. Effects of tolvaptan on physician-assessed symptoms and signs in patients hospitalized with acute heart failure syndromes: analysis from the efficacy of vasopressin antagonism in heart failure outcome study with tolvaptan (EVEREST) trials. Am Heart J. 2011;161(6):1067-72.
26. Fonarow GC, Stough WG, Abraham WT, et al. Characteristics, treatments, and outcomes of patients with preserved systolic function hospitalized for heart failure: a report from the OPTIMIZE-HF Registry. J Am Coll Cardiol. 2007;50(8):768-77.
27. Zile MR, Bennett TD, St John Sutton M, et al. Transition from chronic compensated to acute decompensated heart failure: pathophysiological insights obtained from continuous monitoring of intracardiac pressures. Circulation. 2008;118(14):1433-41.
28. Chun S, Tu JV, Wijeysundera HC, et al. Lifetime analysis of hospitalizations and survival of patients newly admitted with heart failure. Circ Heart Fail. 2012;5(4):414-21.
29. Meta-analysis Global Group in Chronic Heart Failure (MAGGIC). The survival of patients with heart failure with preserved or reduced left ventricular ejection fraction: an individual patient data meta-analysis. Eur Heart J. 2012;33(14):1750-7.
30. Burkhoff D. Mortality in heart failure with preserved ejection fraction: an unacceptably high rate. Eur Heart J. 2012;33(14):1718-20.

31. Shah SJ, Gheorghiade M. Heart failure with preserved ejection fraction: treat now by treating comorbidities. JAMA. 2008;300(4):431-3.
32. Borlaug BA, Paulus WJ. Heart failure with preserved ejection fraction: pathophysiology, diagnosis, and treatment. Eur Heart J. 2011;32(6):670-9.
33. Borlaug BA, Redfield MM. Diastolic and systolic heart failure are distinct phenotypes within the heart failure spectrum. Circulation. 2011;123(18):2006-13.
34. Harinstein ME, Flaherty JD, Fonarow GC, et al. Clinical assessment of acute heart failure syndromes: emergency department through the early post-discharge period. Heart. 2011;97(19):1607-18.
35. Gheorghiade M, Braunwald E. A proposed model for initial assessment and management of acute heart failure syndromes. JAMA. 2011;305(16):1702-3.
36. O'Connor CM, Abraham WT, Albert NM, et al. Predictors of mortality after discharge in patients hospitalized with heart failure: an analysis from the Organized Program to Initiate Lifesaving Treatment in Hospitalized Patients with Heart Failure (OPTIMIZE-HF). Am Heart J. 2008;156(4):662-73.
37. Abraham WT, Fonarow GC, Albert NM, et al. Predictors of in-hospital mortality in patients hospitalized for heart failure: insights from the Organized Program to Initiate Lifesaving Treatment in Hospitalized Patients with Heart Failure (OPTIMIZE-HF). J Am Coll Cardiol. 2008;52(5):347-56.
38. Gheorghiade M, Vaduganathan M, Ambrosy A, et al. Current management and future directions for the treatment of patients hospitalized for heart failure with low blood pressure. Heart fail Rev. 2013;18(2):107-22.
39. Felker GM, Shaw LK, O'Connor CM. A standardized definition of ischemic cardiomyopathy for use in clinical research. J Am Coll Cardiol. 2002;39(2):210-8.
40. Reynolds HR, Hochman JS. Cardiogenic shock: current concepts and improving outcomes. Circulation. 2008;117(5):686-97.
41. Januzzi JL, Filippatos G, Nieminen M, et al. Troponin elevation in patients with heart failure: on behalf of the third Universal Definition of Myocardial Infarction Global Task Force: Heart Failure Section. Eur Heart J. 2012;33(18):2265-71.
42. Gurbel PA, Gattis WA, Fuzaylov SF, et al. Evaluation of platelets in heart failure: is platelet activity related to etiology, functional class, or clinical outcomes? Am Heart J. 2002;143(6):1068-75.
43. Metra M, Nodari S, Parrinello G, et al. The role of plasma biomarkers in acute heart failure. Serial changes and independent prognostic value of NT-proBNP and cardiac troponin-T. Eur J Heart Fail. 2007;9(8):776-86.
44. Schulz R, Rose J, Martin C, et al. Development of short-term myocardial hibernation. Its limitation by the severity of ischemia and inotropic stimulation. Circulation. 1993;88(2):684-95.
45. Felker GM, Benza RL, Chandler AB, et al. Heart failure etiology and response to milrinone in decompensated heart failure: results from the OPTIME-CHF study. J Am Coll Cardiol. 2003;41(6):997-1003.
46. Flaherty JD, Bax JJ, De Luca L, et al. Acute heart failure syndromes in patients with coronary artery disease early assessment and treatment. J Am Coll Cardiol. 2009;53(3):254-63.
47. Kociol RD, Pang PS, Gheorghiade M, et al. Troponin elevation in heart failure prevalence, mechanisms, and clinical implications. J Am Coll Cardiol. 2010;56(14):1071-8.
48. Rossi JS, Flaherty JD, Fonarow GC, et al. Influence of coronary artery disease and coronary revascularization status on outcomes in patients with acute heart failure syndromes: a report from OPTIMIZE-HF (Organized Program to Initiate Lifesaving Treatment in Hospitalized Patients with Heart Failure). Eur J Heart Fail. 2008;10(12):1215-23.

49. Wilcox JE, Fonarow GC, Yancy CW, et al. Factors associated with improvement in ejection fraction in clinical practice among patients with heart failure: findings from IMPROVE HF. Am Heart J. 2012;163(1):49-56.e2.
50. Bonow RO, Maurer G, Lee KL, et al. Myocardial viability and survival in ischemic left ventricular dysfunction. N Engl J Med. 2011;364(17):1617-25.
51. Velazquez EJ, Lee KL, Deja MA, et al. Coronary-artery bypass surgery in patients with left ventricular dysfunction. N Engl J Med. 2011;364(17):1607-16.
52. Kjekshus J, Apetrei E, Barrios V, et al. Rosuvastatin in older patients with systolic heart failure. N Engl J Med. 2007;357(22):2248-61.
53. Brandimarte F, Vaduganathan M, Mureddu GF, et al. Prognostic implications of renal dysfunction in patients hospitalized with heart failure: data from the last decade of clinical investigations. Heart Fail Rev. 2013;18(2):167-76.
54. Damman K, Navis G, Voors AA, et al. Worsening renal function and prognosis in heart failure: systematic review and meta-analysis. J Cardiac Fail. 2007;13(8):599-608.
55. Felker GM, Lee KL, Bull DA, et al. Diuretic strategies in patients with acute decompensated heart failure. N Engl J Med. 2011;364(9):797-805.
56. Blair JE, Pang PS, Schrier RW, et al. Changes in renal function during hospitalization and soon after discharge in patients admitted for worsening heart failure in the placebo group of the EVEREST trial. Eur Heart J. 2011;32(20):2563-72.
57. Metra M, Davison B, Bettari L, et al. Is worsening renal function an ominous prognostic sign in patients with acute heart failure? The role of congestion and its interaction with renal function. Circ Heart Fail. 2012;5(1):54-62.
58. Ambrosy A, Wilcox J, Nodari S, et al. Acute heart failure syndromes: assessment and reconstructing the heart. J Cardiovasc Med (Hagerstown). 2011;12(4):258-63.
59. Khand AU, Rankin AC, Martin W, et al. Carvedilol alone or in combination with digoxin for the management of atrial fibrillation in patients with heart failure? J Am Coll Cardiol. 2003;42(11):1944-51.
60. Wang NC, Bhattacharya S, Gheorghiade M. The potential role of cardiac resynchronization therapy in acute heart failure syndromes. Heart Fail Rev. 2011;16(5):481-90.
61. Wang NC, Piccini JP, Konstam MA, et al. Implantable cardioverter-defibrillators in patients hospitalized for heart failure with chronically reduced left ventricular ejection fraction. Am J Ther. 2010;17(4):e78-87.
62. Chatterjee NA, Lewis GD. What is the prognostic significance of pulmonary hypertension in heart failure? Circ Heart Fail. 2011;4(5):541-5.
63. Taegtmeyer H, Harinstein ME, Gheorghiade M. More than bricks and mortar: comments on protein and amino acid metabolism in the heart. Am J Cardiol. 2008;101(11A):3E-7E.
64. Soukoulis V, Dihu JB, Sole M, et al. Micronutrient deficiencies an unmet need in heart failure. J Am Coll Cardiol. 2009;54(18):1660-73.
65. McMurray JJ, Dunselman P, Wedel H, et al. Coenzyme Q10, rosuvastatin, and clinical outcomes in heart failure: a pre-specified substudy of CORONA (controlled rosuvastatin multinational study in heart failure). J Am Coll Cardiol. 2010;56(15):1196-204.
66. Leslie D, Gheorghiade M. Is there a role for thiamine supplementation in the management of heart failure? Am Heart J. 1996;131(6):1248-50.
67. Pepe S, McLennan PL. Cardiac membrane fatty acid composition modulates myocardial oxygen consumption and postischemic recovery of contractile function. Circulation. 2002;105(19):2303-8.
68. Nodari S, Triggiani M, Campia U, et al. Effects of n-3 polyunsaturated fatty acids on left ventricular function and functional capacity in patients with dilated cardiomyopathy. J Am Coll Cardiol. 2011;57(7):870-9.

69. Senni M, Santilli G, Parrella P, et al. A novel prognostic index to determine the impact of cardiac conditions and co-morbidities on one-year outcome in patients with heart failure. Am J Cardiol. 2006;98(8):1076-82.
70. Mentz RJ, Schmidt PH, Kwasny MJ, et al. The impact of chronic obstructive pulmonary disease in patients hospitalized for worsening heart failure with reduced ejection fraction: an analysis of the EVEREST Trial. J Cardiac Fail. 2012;18(7):515-23.
71. Mentz RJ, Fiuzat M, Wojdyla DM, et al. Clinical characteristics and outcomes of hospitalized heart failure patients with systolic dysfunction and chronic obstructive pulmonary disease: findings from OPTIMIZE-HF. Eur J Heart Fail. 2012;14(4):395-403.
72. Khayat R, Abraham W, Patt B, et al. Central sleep apnea is a predictor of cardiac readmission in hospitalized patients with systolic heart failure. J Cardiac Fail. 2012;18(7):534-40.
73. O'Connor CM, Miller AB, Blair JE, et al. Causes of death and rehospitalization in patients hospitalized with worsening heart failure and reduced left ventricular ejection fraction: results from Efficacy of Vasopressin Antagonism in Heart Failure Outcome Study with Tolvaptan (EVEREST) program. Am Heart J. 2010;159(5):841-9.e1.
74. Gheorghiade M, Peterson ED. Improving postdischarge outcomes in patients hospitalized for acute heart failure syndromes. JAMA. 2011;305(23):2456-7.

CHAPTER 7

Traditional Mechanical Support

Raphael E Bonita, Kariann Abbate

VENTRICULAR ASSIST DEVICES FOR INTERMEDIATE OR LONG-TERM USE

Whether left ventricular assist device (LVAD) is being used as bridge-to-transplant or destination therapy, the goals of device implantation are to maintain and improve end-organ function, enhance quality of life, and increase the patient's activity level as much as possible. When deciding upon a device for this patient's population, important considerations include simplicity that allow patients and families to manage the devices at home, size of the device, noise level, and durability. Small drivelines are preferable to reduce the chance of driveline and pocket infection.

Pulsatile-Flow Devices

First-generation LVADs for long-term use were pulsatile-flow devices. HeartMate XVE (Thoratec Corporation, Pleasanton, California) is approved for both bridge-to-transplant and destination therapy (Fig. 1). It is a positive-displacement pump that is made of titanium with a polyurethane diaphragm and a pusher-plate actuator. Cannulation involves a left ventricular (LV) apical cannula through which blood flows by way of a Dacron conduit in which a 25 mm porcine valve is suspended. The blood is returned through a 20 mm Dacron outflow graft (also protected by a porcine valve) that ultimately is anastomosed to the proximal ascending aorta. It is powered by an electric motor that rotates and displaces the pusher plate. Air that is displaced by the diaphragm is "vented" to the atmosphere by way of the percutaneous driveline into which it is incorporated, and may be used for venting or pneumatic actuation if necessary. Two external batteries and an external controller that weighs less than 300 g supply power.[1] HeartMate XVE can produce between 4 L/min and 10 L/min of flow. This device has a unique blood-pumping surface that is resistant to thrombogenesis. Hence, unlike other LVADs, there is no need for anticoagulation. Antiplatelet agents are recommended. Unfortunately, this surface is immunologically active, which may limit transplant candidacy because of increased

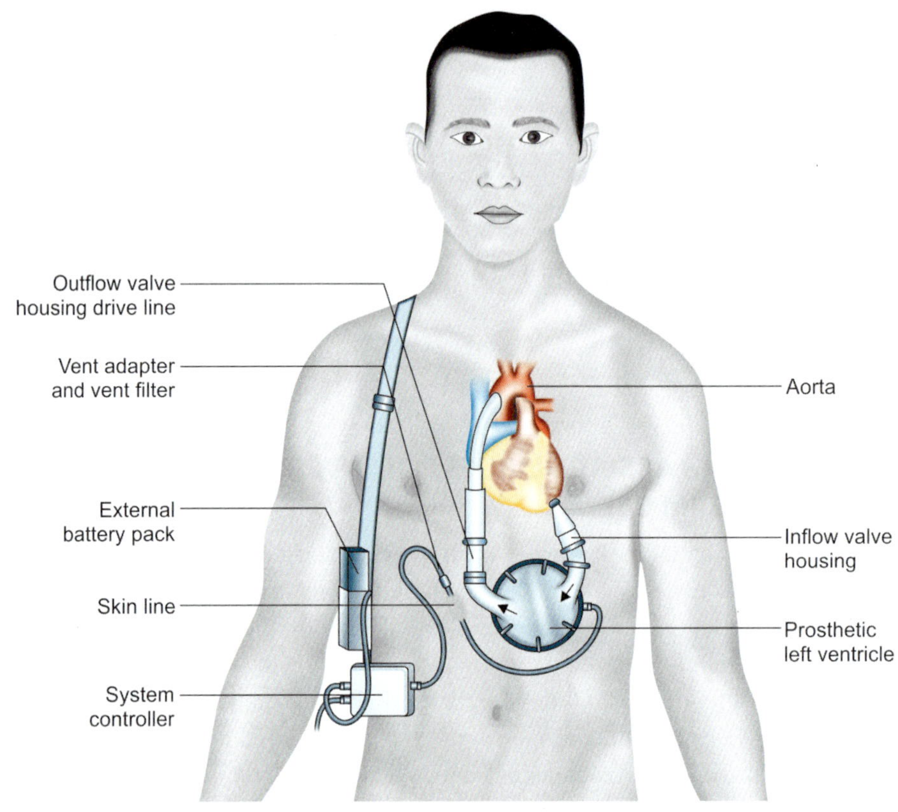

Figure 1: HeartMate XVE.

Source: *From* Rose EA, Gelijns AC, Moskowitz AJ, et al. Long-term use of a left ventricular assist device for end-stage heart failure. N Engl J Med. 2001; 345(20):1435-43, *with permission*.

immunologic reactivity. Other disadvantages of HeartMate XVE are its large size (a body surface area of more than 1.5 m^2 is necessary), durability (incidence of device failure was on the order of 31–35% at 24 months, largely due to internal bearing wear, and degradation of the valved inflow cannula), and driveline infections. The large blood reservoir of the HeartMate XVE is implanted into the peritoneum cavity and often causes a sensation of early satiety. Because of these significant limitations and the benefits of second-generation axial-flow devices, HeartMate XVE is rarely used today. They will no longer be manufactured as of 2012.

Axial-Flow Devices

When LVAD technology was in its beginning phases, many felt the pulsatile flow was necessary to simulate normal physiology. However, with the advent and adaptation of axial-flow devices, we now know that pulsatile flow is not necessary for adequate organ perfusion.

Axial-flow devices have only one moving part (the impeller) which is a major advantage that these devices have over the pulsatile ventricular assist devices (VADs). The impeller is a rotor with helical blades that curve around a central shaft. The spinning of the impeller draws blood from the inflow cannula through the device to the outflow cannula, resulting in nonpulsatile flow. An external driveline provides electrical power to a motor that drives the rotation of the impeller by electromagnetic induction. Axial-flow devices do not require a reservoir, so the devices are significantly smaller than the pulsatile, volume displacement LVADs. These devices can be implanted in women and children. This device still requires an external driveline that is susceptible to infection, but it is much smaller in caliber than the driveline of the first-generation LVADs. Because the axial-flow devices only have one moving part, these devices are more durable than the first-generation pulsatile-flow devices. The ball bearings, which are the components of a device most susceptible to wear, have demonstrated remarkable durability in the HeartMate II lasting more than 7 years in some patients. Slaughter et al. conducted a randomized control trial comparing axial-flow versus pulsatile-flow devices. A total of 200 patients who had advanced heart failure and were ineligible for transplantation were randomly assigned to receive either the axial-flow LVAD or the pulsatile-flow LVAD. The primary end-point was event-free survival at 2 years, with the events being disabling stroke and reoperation for device repair or replacement. Patients who had been assigned to receive the axial-flow device fared better than those assigned to receive the pulsatile-flow device, with 46% and 11%, respectively, reaching the composite primary end-point (Fig. 2). This finding was driven largely by the reduced need for device replacement in the continuous-flow group. One third of the pulsatile-flow pumps required replacement over the 2-year study period [similar to the fraction in the Randomized Evaluation of Mechanical Assistance for the Treatment of Congestive Heart Failure (REMATCH trial)] as compared with only 10% of the continuous-flow pumps. Survival was significantly increased with the continuous-flow device (58%) as compared with the pulsatile-flow device (24%) (P = 0.008). Quality of life measures were also improved to a similar degree in the two treatment groups. Adverse events, including sepsis, right heart failure (RHF), and repeat hospitalization, were less common with the continuous-flow pump.[2]

HeartMate II

HeartMate II is the second-generation LVAD designed by Thoratec Corporation (Pleasanton, California), (Fig. 3). It is the only axial-flow LVAD approved for both bridge-to-transplant and destination therapy in the United States. It is implanted via a median sternotomy below the left costal margin. The inflow cannula exits the LV apex and is aligned parallel to the interventricular septum with the cannula pointed toward the mitral valve. It crosses the diaphragm at the costophrenic angle

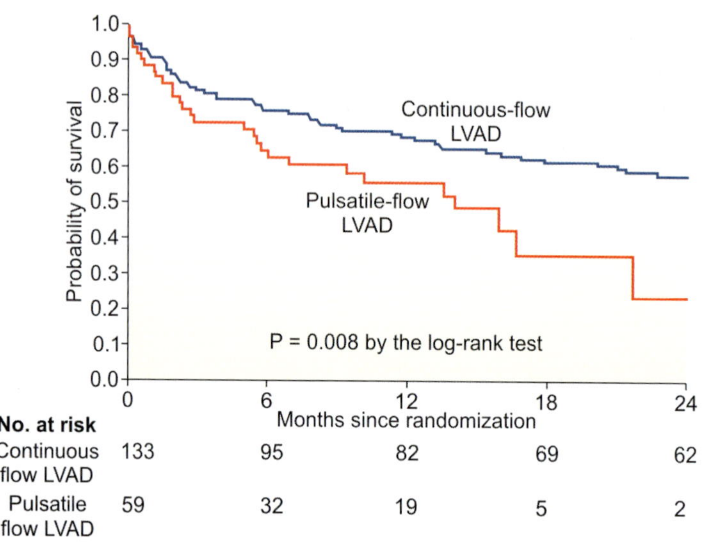

Figure 2: Kaplan-Meier estimates of survival from the as-treated analysis, according to treatment group.[2] LVAD, left ventricular assist device.

Source: *From* Slaughter MS, Rogers JG, Milano CA, et al. Advanced heart failure treated with continuous-flow left ventricular assist device. N Engl J Med. 2009;361(23):2241-51, *with permission*.

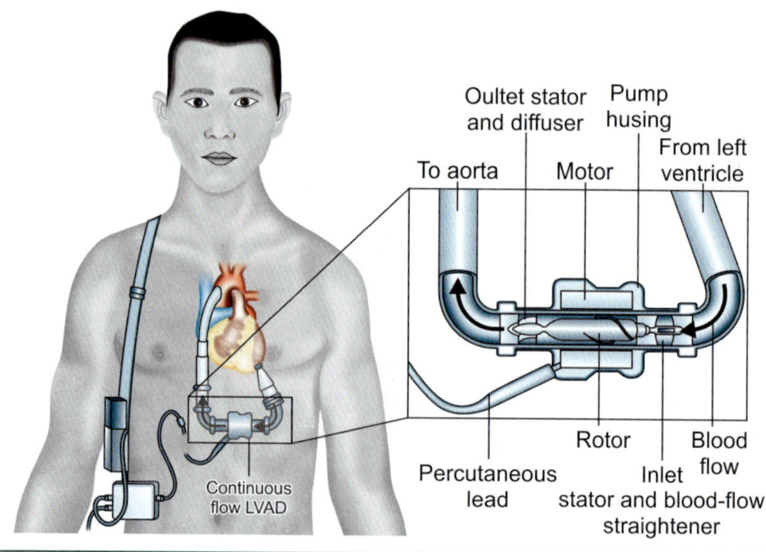

Figure 3: HeartMate II.[2] LVAD, left ventricular assist device.

Source: *From* Slaughter MS, Rogers JG, Milano CA, et al. Advanced heart failure treated with continuous-flow left ventricular assist device. N Engl J Med. 2009;361(23):2241-51, *with permission*.

and enters a pocket under the left rib margin to attach to the pump. The pump lies parallel to the diaphragm. The outflow cannula is anastomosed to the ascending aorta. The percutaneous driveline is tunneled through the abdominal wall and exits the right upper quadrant. The driveline is connected to an external power source.[1] The HeartMate II is usually performed using cardiopulmonary bypass but can be performed off-pump.

Anticoagulation is recommended for patients with HeartMate II devices.

Jarvik 2000

The Jarvik 2000 is an axial-flow device that provides continuous flow from the left ventricle to the descending thoracic aorta. The system consists of a blood pump, outflow graft, percutaneous power cable, pump-speed controller, and direct-current power supply (Fig. 4). Unlike other axial-flow devices, the Jarvik 2000 can be placed within the left ventricle without the need of an inlet cannula. It can be placed via a left thoracotomy, sparing patients a median sternotomy surgery. It is approved as bridge to transplant in the United States. The Jarvik 2000 pump is small, comparable in size to a "C" battery. Similar to the HeartMate II, the Jarvik 2000 has only one moving part (the impeller) that pumps blood from the heart at up to 7 L/min. The goal of the

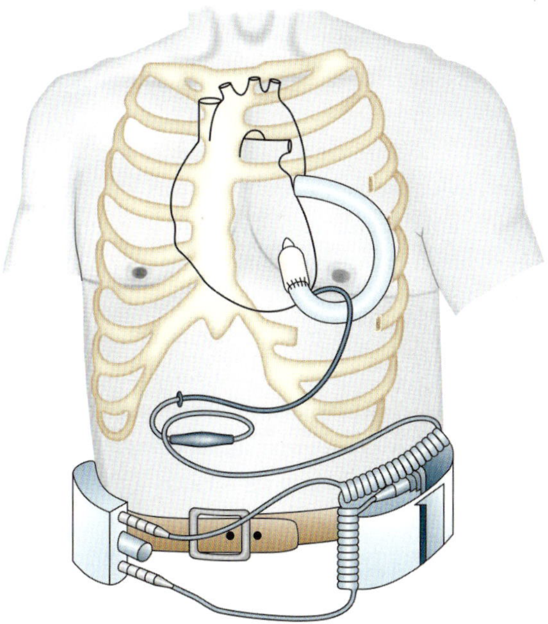

Figure 4: Jarvik 2000.[3]

Source: Jarvik Heart® (2000). The Jarvik 2000 [online]. Available from: www.jarvikheart.com/basic.asp?section=Jarvik+2000. [Accessed April, 2013].

Jarvik 2000 is not to completely take over the function of the biological heart, but to augment the weakened heart's blood output to help restore a normal cardiac output throughout the body. The Jarvik 2000 performs optimally when it acts as a true assist device. To date, not a single mechanical failure of the mechanical blood pump has occurred in any of the more than 200 patients who have received the Jarvik 2000.[3] Unfortunately, driveline fracture is not uncommon. Haj-Yahia et al. described their experiences with 23 patients who received the Jarvik 2000 LVADs and noted driveline failure/fractures in three patients. Each driveline complication occurred after more than 293 days of LVAD support and none of the events led to fatality.[4]

Complications of Axial-Flow Left Ventricular Assist Devices

The major complications noted with axial-flow devices are bleeding and thrombotic events. It is recommended that antiplatelet and anticoagulation agents can be used with all axial-flow devices which predispose patients to bleeding. The international normalized ratio (INR) goal for patients with HeartMate II LVADs differs among different centers, but is usually between 1.5 and 2.5. Additionally, patients with axial-flow LVADs always develop acquired von Willebrand disorder. Uriel et al. conducted a retrospective study of 79 patients with HeartMate II devices with the goal of determining the prevalence of bleeding during continuous-flow LVAD support and to identify potential mechanisms for those bleeding events. Anticoagulation included warfarin in 68.3%, aspirin in 55.7%, and dipyridamole in 58.2% of the patients. Of these patients, nearly half had bleeding episodes at 112 days after LVAD implantation, with 50% of the total patients with bleeding events experiencing an event within 2 months. Gastrointestinal (GI) bleeding was the most frequent event. At the index event, the INR averaged 1.67, which was less than what is traditionally considered "therapeutic anticoagulation". The platelet count was within the normal range in the majority of patients with bleeding events (237 ± 119 × 109/l). Transfusion requirements at the time of heart transplantation of 35 HeartMate II patients compared with 62 HeartMate XVE patients demonstrated twice the transfusion requirements in HeartMate II patients. High molecular weight von Willebrand factor multimers were measured in 31 HeartMate II patients and were reduced in all patients, with 18 of these 31 (58%) patients had bleeding.[5] It is hypothesized that von Willebrand multimers that are necessary for adequate platelet function are broken down by the axial-flow pump.[6]

Arteriovenous malformations (AVMs) of the GI tract are a common source of bleeding in patients with axial-flow LVADs. In a study 30 of 172 patients receiving axial-flow support, 31% of GI tract bleeding events were caused by AVMs. The same mechanisms responsible for AVM formation in aortic stenosis are plausible in patients treated with axial-flow devices given the chronic low pulse pressure associated with the pump.

Although the risk of thrombotic events with axial devices is low, they can be a devastating complication for patients with LVADs. Boyle et al. conducted a retrospective study of 331 patients discharged with HeartMate II devices. Ten had thrombotic events (9 ischemic strokes, and 3 pump thrombosis) and 58 had hemorrhagic events (7 strokes, 4 hemorrhages requiring surgery, and 102 requiring transfusions). The median INR was 2.1 at discharge and 1.90 at 6 months. Although the incidence of stroke was low, 40% of ischemic strokes occurred in patients with INRs less than 1.5 and 33% of hemorrhagic strokes were in patients with INRs more than 3.0. The highest incidence of bleeding was at INRs more than 2.5.[7] Because bleeding complications occur frequently in patients with axial-flow devices, anticoagulation and/or antiplatelet therapy is often held or stopped. In this setting, patients are predisposed to thrombotic events.

Right ventricular (RV) failure is a complication after LVAD implantation and can be a major cause of morbidity and mortality. It leads to underfilling of the left ventricle, resulting in poor LVAD output. Patients suffering from RHF often require additional RV support in the form of inotropes or a right-sided mechanical device. When RV failure occurs, the perioperative mortality of LVAD surgery increases to 19–43% and patients tend to have higher mortality after cardiac transplant.[8] Dang et al. described experience with RHF in chronic congestive heart failure (CHF) patients at Columbia Presbyterian Hospital between 1996 and 2004. One hundred eight patients with chronic CHF who underwent HeartMate LVAD implantation were identified. Right heart failure was defined as the need for a subsequent right ventricular assist device (RVAD), more than or equal to 14 days of intravenous inotropes/pulmonary vasodilators or both. Forty-two (38.9%) RHF patients were identified. Fourteen of these required RVAD insertion. Outcome parameters measured included mortality within the first 30 days, intensive care unit (ICU) length of stay, incidence of reoperation for bleeding and acute renal failure and stroke, bridge-to-transplantation rate, and post-transplantation survival rate. Female sex was found to be a risk factor for RHF (73.3% vs. 26.7%, P = 0.003). Right heart failure patients had a higher early mortality rate, greater ICU length of stay, higher rates of reoperation for bleeding and renal failure, and lower bridge-to-transplantation rate than non-RHF patients. Fourteen (33.3%) RHF patients required RVAD insertion. Elevated intraoperative central venous pressure (CVP) was also found to be an independent predictor of post-LVAD RHF. Overall, bridge-to-transplantation rate for the entire study cohort was 73.1%. Deng et al. concluded that the development of RHF after LVAD insertion confers significant morbidity and mortality. Clinicians should not hesitate to initiate inotropes and pulmonary vasodilators and timely RVAD insertion, if necessary, to support patients with evidence of RHF after LVAD insertion.[9]

There are several methods clinicians can use to predict which patients will develop RHF following LVAD placement, but none are perfect. An elevated

Table 1 **Right ventricular failure risk score and likelihood of right ventricular failure by score strata[8]**

Risk score	n	RV failure (n)	No RV failure (n)	Likelihood ratio (95% CI)
3.0 < 3.0	142	29	113	0.49 (0.37–0.64)
4.0–5.0	25	15	10	2.8 (1.4–5.9)
5.5 > 5.5	30	24	6	7.6 (3.4–17.1)

CI, confidence interval; RV, right ventricular.
*Risk score is derived by summing points awarded for the presence of a vasopressor requirement (4 points), aspartate aminotransferase (AST) more than or equal to 80 IU/L (2 points), bilirubin more than or equal to 2.0 mg/dL (2.5 points) and creatinine more than or equal to 2.3 mg/dL (3 points).

transpulmonary gradient may be predictive of post-LVAD RHF. Echo parameters can also be useful in predicting poor RV function following VAD including a dilated and hypokinetic RV. Matthews et al. developed a right ventricular failure risk score (RVFRS) to help identify LVAD candidates at risk for RV failure (Table 1). Data on LVAD candidates were prospectively evaluated for preoperative clinical, laboratory, echocardiographic, and hemodynamic predictors of RV failure. Right ventricular failure was defined as the need for postoperative intravenous inotrope support for more than 14 days, inhaled nitric oxide for 48 hours, right-sided circulatory support or hospital discharge on an inotrope. Of 197 LVADs implanted, 35% were complicated by postoperative RV failure. A vasopressor requirement (4 points), aspartate aminotransferase (AST) more than or equal to 80 IU/L (2 points), bilirubin more than or equal to 2.0 mg/dL (2.5 points), and creatinine more than or equal to 2.3 mg/dL (3 points) were independent predictors of RV failure. The authors concluded that the RVFRS can be easily incorporated in usual care and effectively stratifies the risk of RV failure and death after LVAD implantation.[8] The right ventricular Stroke Work Index (RVSWI) can be used to predict right heart failure following LVAD implantation. The RVSWI = (mean pulmonary artery pressure - the meain right atrial pressure) divided by the stroke volume index. Stroke volume can be calculated by dividing the cardiac index by the heart rate.[9]

Total Artificial Heart

Total artificial heart (TAH) is a mechanical device that replaces the heart. There are two main TAHs on the market today: CardioWest™ device (SynCardia, Fig. 5) and the AbioCor® (Abiomed, Fig. 6).

CardioWest™ Total Artificial Heart

The CardioWest™ TAH is a biventricular, pneumatic, pulsatile blood pump that completely replaces the patient's native ventricles and all four cardiac valves orthotopically. It weighs 160 g and displaces 400 mL of volume. It delivers a cardiac output of more than 9 L/min. As of 2012 in the United States, the device is

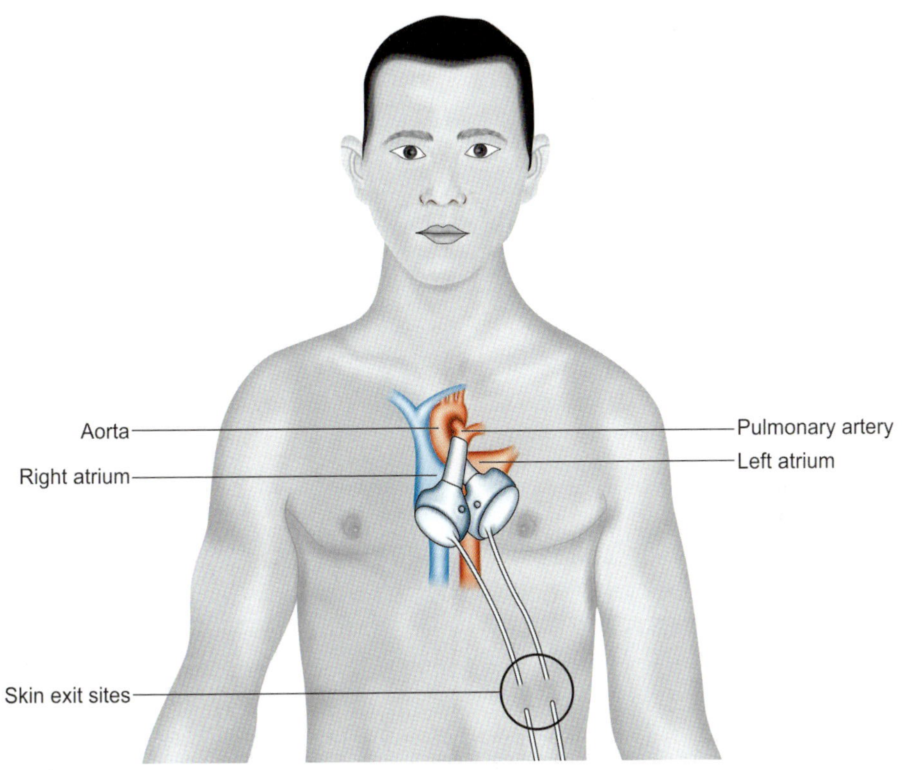

Figure 5: CardioWest™ total artificial heart.[10]

Source: *From* Copeland JG, Smith RG, Arabia FA, et al. Cardiac replacement with a total artificial heart as a bridge to transplantation. N Engl J Med. 2004; 351(9):859-67, *with permission.*

powered by a large console on wheels that prevents hospital discharge. However, home discharge is a viable option for patients in Europe as portable drivers are available. The device may be useful in patients, for whom LVADs and bi-VADs are contraindicated, including patients with aortic insufficiency, cardiac arrhythmias, a LV thrombus, an aortic prosthesis, an acquired ventricular septal defect, or irreversible biventricular failure requiring high pump outputs.[10] Copeland et al. conducted a prospective randomized study evaluating the safety and efficacy of the CardioWest™ TAH in transplant-eligible patients at risk for imminent death from irreversible biventricular cardiac failure and compared them to historical controls. The primary end-points included the rates of survival to heart transplantation and of survival after transplantation. Survival to transplantation was achieved in 79% of the patients who received a TAH according to protocol as compared with 46% of the controls ($P < 0.001$). The meantime from entry into the study to transplantation or death was 79.1 days among all the patients who received an implant and 8.5 days among the controls ($P < 0.001$). Bleeding, infection, device malfunction,

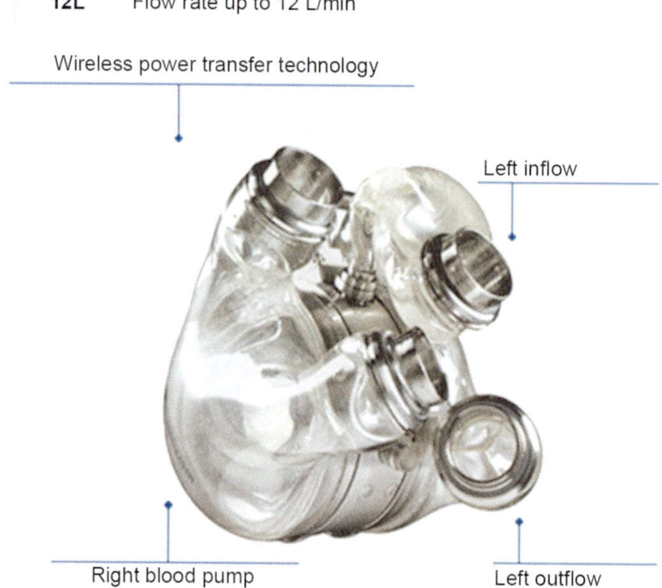

Figure 6: AbioCor®[11]

Source: Abiomed. (2013). AbioCor® [online]. Available from: www.abiomed.com/products/heart-replacement/. [Accessed April, 2013].

hepatic dysfunction, neurologic events, peripheral thromboembolism, and need for reoperation were the most common adverse events in the CardioWest™ TAH group. The authors concluded that implantation of the CardioWest™ TAH was a successful bridge to transplantation in patients with heart failure in whom inotropic therapy had failed and who were not candidates for the use of LVAD. Implantation of the TAH helped to restore hemodynamic function, promoted end-organ recovery and mobility, and was associated with a posttransplantation survival rate similar to national survival rates 5 years after transplantation. The CardioWest™ TAH is a nice option as a bridge-to-transplant for patients who have failed optimal medical therapy and who are not candidates for LVAD therapy.[11]

AbioCor® (Abiomed)

The AbioCor® is the first completely self-contained, internal artificial heart. It weighs approximately 2 pounds and consists of two artificial ventricles, two artificial valves, and a hydraulic pumping system. It operates using both internal and external lithium batteries. The internally implanted battery is continually recharged from an external power source or from a basic patient-carried external battery pack using transcutaneous energy transmission. The AbioCor® is intended for use with patients who suffer from biventricular heart failure and for whom heart transplantation is not an option. It received Food and Drug Administration (FDA) approval under a humanitarian device exemption (HDE) on September 5, 2006. As of April 2011, 14 patients have been implanted with the AbioCor®, with one patient living for 512 days.[12]

Third-Generation Left Ventricular Assist Device—HeartWare® Ventricular Assist Device

The HeartWare® ventricular assist system (VAS) is a miniaturized implantable centrifugal blood pump that draws blood from the left ventricle and propels it through an outflow graft connected to the patient's ascending aorta (Fig. 7). It can generate a cardiac output up to 10 L/min. Because of its small size, the pump is able to be implanted in the pericardial space, decreasing the surgical morbidity. The impeller is the only moving part of the HeartWare® device, which spins at rates between 2,400 revolutions/min and 3,200 revolutions/min. The impeller is suspended within the pump housing through a combination of passive magnets and hydrodynamic thrust bearings. When the impeller spins, blood flows across inclined surfaces, creating a "cushion" between the impeller and the pump housing. There are no mechanical bearings or any points of contact between the impeller and the pump housing.[13]

HeartWare® is conducting an ongoing study called the Evaluation of the HeartWare Left Ventricular Assist Device for the Treatment of Advanced Heart Failure (ADVANCE). Preliminary results were presented at the Scientific Sessions at the American Heart Association meeting in 2010. The study was designed to compare

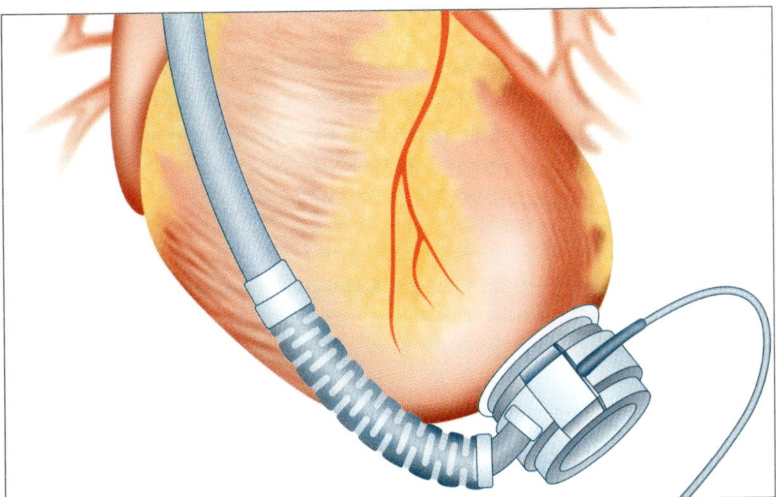

Figure 7: HeartWare® ventricular assist system.[14]

Source: HeartWare. (2012). Clinical trials [online]. Available from: www.heartware.com.au/clinicians/clinical-trials. [Accessed April, 2013].

HeartWare® to HeartMate II as a bridge to heart transplant. One hundred forty patients who received a HeartWare® device (treatment group) were compared with patients in the Interagency Registry for Mechanically Assisted Circulatory Support (INTERMACS™) registry who had received HeartMate II devices (control group). The primary end-point was survival on the originally implanted device, transplant, or explant for ventricular recovery at 180 days. Secondary end-points included a comparison of survival between treatment and control groups, functional and quality of life outcomes and adverse events. HeartWare® VAD met criteria for noninferiority, but not superiority. The success rate of the treatment group was 92% compared to 90% in the control group. There appeared to be less bleeding and infection with the HeartWare® device, but a higher incidence of stroke than expected.[13]

In June 2010, the FDA granted HeartWare® conditional approval to begin enrollment in an investigational device exemption (IDE) destination therapy clinical study for the HeartWare® VAS. The study was designed to enroll 450 patients at 50 United States hospitals. It is a noninferiority study entitled "A Clinical Trial to Evaluate the HeartWare® Ventricular Assist System (ENDURANCE)". The trial is a randomized, controlled, unblinded, multicenter clinical trial to evaluate the use of the HeartWare® VAS as a destination therapy in advanced heart failure patients. The study population will be selected from patients with end-stage heart failure who have not responded to standard medical management and who are ineligible for cardiac transplantation.[14] Pagani et al. are also conducting a study comparing HeartWare® VAS to optimal medical therapy in patients with advanced heart failure who do not yet qualify for transplantation or LVAD therapy using currently approved guidelines. The study is entitled "The Evaluation of VAD InterVEntion before Inotropic Therapy (REVIVE-IT)" and enrollment is scheduled to begin in 2012.

An exciting feature of the HeartWare® VAS is transcutaneous electrical transfer (TET). This technology allows batteries to be surgically placed and can be recharged transcutaneously. This eliminates the need for a driveline, which will significantly decrease the chance of infection. Currently, the available time between battery charges is limited to approximately 3 hours, but hopefully as technology improves; the timeframe between required battery charges will lengthen.

Thoratec is also working on a third-generation axial-flow device that is smaller than the HeartMate II. It will use a magnetically levitated impeller. Other exciting future prospects for LVADs include devices placed percutaneously, eliminating the need for major cardiac surgery.

SUMMARY

Mechanical circulatory support provides rescue in the setting of cardiogenic shock complicated by acute myocardial infarction, myocarditis, or dilated cardiomyopathy in patients failing medical therapy. Mechanical assistance corrects hemodynamic derangement allowing for restoration of end-organ dysfunction and possibly recovery of the myocardium. The duration of mechanical support required as well as the presence of primarily left, right, or biventricular dysfunction are some of the major factors taken into consideration when deciding on the type of mechanical support needed. Despite the benefits of device therapy, they are not perfect, and expose the patient to potential complications that can result in significant morbidity, even mortality. Future device development will hopefully improve upon current complication rates. When these devices are implanted as destination therapy, it will be important that the medical teams caring for these patients consider having palliative care discussions from the beginning as long-term survival remains limited when compared to heart transplantation.

REFERENCES

1. Frazier OH, Kirklin J. ISHLT Monograph Series: Mechanical Circulatory Support. New York, USA: Elsevier; 2006.
2. Slaughter MS, Rogers JG, Milano CA, et al. Advanced heart failure treated with continuous-flow left ventricular assist device. N Engl J Med. 2009;361(23):2241-51.
3. Jarvik Heart®. (2000). The Jarvik 2000. [online] Available from www.jarvikheart.com/basic.asp?section=Jarvik+2000. [Accessed April, 2013].
4. Haj-Yahia S, Birks EJ, Rogers P, et al. Midterm experience with the Jarvik 2000 axial flow left ventricular assist device. J Thorac Cardiovasc Surg. 2007;134(1):199-203.
5. Uriel N, Pak S, Jorde UP, et al. Acquired von Willebrand syndrome after continuous-flow mechanical device support contributes to a high prevalence of bleeding during long-term support and at the time of transplantation. J Am Coll Cardiol. 2010;56(15):1207-13.
6. Suarez J, Patel CB, Felker GM, et al. Mechanisms of bleeding and approach to patients with axial-flow left ventricular assist devices. Circ Heart Fail. 2011;4(6):779-84.
7. Boyle AJ, Russell SD, Teuteberg JJ, et al. Low thromboembolism and pump thrombosis with the HeartMate II left ventricular assist device: analysis of outpatient anti-coagulation. J Heart Lung Transplant. 2009;28(9):881-7.
8. Matthews JC, Koelling TM, Pagani FD, et al. The right ventricular failure risk score: a pre-operative tool for assessing the risk of right ventricular failure in left ventricular assist device candidates. J Am Coll Cardiol. 2008;51(22):2163-72.
9. Fukamachi K, McCarthy PM, Gmedira NG, et al. Preoperative risk factors for right ventricular failure after implantable left ventricular assist device insertion. Ann Thorac Surg. 1999;68(6):2181-4.
10. Dang NC, Topkara VK, Mercando M, et al. Right heart failure after left ventricular assist device implantation in patients with chronic congestive heart failure. J Heart Lung Transplant. 2006;25(1):1-6.
11. Copeland JG, Smith RG, Arabia FA, et al. Cardiac replacement with a total artificial heart as a bridge to transplantation. N Engl J Med. 2004;351(9):859-67.
12. Abiomed. (2013). AbioCor®. [online] Available from: www.abiomed.com/products/heart-replacement/. [Accessed April, 2013].
13. Zoler ML. (2010). Third-generation LVAD shows good efficacy, safety. [online] Available from www.ehospitalistnews.com/index.php?id=2050&type=98&tx_ttnews%5Btt_news%5D=19132&cHash=da03e20e36. [Accessed April, 2013].
14. HeartWare. (2012). Clinical trials. [online] Available from www.heartware.com.au/clinicians/clinical-trials. [Accessed April, 2013].

CHAPTER 8

Percutaneous Mechanical Support

Raphael E Bonita, Kariann Abbate

INTRODUCTION

There are approximately 5.8 million people in the United States living with heart failure (HF).[1] These numbers are expected to increase over the next decade due to the aging population. Despite the increasing prevalence of HF, the number of donor hearts available for transplant has remained stagnant. In 2010, there were 2,333 heart transplants performed in the United States.[2] A severe donor shortage has limited the availability of donor hearts resulting in prolonged waits for organs for patients with advanced HF. Furthermore, more than 200,000 patients with heart failure are not eligible for transplant due to age or comorbidities.[3] The advent of mechanical circulatory support has decreased mortality and improved the quality of life for patients awaiting heart transplantation as well as for those ineligible for transplantation.

INDICATIONS FOR MECHANICAL ASSIST DEVICES

Mechanical assist devices are indicated for patients who are failing optimal medical therapy. When patients are exhibiting evidence of end-organ dysfunction despite optimal medical therapy, mechanical assist devices should be considered. Mechanical assist devices are used for both acute and chronic HF. The National Institute of Health has developed profiles using data from Interagency Registry for Mechanically Assisted Circulatory Support (INTERMACS) to assist in clarification of target populations for mechanical assist devices (Table 1). There are three main indications for mechanical assist devices: (1) bridge to myocardial recovery, (2) bridge to cardiac transplantation, and (3) destination therapy.

Bridge to Recovery

Mechanical assist devices are commonly used to support patients suffering from postcardiotomy shock that are unable to be weaned from cardiopulmonary bypass

Table 1 INTERMACS profile description

Clinical presentations	*Time frame for intervention*
Profile 1: Critical cardiogenic shock	
Patients with life-threatening hypotension despite rapidly escalating inotropic support, critical organ hypoperfusion, often confirmed by worsening acidosis and/or lactate levels. "Crash and burn"	Definitive intervention needed within hours
Profile 2: Progressive decline	
Patients with declining function despite intravenous inotropic support may be manifested by worsening renal function, nutritional depletion, inability to restore volume balance, "sliding on inotropes". Also describes declining status in patients unable to tolerate inotropic therapy	Definitive intervention needed within a few days
Profile 3: Stable but inotrope dependent	
Patients with stable blood pressure, organ function, nutrition, and symptoms on continuous intravenous inotropic support (or a temporary circulatory support device or both), but demonstrated repeated failing to wean from support due to recurrent symptomatic hypotension or renal dysfunction "dependent stability"	Definitive intervention elective over a period of weeks to months
Profile 4: Resting symptoms	
Patients can be stabilized close to normal volume status but experiences daily symptoms of congestion at rest or during ADL. Doses of diuretics generally fluctuate at very high levels. More intensive management and surveillance strategies should be considered, which may in some cases reveal poor compliance that would compromise outcomes with any therapy. Some patients may shuttle between 4 and 5	Definitive intervention elective over a period of weeks to months
Profile 5: Exertion intolerance	
Comfortable at rest and with ADL but unable to engage in any other activity, living predominantly within the house. Patients are comfortable at rest without congestive symptoms, but may have underlying refractory elevated volume status, often with renal dysfunction. If underlying nutritional status and organ function are marginal, patient may be more at risk than INTERMACS 4 and require definitive intervention	Variable urgency depends upon maintenance of nutrition, organ function and activity
Profile 6: Exertion limited	
Patient without evidence of fluid overload is comfortable at rest and with activities of daily living and minor activities outside the home but fatigues after the first few minutes of any meaningful activity. Attribution to cardiac limitation requires careful measurement of peak oxygen consumption, in some cases with hemodynamic monitoring to confirm severity of cardiac impairment. "Walking wounded"	Variable urgency depends upon maintenance of nutrition, organ function and activity level
Profile 7: Advanced NYHA III	
A placeholder for more precise specification in future, this level includes patients who are without current or recent episodes of unstable fluid balance, living comfortably with meaningful activity limited to mild physical exertion	Transplantation or circulator support may not currently be indicated

Contd...

Contd...

Modifiers for profiles	Possible profiles to modify
Temporary circulatory support can modify only patients in hospital (other devices would be INTERMACS devices) includes IABP, ECMO, TandemHeart®, Levitronix, BVS 5000 or AB5000, Impella®	1,2,3 in hospital
Arrhythmia (A)—Can modify any profile. Recurrent ventricular tachyarrhythmias that have recently contributed substantially to clinical compromise. This includes frequent ICD shock or requirement for external defibrillator, usually more than twice weekly	Any profile
Frequent Flyer (FF)—Can modify only outpatients, designate a patient requiring frequent emergency visits or hospitalizations for diuretics, ultrafiltration, or temporary intravenous vasoactive therapy	3 if at home, 4, 5, 6. A frequent flyer would rarely be profile 7

INTERMACS, interagency registry for mechanically assisted circulatory support; ADL, activities of daily living; NYHA, New York Heart Association; IABP, Intra-aortic balloon pump; ECMO, extracorporeal membrane oxygenating system; ICD, implantable cardioverter-defibrillator

and hemodynamically unstable patients following acute myocardial infarction (MI) or acute viral myocarditis. These patients are most often in INTERMACS profile 1. Percutaneous, temporary assist devices, such as extracorporeal membrane oxygenating system (ECMO), intra-aortic balloon pump (IABP), TandemHeart®, and Impella® are frequently used in these situations because of their relative ease of insertion. If a patient does not adequately recover with these temporary devices, a more permanent ventricular assist device (VAD) may be considered. Often, a temporary device is used as a "bridge-to-bridge", stabilizing the patient's hemodynamics so that a more definitive VAD can be placed or transplant can be performed. If both right- and left-heart support is needed, devices such as the Thoratec CentriMag or Thoratec VAD system can be used.

Occasionally, patients with chronic HF symptoms, usually due to a nonischemic cardiomyopathy, have a left ventricular assist device (LVAD) placed and recover enough myocardial function to have the LVAD explanted. In a retrospective study conducted by Mancini et al., only 5% of patients fell into this category and had the LVAD successfully explanted. Exercise testing may be a useful modality to identify those patients in whom the device can be explanted.[4]

Bridge to Transplant

This is the most common indication for LVAD placement. Due to long waiting times on the transplant list, especially for patients with blood type O, mechanical assist devices are often used to prevent end-organ damage and improve quality of life while patients are waiting for heart transplant. LVAD placement prior to transplant can improve end-organ function, enhance nutritional status, and allow patients to participate in rehabilitation programs, which can improve post-transplant outcomes.[5] The timing of VAD placement in these patients is sometimes challenging. For patients awaiting transplant, performing multiple sternotomy procedures may predispose patients to adverse outcomes, such as sternal wound infection following their definitive transplant surgery. Conversely, waiting too long for VAD placement may compromise renal and other end-organ function and allow deconditioning and cardiac cachexia to occur, resulting in worse outcomes at the time of transplant. Jarvik 2000 is a continuous flow LVAD approved in the United States for bridge to transplant. This device can be placed via left thoracotomy, which can spare patients a sternotomy procedure. HeartMate II is the most commonly used for bridge to transplant.

Destination Therapy

In 2001, the Randomized Evaluation of Mechanical Assistance for the Treatment of Congestive Heart Failure (REMATCH) group published a landmark study demonstrating a mortality benefit of LVAD versus optimal medical therapy in patients with end-stage heart failure. REMATCH was a multicenter, controlled trial that randomly assigned 129 patients with advanced heart failure who were ineligible for transplant to receive HeartMate XVE LVAD versus optimal medical therapy (including inotropes). Survival analysis showed a reduction of 48% in the risk of death from any cause in the group that received LVADs as compared with the medical-therapy group (relative risk, 0.52; 95% confidence interval, 0.34–0.78; P = 0.001, Fig. 1). The rates of survival at 1 year were 52% in the device group and 25% in the medical-therapy group (P = 0.002), and the rates at 2 years were 23% and 8% (P = 0.09), respectively.[6] REMATCH demonstrated a significant improvement in survival for patients receiving pulsatile flow LVAD compared with medical therapy, but it also revealed limitations of these devices for long-term support. Survival at 1 year was 52% in the LVAD group and at 2 years was only 25%; 65% of patients surviving to 2 years required device replacement due to mechanical failure. Driveline infections were common. Some have questioned whether there was simply a mode switch of death in patients receiving first generation LVADs for destination therapy.[7] Second generation axial flow LVADs have shown improved survival compared to the pulsatile devices studied in REMATCH. Axial flow devices have overcome many of the limitations of pulsatile flow devices. Pulsatile flow devices require a large reservoir to store blood, which limits its utility in small women and children. Axial flow devices are smaller and can be used in a more diverse group of patients. Axial flow devices are quieter and more comfortable. Although driveline infections are still a problem with axial flow devices, they are much less frequent compared to pulsatile devices. Currently, HeartMate II is the only axial flow device approved for destination therapy in the United States. This device was approved based on a study conducted

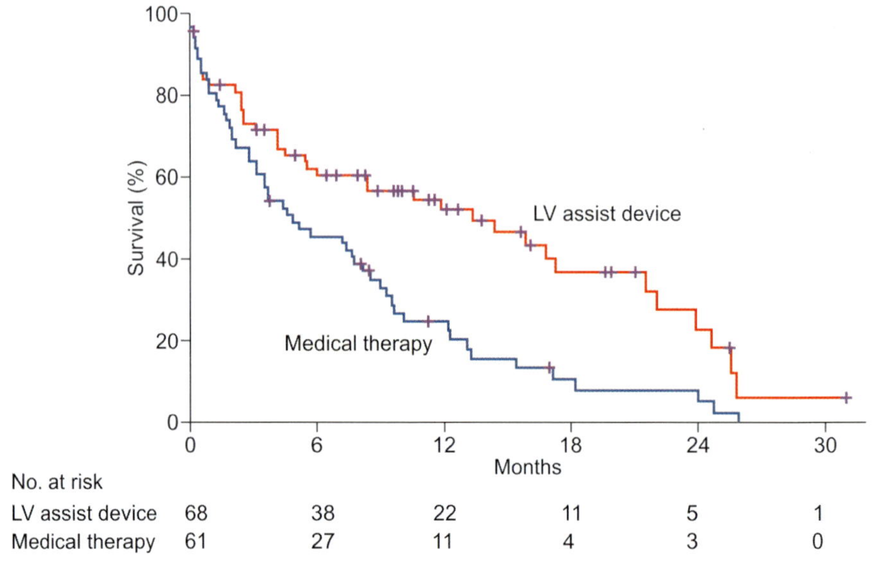

Figure 1: Kaplan-Meier survival curves in patients receiving left ventricular (LV) assist devices versus optimal medical therapy.

Source: *From* Rose EA, Gelijns AC, Moskowitz AJ, et al. Long-term use of a left ventricular assist device for end-stage heart failure. N Engl J Med. 2001;345:1435-45, *with permission*.

by the HeartMate II investigators in 2009. It randomized patients with advanced HF who were ineligible for transplantation, in a 2:1 ratio, to undergo implantation of a continuous-flow device or pulsatile-flow device. The primary composite end- point was, at 2 years, survival-free from disabling stroke and reoperation to repair or replace the device. The primary composite end-point was achieved in more patients with continuous-flow devices than with pulsatile-flow devices [62 of 134 (46%) vs. 7 of 66 (11%); P < 0.001; hazard ratio, 0.38; 95% confidence interval, 0.27–0.54; P < 0.001], and patients with continuous-flow devices had superior actuarial survival rates at 2 years (58% vs. 24%, P = 0.008). Adverse events and device replacements were less frequent in patients with the continuous-flow device.[8]

DEVICES USED FOR SHORT-TERM MECHANICAL CIRCULATORY SUPPORT

The choice of mechanical circulatory support is based on stability of the patient, the amount and type of circulatory support needed, and the expected duration the device will be used. Mechanical circulatory support devices can be placed percutaneously or surgically and can be extracorporeal, paracorporeal, or intracorporeal. For patients in cardiogenic shock, the most effective devices are relatively easy to implant and have a good safety profile.

Percutaneous Devices

The IABP, TandemHeart®, and Impella® are the percutaneous devices that are currently available in the United States. They are most frequently used as rescue devices for patients in cardiogenic shock or to provide support for patients undergoing high-risk percutaneous coronary interventions (PCIs) or surgeries. The advantage of percutaneous devices is that they can be placed with relative ease in the cardiac catheterization laboratory. As with all mechanical circulatory support devices, they carry the risks of bleeding, hemolysis, thrombus formation, infection, and device failure. Percutaneous devices carry the additional risk of peripheral vascular complications. This is particularly important, as many of the patients eligible for these devices are at high risk of peripheral vascular disease. If a percutaneous device is being considered, imaging of the distal aorta, iliac, and femoral vessels with angiography, computed tomography, or magnetic resonance imaging should be considered.[9]

Intra-Aortic Balloon Pump

The IABP consists of a cylindrical polyethylene balloon that sits in the aorta, approximately 2 cm from the left subclavian artery. It deflates in systole increasing cardiac output by reducing afterload and decreases myocardial oxygen consumption. Inflation during diastole increases coronary artery perfusion. Based on American College of Cardiology and American Heart Association Guidelines, IABP is a Class IB indication for patients in cardiogenic shock. It is commonly used following an acute MI and has proven beneficial in patients who suffer from mechanical complications of acute MI, including mitral regurgitation and rupture of the ventricular septum.[10,11] IABP is also used to provide hemodynamic support during high-risk PCI or cardiac surgery and is sometimes placed to assist in weaning patients from cardiopulmonary bypass following cardiac surgery. Although hemodynamics is improved in patients suffering from cardiogenic shock after placement of IABP, it is unclear if placement of IABP provides a mortality benefit. To date, there are no randomized control trials comparing IABP to standard therapy in patients suffering from cardiogenic shock. In 2009, a meta-analysis was performed evaluating the available evidence of IABP in ST segment elevation myocardial infarction (STEMI) with or without cardiogenic shock. The pooled randomized data do not support IABP in patients with high-risk STEMI. The meta-analysis of cohort studies in the setting of STEMI complicated by cardiogenic shock supported IABP therapy adjunctive to thrombolysis. In contrast, the observational data did not support IABP therapy adjunctive to primary PCI. These findings should be taken with caution, as the authors noted that currently available observational data concerning IABP therapy in the setting of cardiogenic shock is hampered by bias and confounding.[12]

Contraindications to the use of IABP include severe aortic valve insufficiency, aortic dissection, severe peripheral vascular disease, and irreversible brain damage. Inflation and deflation of the intra-aortic balloon is timed with the electrocardiogram (EKG), rendering IABP ineffective in unstable rhythms.

The complication rate for IABP placement ranges from 8.7% to 29% and averages 15%.[13-15] Most complications are vascular in nature with the most severe complications being arterial thrombosis and limb loss. Other vascular complications include compartment syndrome, arterial dissection, hematoma, and retroperitoneal bleeding. Infectious complications can occur, especially in situations where IABP is used for a long duration. Risk factors for complications include peripheral vascular disease, female sex, and diabetes.[9]

TandemHeart®

TandemHeart® is manufactured by CardiacAssist, Pittsburgh, Pennsylvania. It is comprised of three components: (1) a centrifugal continuous flow pump, (2) a microprocessor-based controller, and (3) a 21-French transseptal cannula (Fig. 2). The inflow catheter can be placed percutaneously in the left atrium through a transseptal approach and whose outflow cannula is placed in the femoral artery. TandemHeart can provide up to 5 L of flow per minute when placed percutaneously. If placed in the or using direct surgical cannulation technique, TandemHeart® can provide up to 8 L per minute of flow. The indications for TandemHeart® are similar to the indications for IABP support: cardiogenic shock due to acute MI, postcardiotomy, or decompensated heart failure. Because TandemHeart® is capable of providing 5 L of flow per minute, it may be preferred to IABP in patients with severe cardiogenic shock. However, TandemHeart® is more technically challenging to place compared to an IABP. Thiele et al. conducted a randomized control trial in 2005 comparing IABP to TandemHeart for patients presenting with cardiogenic shock and acute MI. They found that the hemodynamic and metabolic parameters in cardiogenic shock were reversed more effectively with TandemHeart® compared to IABP treatment. However, there were more complications encountered with the TandemHeart® including severe bleeding and limb ischemia. The study was not powered to detect a mortality difference. The authors speculate that the complications associated with VAD therapy may be due to a systemic inflammatory response triggered by the extracorporeal circulation. This response may play a role in triggering disseminated intravascular coagulation (DIC). In patients treated with VAD for more than 2 days, nearly all patients required a blood transfusion as a consequence of DIC. The VAD took 25 minutes to place, compared to 11.5 minutes for placement of IABP.[16]

Given the higher complication rate with TandemHeart® compared to IABP, TandemHeart® is usually considered only after a patient suffering from cardiogenic shock has failed medical therapy and IABP support. TandemHeart® is used as first

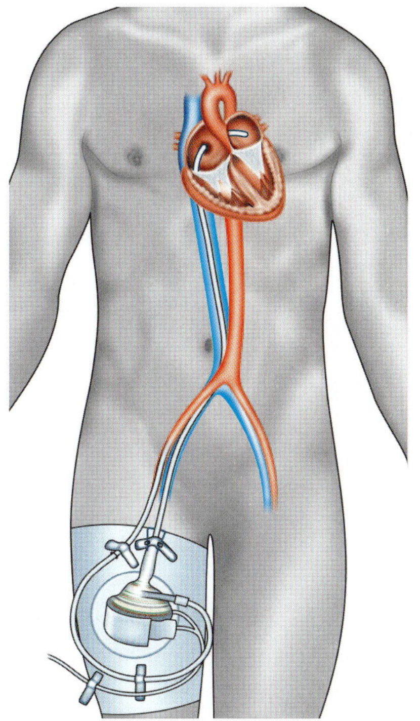

Figure 2: Tandem heart.

Source: CardiacAssist, Inc. [online] Available from: http://www.cardiacassist.com. [Accessed April, 2013].

line support in patients who are predicted to require more than 3 L of additional cardiac output.

TandemHeart® is contraindicated in patients with predominant right ventricular (RV) failure because the low left atrial pressure does not permit adequate pumping. It is also relatively contraindicated in patients with a ventricular septal defect due to the risk of hypoxemia secondary to right-to-left shunting. Other contraindications include aortic insufficiency and severe peripheral arterial disease.[17]

Impella 2.5

Impella 2.5 (Abiomed Europe GmbH, Aachen, Germany) is a catheter-based, impeller-driven axial flow pump with a maximal flow rate of 2.5 L/minute from the left ventricle to the ascending aorta (Fig. 3). It can be implanted percutaneously. Impella 5.0 is capable of generating 5 L/minute of flow, but must be placed in the OR. The Placebo-controlled Randomized Study of the Selective A1 Adenosine Receptor Antagonist Rolofylline for Patients Hospitalized with Acute Decompensated Heart Failure and Volume Overload to Assess Treatment Effect on Congestion and Recent

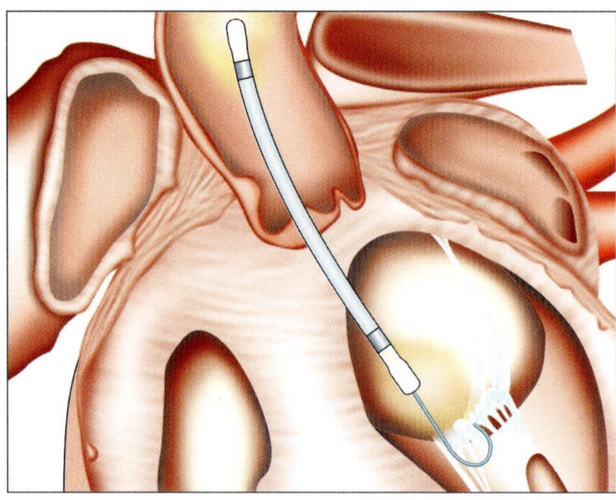

Figure 3: Impella 2.5.

Source: ABIOMED [online]. Available from: www.abiomed.com [Accessed April, 2013].

Function (PROTECT 1) trial was a randomized control trial that demonstrated improved hemodynamics, safety, and efficacy of Impella 2.5 in use prior to high risk PCI. The Impella LP 2.5 vs. IABP in Cardiogenic Shock (ISAR-SHOCK) trial was a randomized control trial that demonstrated that Impella 2.5 improved hemodynamics, increased cardiac output, and was safe in patients receiving Impella for acute MI. Seyfarth et al. published a randomized control study in 2008 comparing Impella LP 2.5 to IABP in patients suffering from cardiogenic shock secondary to acute MI. The study was not powered to detect mortality. The investigators found that hemodynamics including cardiac index were statistically significantly improved in the Impella group compared to the IABP group. There was no increased risk of major bleeding, distal limb ischemia, arrhythmia, or infection in the Impella group. Transient hemolysis was noted in the Impella group. USpella is a United States multicenter registry of Impella 2.5 patients evaluating the safety and feasibility of left ventricular support with the Impella 2.5 during high-risk PCI and treatment of acute MI. It examined approximately 181 patients. In situations where Impella 2.5 was used to facilitate high-risk PCI, the registry showed that overall major adverse event rate was low at 6% and 30-day survival rate was 97%. In patients who received an Impella for acute MI, Impella improved hemodynamics by increasing cardiac index from 1.9 to 2.5 L/min/m^2 and mean arterial pressure from 62 to 87 mmHg. It was able to successfully lower wedge pressure from 28 to 20 mmHg and systemic vascular resistance (SVR). After Impella 2.5 support, overall ejection fraction in AMI patients improved from 29 to 37%. Impella successfully supported AMI refractory shock patients with 69% survival to the next therapy or on to recovery. Also, 58% of AMI shock patients and 89% of AMI patients with no shock were discharged.[18]

Contraindications to Impella 2.5 include prosthetic aortic valves, moderate to severe aortic insufficiency, heavily calcified aortic valves, documented left ventricular thrombus, severe peripheral vascular disease, and in patients who are unable to tolerate anticoagulation.

The most commonly reported complications of Impella 2.5 placement and support include limb ischemia, vascular injury, and bleeding requiring blood transfusion. Hemolysis has been reported. Other potential complications include aortic valve damage, displacement of the distal tip of the device into the aorta, infection, and sepsis.[19]

Impella 2.5 is most commonly used in patients with cardiogenic shock who have failed IABP or in patients with cardiogenic shock or prior to high-risk PCI who are anticipated to require more hemodynamic support than an IABP can provide.

Extracorporeal Membrane Oxygenation

Extracorporeal membrane oxygenation is similar to cardiopulmonary support provided during cardiac surgery but can be delivered for a more prolonged period. There are two types of ECMO: (1) venovenous (VV) and (2) venoarterial (VA). Both provide respiratory support, but only VA ECMO can provide hemodynamic support. Although there are data to support a mortality benefit with the use of VV ECMO for acute respiratory failure, the literature supporting the use of VA ECMO for patients in cardiogenic shock is less robust. To date, no randomized control trials have been conducted to determine the efficacy of this modality in hemodynamically unstable patients.

Venoarterial extracorporeal membrane oxygenation is comprised of a cannula that is inserted into the femoral artery and a cannula that is inserted into the femoral vein. The ECMO circuit is based on a centrifugal pump and a hollow-fiber membrane oxygenator. All circuit components are heparin surface coated. During ECMO, blood is extracted from the native vascular system and circulated outside the body by a mechanical pump. The blood passes through an oxygenator and heat exchanger, where the hemoglobin becomes fully saturated with oxygen and carbon dioxide is removed. The blood is then reinfused into the native vascular system. VA ECMO has the capability of providing as much augmentation to cardiac output as an LVAD but can be placed quickly and less invasively. ECMO is often placed percutaneously. It can provide hemodynamic support to both the right and left hearts. It has become a popular option for patients in cardiogenic shock who require rapid implementation of hemodynamic and/or respiratory support. Indications for VA ECMO include support after cardiac arrest, inability to wean from cardiopulmonary bypass following cardiac surgery, cardiogenic shock following acute MI, bridge-to-decision or bridge-to-transplant in advanced heart failure patients, and cardiogenic shock associated with myocarditis, poisoning or hypothermia. ECMO has proven successful in supporting patients with fulminant myocarditis (FM). Chen and Yu described their experience with ECMO in patients with FM in 2004. From 1995 to 2001, they used ECMO as first-line mechanical support to treat 15 FM patients with shock, including five under external cardiopulmonary resuscitation (CPR) and ten with high-degree atrioventricular block. Their results revealed 93.3% (14/15) in successful weaning rate and 73.3% (11/15) in discharge survival rate. The average ECMO support time was 129 ± 50 hours (127 ± 83 hours for the survivors). As compared with ABIOMED BiVAD use for FM, ECMO group had lower morbidity rate than VAD group: mechanical related thromboembolism was 6.7% in ECMO group and 40–27.3% in VAD group; re-exploration for hemostasis was 20% in ECMO group and 45.5% in VAD group. They pointed out that since FM tends to recover within 2 weeks, ECMO is an appropriate option for this relatively short duration. ECMO is easier to wean off than VAD, and ECMO can be converted to VAD at any time if necessary.[20]

Since anticoagulation is necessary to prevent blood from clotting in the ECMO circuit, ECMO is contraindicated in patients who are not candidates for anticoagulation, such as patients with active bleeding issues, recent surgery, and recent intracranial injury. ECMO is also relatively contraindicated in patients with irreversible cardiac failure who are not candidates for transplant or more permanent VADs. Other factors to consider before implementing ECMO include age, body mass index, neurological function, and prior functional status.

The most frequent complication of ECMO is bleeding. Patients on ECMO are predisposed to bleeding due to the need to receive a continuous infusion of heparin or a similar anticoagulant and platelet dysfunction that is caused by the ECMO circuit. Thromboembolism due to thrombus formation in the ECMO circuit is another serious complication. Vascular complications can result from cannula placement, such as limb ischemia, vessel perforation, and/or vessel dissection. Complications specific to VA ECMO include pulmonary hemorrhage, pulmonary infarction, aortic thrombosis, coronary ischemia, and stroke.

Centrifugal Ventricular Assist Device

A centrifugal assist device is an extracorporeal cone-shaped rotor contained within a plastic or metal housing. Blood flows into the pump at the cone's apex and exits at the edge of the base. The spinning of the rotor creates a centrifugal force that is imparted to the blood, generating a constant, nonpulsatile flow. These devices are indicated for short-term support including cardiopulmonary bypass surgery, postcardiotomy shock, and bridge-to-bridge situations. Centrifugal pumps can also be used to provide RV support after cardiac transplant (Fig. 4). These devices can

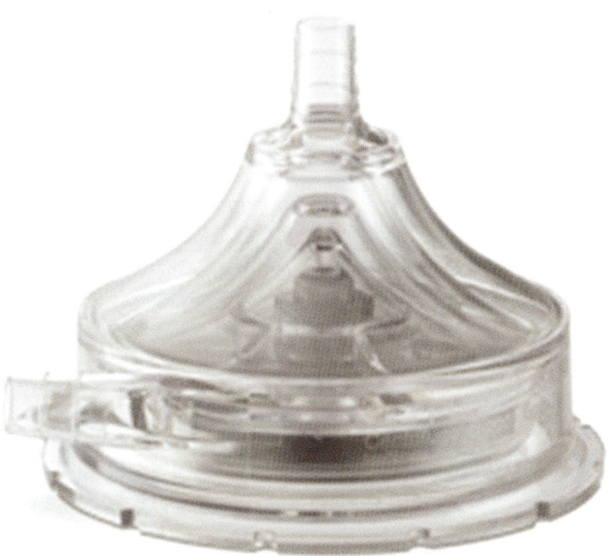

Figure 4: BPX-80 BIO Pump plus centrifugal blood pump.

Source: [online] Available from: http://www.medtronic.com/for-healthcare-professionals/products-therapies/cardiovascular/cardiopulmonary-products/bpx-80-bio-pump-plus-centrifugal-blood-pump/index.htm [Accessed April 2013].

provide up to 10 L/min of flow. The most commonly used centrifugal device is Bio-Medicus Perfusion System (Medtronic).

Pulsatile Assist Devices for Short-term Use

Pulsatile flow devices consist of plastic or metal housing with a mechanically driven volume displacement chamber that fills either passively or by suction applied during chamber expansion. Blood enters through an inflow valve and fills the chamber as it expands. The blood is then forced out through an outflow valve as the chamber contracts. These pumps mimic the cyclic systole and diastole of the heart and generate pulsatile blood flow. The inflow valve (bioprosthetic or mechanical) allows unidirectional flow into the device and prevents regurgitation during mechanical systole and the outflow valve prevents regurgitation during mechanical relaxation.

Abiomed AB5000 is a pulsatile assist device that can supply one or both sides of the heart. The AB5000 ventricle is vacuum-assisted technology with clear housing to allow clinicians a view into the device. Regardless of whether the device is supporting one or both ventricles, the AB5000 only requires one driver. The AB Portable Driver is designed to allow patients to leave their hospital rooms and walk within the hospital and on hospital grounds.

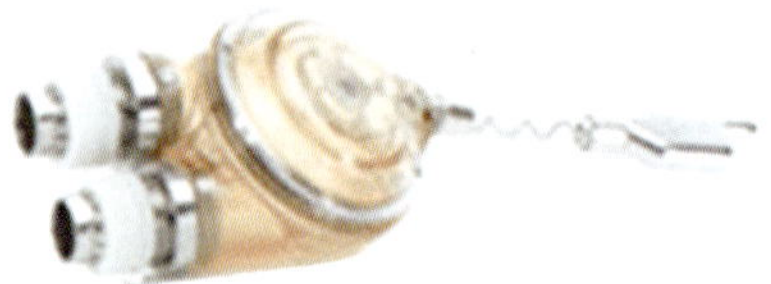

Figure 5: Thoratec percutaneous ventricular assist device.

Source: Thoratec Corporation [online]. Available from: http://www.thoratec.com/medical-professionals/vad-product-information/thoratec-pvad.aspx [Accessed April, 2013].

Right Ventricular Assist Devices and Biventricular Assist Devices

Right ventricular failure presents a unique challenge when considering VADs. Because the right ventricle is less muscular and thinner than the left ventricle, it is more difficult to canalize the right ventricle. There is greater risk of complications when the right ventricle is canalized, such as right ventricular perforation or displacement of the cannula. Because of the tenuous nature of RVADs and BiVADs, most patients who require these devices are confined to the hospital. Abiomed AB5000 (as discussed above) is an example of a device that can provide biventricular support. Other biventricular VADs include Thoratec percutaneous ventricular assist device [(PVAD) Fig. 5], Thoratec CentriMag Blood Pump, and the Thoratec IVAD. The Thoratec IVAD is the only biventricular device that allows patients to be discharged home. Indications for RVADs or BiVADs are bridge to recovery or bridge to transplant.

REFERENCES

1. Lloyd-Jones D, Adams RJ, Brown TM, et al. Heart disease and stroke statistics—2010 update: a report from the American Heart Association. Circulation. 2010;121(7): e46-215.
2. Transplant: Transplant Year (2009-2010) by Organ US Transplants Performed: January 1, 1988-September 30, 2011 Based on OPTN Data as of December 23, 2011. Available from: http://optn.transplant.hrsa.gov/latestData/rptData/asp. Accessed on December 31, 2011.
3. Ammar KA, Jacobsen SJ, Mahoney DW, et al. Prevalence and prognostic significance of heart failure stages: application of the American College of Cardiology/American Heart Association heart failure staging criteria in the community. Circulation. 2007;115:1563-70.
4. Mancini DM, Beniaminovitz A, Levin H, et al. Low incidence of myocardial recovery after left ventricular assist device implantation in patients with chronic heart failure. Circulation. 1998;98:2383-9.
5. Ashton RC, Goldstein DJ, Rose EA, et al. Duration of left ventricular assist device support affects transplant survival. J Heart Lung Transplant. 1996;15:1151-7.
6. Rose EA, Gelijns AC, Moskowitz AJ, et al. Long-term use of a left ventricular assist device for end-stage heart failure. N Engl J Med. 2001;345:1435-43.
7. Deng MC, Naka Y. Mechanical circulatory support therapy in advanced heart failure. London: Imperial College Press; 2007.

8. Slaughter MS, Rogers JG, Milano CA, et al. Advanced heart failure treated with continuous-flow left ventricular assist device. N Engl J Med. 2009;361:2241-51.
9. Feldman AM. Heart failure: device management. Oxford: Blackwell Publishing; 2010.
10. Decker AL, Reesink KD, Van Der Veen FH, et al. Intra-aortic balloon pumping in acute mitral regurgitation reduces aortic impedance and regurgitrant fraction. Shock. 2003;19:334-8.
11. Bouchart F, Bessou JF, Tabley A, et al. Urgent surgical repair of postinfarction ventricular septal rupture: early and late outcomes. J Cardiac Surg. 1998;12:104-12.
12. Sjaw KD, Engstrom AE, Vis MM, et al. A systematic review and meta-analysis of intra-aortic balloon pump therapy in ST-elevation myocardial infarctions: should we change the guidelines? Eur Heart J. 2009;30(4):459-68.
13. Arafa OE, Pedersen TH, Svennevig JL, et al. Vascular complications of the intra-aortic balloon pump in patients undergoing open-heart operations: 15-year experience. Ann Thorac Surg. 1999;67:645-51.
14. Cohen M, Dawson MS, Kopistansky C, et al. Sex and other predictors of intra-aortic balloon counterpulsation-related complications: prospective study of 1119 consecutive patients. Am Heart J. 2000;139:282-7.
15. Cook L, Pillar B, McCord G, et al. Intra-aortic balloon pump complications: A five-year retrospective study of 283 patients. Heart Lung. 1999;28:195-202.
16. Thiele H, Sick P, Boudriot E, et al. Randomized comparison of intra-aortic balloon support with a percutaneous left ventricular assist device in patients with revascularized acute myocardial infarctions complicated by cardiogenic shock. Eur Heart J. 2005;26:1276-83.
17. De Suoza CF, de Suoza Brito F, De Lima VC, et al. Percutaneous mechanical assistance for the failing heart. J Interv Cardiol. 2010;23:195-202.
18. Cath Lab Digest [Internet] Available from: http://www.cathlabdigest.com/Abiomed-Presents-Results-From-Two-Studies-USpella-and-MACH-II.
19. McCulloch B. Use of Impella 2.5 in high-risk percutaneous coronary intervention. Crit Care Nurse. 2011;31:e1-16.
20. Chen YS, Yu HY. Choice of mechanical support for fulminant myocarditis: ECMO vs. VAD? Eur J Cardiothorac Surg. 2005;27:931-2.

CHAPTER

9 Cardiac Resynchronization Therapy

Toshimasa Okabe, Behzad B Pavri

INTRODUCTION

Cardiac resynchronization therapy (CRT), also known as biventricular (BiV) pacing, has revolutionized the treatment of chronic drug-refractory heart failure (HF). The American College of Cardiology (ACC)/American Heart Association (AHA)/Heart Rhythm Society (HRS) 2008 guidelines for device-based therapy provide a Class I indication for CRT in New York Heart Association (NYHA) Class III or ambulatory IV HF patients with left ventricular ejection fraction (LVEF) less than or equal to 35% and QRS duration greater than or equal to 120 ms who are already on optimal recommended medical therapy.[1] In this population, CRT is capable of improving exercise tolerance and NYHA functional class and reducing both mortality and HF hospitalization. As an adjunct therapy, CRT has proved to be as powerful as other established HF pharmacotherapy including beta-blockade and renin-angiotensin-aldosterone inhibition.[2]

Benefits of CRT have also been studied in less symptomatic HF (NYHA Class I and II HF), HF patients with atrial fibrillation (AF), patients with bradycardia requiring frequent right ventricular (RV) pacing, and HF patients with narrow QRS complex. Investigational efforts have also been aimed at improving response rates in patients who do not respond to CRT and methods to optimize the response to CRT.

This chapter summarizes:

1. Rationale for CRT.
2. Review of major CRT trials.
3. Effects of CRT.
4. Emerging indications and expanding roles of CRT.
5. CRT nonresponders and methods to improve response.
6. Complications of CRT.
7. Future directions.

RATIONALE FOR CARDIAC RESYNCHRONIZATION THERAPY

Widening of the QRS complex is seen in up to 30% of patients with HF, most commonly as a left bundle branch block (LBBB) pattern, and is associated with increased 1-year sudden and total mortality rate.[3] Clinically, LBBB has been associated with higher event rates in HF patients, and is also a risk factor for developing future HF in asymptomatic patients.[4,5] LBBB may itself cause a form of dilated cardiomyopathy related to abnormal electrical propagation and resulting mechanical [interventricular (V-V) and intraventricular] dyssynchrony.[6-8] Animal and human studies have shown that an abnormal ventricular activation with LBBB is associated with abnormal systolic septal movement, alterations in regional myocardial perfusion, increased energy utilization, structural changes, and impaired cardiac performance.

Similar adverse hemodynamic effects are also seen in RV pacing. Similar to the activation sequence of LBBB, RV pacing results in earlier activation of the RV and the left ventricular (LV) septum contracts before the lateral wall of the LV.[9] The resulting mechanical dyssynchrony not only reduces systolic function, but also impairs cardiac energetics as demonstrated in canine asynchronous ventricular pacing models.[10,11]

Various repercussions of conduction disturbance, including LBBB, right bundle branch block (RBBB) and nonspecific intraventricular conduction delay (IVCD), are also seen at cellular levels, including regional alteration in protein expression, myocyte hypertrophy, apoptosis, and fibrosis. Finally, a canine model of LBBB has demonstrated that there are a variety of electrophysiologic effects of dyssynchrony, including reduced conduction velocity, action potential duration, and refractory periods in late-activated lateral LV segments.[12] In this model, distribution of connexin 43 was altered from intercalated disks to lateral myocyte membranes. In addition, the normal gradient in conduction velocity from epicardium to endocardium was reversed. These profound mechanical, electrophysiologic, and clinical abnormalities seen in dyssynchronous ventricles provide the rationale for CRT.

Cardiac resynchronization therapy was first described in 1983 by de Teresa et al. at the 7th World Symposium on Cardiac Pacing. The authors described four patients with LBBB who underwent aortic valve replacement and atrial synchronous "epicardial" LV pacing. The atrioventricular (AV) delay was adjusted to allow for fusion beat between native conduction through a right bundle branch and epicardial LV pacing, causing resynchronization of the two ventricles. There was an impressive 25% increase in LVEF and improvement in dyssynchrony based on angioscintigraphy.[13] The importance of these observations went unappreciated for almost a decade.

In history of pacing therapy in HF, initial efforts were focused on resynchronization of AV timing. Prolonged AV conduction time (commonly seen in HF patients) results in atrial systole occurring too early in diastole, leading to an ineffective contribution of atrial contraction to ventricular filling. By programming a shorter

AV, AV resynchronization resulted in virtually 100% RV pacing. Initial enthusiasm for AV resynchronization by way of dual chamber rate adaptive pacemaker (DDDR) pacing, however, was hampered by an unexpected increase in new or worsening HF and death in major pacing mode trials.[14,15]

In 1994, Cazeau et al. reported the first use of CRT in a patient with alcohol-induced dilated cardiomyopathy; LBBB, prolonged PR interval, and NYHA Class IV symptoms, which were clinically deteriorating despite optimal medical therapy.[16] M-mode echocardiography demonstrated significant septal-to-posterior wall contraction delay. To correct the conduction abnormalities, the authors implanted a four-chamber pacer (transvenously placed right atrial, left atrial, RV leads, and epicardially placed LV via thoracotomy). The patient experienced acute improvements in pulmonary capillary wedge pressure, and cardiac output, and QRS duration. Six weeks after the implantation, the patient's functional class improved from NYHA Class IV to Class II. Shortly after this report, several small case series of the acute benefits of ventricular resynchronization utilizing epicardial LV leads were reported.[6,17,18]

In 1998, Daubert et al. described the first transvenous insertion of an LV lead into a branch of the coronary sinus and this has become the standard implantation technique.[19] This approach to LV lead placement simplified the implanting procedure, enabled nonsurgeon operators to implant the device in non-OR setting with lower operative risks.

These initial small reports provided the foundation for the larger clinical trials that followed. In 2001, the Food and Drug Administration (FDA) approved the first BiV pacemaker for treating drug-refractory HF. Subsequently, CRT was incorporated into defibrillators, thereby increasing the therapeutic potential of these devices.

REVIEW OF MAJOR CARDIAC RESYNCHRONIZATION THERAPY TRIALS

The short-term clinical response to CRT has been examined in numerous studies.[20-27] Consistently, these studies showed improved symptoms and functional capacity in patients with severe HF symptoms (NYHA Class III or IV), LVEF less than 35% and widened QRS (Table 1). The Multicenter InSync Randomized Clinical Evaluation (MIRACLE) study was the first large randomized double-blinded study comparing optimal medical management and CRT in 453 patients.[23] Over a 6-month follow-up, the study found significant improvement in NYHA functional class, 6-minute walk distances (6MWDs) and quality-of-life (QoL) scores in patients randomized to CRT. Furthermore, patients assigned to CRT had significantly greater improvements in LVEF, increase in measured maximum aerobic/exercise capacity (VO_2 max), decrease in mitral regurgitation (MR), and decrease in left ventricular end-diastolic dimensions (LVEDDs). These favorable responses were seen within 1 month after

Table 1 Major cardiac resynchronization therapy trials

Trial, year published (reference)	Number of patients (CRT/ control)	Inclusion criteria			Mean QRS duration (ms)/ follow-up duration (months)	Statistically significant improvements
		NYHA class	LVEF cut-off (%)	QRS duration cut-off (ms)		
CONTAK® CD, 2003[20]	245/245	II–IV	35	120	158/3–6	LV dimensions and LVEF
MUSTIC, 2001[22]	58 (crossover)-	III	35	150	176/6	6MWD, QoL score, $VO_{2\ max}$
MIRACLE, 2002[23]	228/225	III, IV	35	130	166/6	6MWD, QoL score, NYHA class, LVEF
Meta-analysis of CONTAK CD, MUSTIC, MIRACLE, and InSync ICD, 2003[24]	809/825	II–IV	35	120–150	158–76/ 3–6	Death from HF, HF hospitalization
COMPANION, 2004[25]	CRT-P 617; CRT-D 595/ control 308	III, IV	35	120	159/12	Death or HF hospitalization, all-cause mortality
CARE-HF, 2005[26]	409/404	III, IV	35	120	160/29.4	Death or cardiovascular hospitalization, all-cause mortality
InSync® ICD, 2002[27]	186/176	II–IV	35	130	165/6	QoL score, NYHA class, 6MWD

CRT, cardiac resynchronization therapy; NYHA class, New York Heart Association Functional Classification; LVEF, left ventricular ejection fraction; LV, left ventricular; ICD, implantable cardioverter defibrillator; QoL, quality of life; 6MWD, six-minute walk distance; MUSTIC, Multisite Stimulation in Cardiomyopathies; $VO_{2\ max}$, maximum aerobic/exercise capacity; MIRACLE, Multicenter InSync Randomized Clinical Evaluation Study; HF, heart failure; COMPANION, Comparison of Medical Therapy, Pacing, and Defibrillation in Heart Failure Trial; CRT-P, cardiac resynchronization therapy pacemaker; CRT-D, cardiac resynchronization therapy defibrillator; CARE-HF, Cardiac Resynchronization in Heart Failure Trial.

device implantation in the majority of patients, and were sustained at 6-month and 1-year follow-up.

The Comparison of Medical Therapy, Pacing, and Defibrillation in Heart Failure (COMPANION)[25] and Cardiac Resynchronization in Heart Failure (CARE-HF)[26] trials were designed to test mortality benefit of CRT. The largest study to date, COMPANION, randomized 1,520 patients with NYHA Class III or IV HF, LVEF less than or equal to 35%, QRS greater than or equal to 120 msec and sinus rhythm to cardiac resynchronization therapy pacemaker (CRT-P) (BiV pacing only), cardiac resynchronization therapy defibrillator (CRT-D) (defibrillator with BiV pacing), or optimal medical therapy in a 1:2:2 ratio. Over a follow-up period of 12 months, both CRT-P and CRT-D arms showed a comparable and statistically significant improvement in the primary end-point of death or hospitalization from any cause [CRT-P versus medical therapy: hazard ratio (HR) = 0.81, P = 0.014; CRT-D versus medical therapy: HR = 0.80, P = 0.01]. While CRT-P did not reach a statistically significant reduction in death (P = 0.059), there was a significant reduction in the risk of death in the CRT-D arm (P = 0.003) likely due to aborted sudden cardiac deaths.

Cardiac Resynchronization in Heart Failure trial compared CRT-P (BiV pacing without a defibrillator) and optimal medical management in 813 patients over a mean follow-up duration of 29.4 months. Eligible patients had to have sinus rhythm, NYHA Class III or IV HF, LVEF less than or equal to 35%, LVEDD greater than or equal to 30 mm, and QRS greater than or equal to 120 ms. Additionally, patients with QRS duration between 120 and 149 ms were required to meet two of three indices of echocardiographic dyssynchrony. CARE-HF was the first trial to demonstrate a significant survival benefit with CRT-P compared with medical management (P < 0.002). Both COMPANION and CARE-HF confirmed prior findings of significant improvements in clinical symptoms and LV reverse remodeling.

EFFECTS OF CARDIAC RESYNCHRONIZATION THERAPY

Improvements in cardiac hemodynamics are often seen shortly after the initiation of BiV pacing. Hemodynamic monitoring during CRT device implantation demonstrated acute improvements in systolic blood pressure, cardiac output, peak rate of pressure change in the ventricle (*dP/dt*) and LVEF, accompanied by a decline in pulmonary capillary wedge pressure.[28-31] Mechanisms for these acute improvements include changes in loading conditions, reduced MR and enhanced contractile function. Importantly, these changes occur without an increase in myocardial oxygen consumption (VO_2), suggesting improved cardiac efficiency as the predominant acute effect of CRT.[31]

Numerous studies have reported decrease in functional MR.[22,23,26,32,33] The mechanisms for this improvement are multifactorial,[33] including improved ventricular contractile function and increased transmitral gradient, enabling earlier mitral valve closure,[34] restoration of coordinated papillary muscle activation, and reduction in mitral annular dilatation due to favorable LV reverse remodeling.[34-36] A patient with nonischemic cardiomyopathy (NICM), a nondilated LV (LVEDD <75 mm), and mild-to-moderate MR would have a greater than 90% predicted probability of favorable response to CRT.[37] However, a patient with marked MR prior to CRT may not show improvement.[37,38]

Favorable cardiac remodeling effects of CRT are also seen at the atrial level. Improved atrial systolic function, atrial compliance, and atrial dimensions have been observed in patients after CRT.[39]

Cardiac resynchronization therapy also benefits the maladaptive neurohormonal responses seen in HF. Studies suggest that sympathetic nerve activity is reduced after CRT (greater than the reduction seen with optimal medical therapy alone) and sustained after CRT is turned off, as reflected by improved cardiac ^{123}I-meta-iodobenzylguanidine (^{123}I-MIBG) uptake.[40,41] The CARE-HF trial also demonstrated a large reduction in N-terminal brain natriuretic peptide (BNP)[26] and several studies have shown significant improvement in heart rate variability and heart rate profiles after initiation of CRT. Cardiac resynchronization therapy shifts the neurohormonal balance away from sympathetic excess that is ubiquitous in HF.[42]

Recent data have shed light on numerous beneficial effects of BiV pacing beyond improvement in LV systolic function including improvements in sleep apnea,[43] pulmonary hypertension,[30] RV function, tricuspid regurgitation,[29,44] augmentation of coronary flow,[45] and His-Purkinje conduction system (so-called "electrical remodeling").[46]

EMERGING INDICATIONS AND EXPANDING ROLES OF CARDIAC RESYNCHRONIZATION THERAPY

Patients with Mild Heart Failure

Based on the mortality and morbidity benefits of CRT in patients with NYHA Class III or IV HF, CRT was tested in patients with reduced LV function and wide QRS complexes, but milder (NYHA Class I and II) HF symptoms. Three major randomized trials and one meta-analysis demonstrated convincing morbidity and mortality benefits of CRT in patients with mild HF symptoms.[47-50]

The Resynchronization Reverses Remodeling in Systolic Left Ventricular Dysfunction (REVERSE) trial showed that CRT was associated with positive LV remodeling and delayed progression to symptomatic HF at 1 year,[47] most notably in patients with the widest QRS complexes (>150 ms) and in patients with nonischemic cardiomyopathy.[51] The Multicenter Automatic Defibrillator Implantation Trial with Cardiac Resynchronization Therapy (MADIT-CRT) trial also showed reduced HF event after 2.4 years with CRT, along with significant improvement in LV volumes and LVEF (11% increase in the CRT-D group vs. 3% increase without CRT, $P < 0.001$).[52] As in the REVERSE trial, clinical benefit in MADIT-CRT was mainly seen in patients with a QRS greater than or equal to 150 ms and LBBB morphology.[53] Finally, the Resynchronization-Defibrillation for Ambulatory Heart Failure Trial (RAFT) investigators showed that after 40 months, the primary end-point of death from any cause or HF hospitalization was lower in the CRT-D group (HR = 0.75, P = 0.003), as were the secondary end-points of all-cause mortality, cardiovascular death, and HF hospitalization.[49] Once again, the subgroup of patients with an intrinsic QRS greater than or equal to 150 ms and with LBBB morphology derived the greatest benefit.

A recent meta-analysis of randomized controlled CRT trials in adults with HF and LVEF less than or equal to 40% concluded that in patients with NYHA Class I and II HF, CRT reduced all-cause mortality [95% confidence interval (CI), 0.72–0.96] and HF hospitalization (95% CI, 0.57–0.87) without improving functional class or QoL.[50] The authors concluded that CRT was beneficial for patients with symptomatic HF, reduced LVEF and prolonged QRS, "regardless of NYHA class". A small observational study concluded that CRT resulted in greater improvements in general health and social functioning in patients with NYHA Class II HF as compared to patients with NYHA Class III HF.[54]

Based on these data, the recently updated guidelines of the European Society of Cardiology extended recommendations for CRT to include patients with mild HF and a QRS duration greater than or equal to 150 ms.[55] In 2010, the FDA approved use of a CRT device in patients with mild or asymptomatic HF and LBBB.[56]

Patients with Atrial Fibrillation

Atrial fibrillation is a common occurrence with HF and the prevalence of AF increases with the severity of HF from 6% in patients with mild HF to more than 40% in patients with advanced HF.[57,58] However, most of the major clinical trials on CRT have excluded patients with AF. The use of CRT in AF is a Class IIA recommendation in the ACC/AHA/HRS 2008 guidelines in patients with NYHA Class III or ambulatory Class IV, LVEF less than or equal to 35%, and QRS greater than or equal to 120 ms.[1] Atrial fibrillation, in addition to eliminating normal AV synchrony, is particularly problematic when ventricular rates are rapid (faster than the programmed pacing rate). This prevents delivery of BiV pacing, and blunts the benefits of CRT. Recent data suggest that the greatest mortality benefit from CRT is observed when the percentage of true BiV pacing is greater than 98%.[59]

Cardiac resynchronization therapy recipients with AF may be subdivided into two groups. The first group includes "AF patients who have bradycardia" (AV block, either spontaneous or as a result of AV node ablation, and patients who have slow ventricular rates in AF). With conventional (RV only) pacing, such patients would become 100% dyssynchronously paced. The second subgroup consists of "AF patients without bradycardia", in whom conventional pacing is not indicated, but who have a wide QRS complex, and therefore could benefit from CRT.

Several small trials have reported on AF patients who had previously undergone AV nodal ablation or had high RV pacing burden due to standard pacing indications, and tested the efficacy of CRT in comparison to conventional RV pacing.[60-63] In these studies, CRT appeared to be superior to conventional RV pacing in terms of improvements in functional class and LV function. These favorable outcomes led to a larger randomized single-blind study in patients with symptomatic HF and chronic AF (>30 days) undergoing AV node ablation. Patients were assigned to receive CRT or a RV pacing system.[64] At 6 months, CRT provided a significant improvement in 6MWD and LVEF compared to RV pacing, with the greatest benefits in patients with LVEF less than or equal to 45% or NYHA Class II or III HF; there was no mortality benefit during a 6-month follow-up. More recently, the assessment of Cardiac Resynchronization Therapy in Patients with Permanent Atrial Fibrillation (APAF) trial[65] enrolled patients with permanent AF who were undergoing AV node ablation for either (1) rapid ventricular rates or (2) drug-refractory HF with reduced LVEF. All patients underwent AV node ablation and implantation of a CRT device, and were randomized to CRT or RV apical pacing. During a median follow-up of 20 months, the primary composite end-point of death from HF, HF hospitalization or worsening HF occurred in 11% in the CRT group and 26% in the RV pacing group (HR = 0.37, P = 0.005); once again, there was no difference in mortality. The role of CRT in HF patients with relatively preserved LVEF, HF patients with different types of AF (paroxysmal or persistent) and demonstration of mortality benefit await future studies.

Far fewer data exist on the benefit of CRT in patients with AF but without a standard pacing indication. Several studies have reported on the efficacy of CRT in patients with AF (whether heart rate was controlled pharmacologically or via AV node ablation) in comparison to patients without AF.[66-69] A recent meta-analysis showed that the presence of AF itself was associated with an increased probability of nonresponse and greater all-cause mortality among CRT recipients.[70] Recent data from the Multicenter Longitudinal Observational Study (MILOS) group registry suggest that when rate control is not attained pharmacologically (as assessed by less than 86% true BiV pacing), ablation of the AV junction (with resultant increase in BiV pacing) improves all-cause mortality, cardiac mortality, and HF mortality at a median follow-up of 34 months.[69]

In conclusion, the benefit of CRT may be reduced in patients with AF, especially in the setting of rapid ventricular rates. Patients with AF who undergo AV node ablation and receive 100% BiV pacing appear to derive similar CRT benefit compared with patients in sinus rhythm, although a prospective randomized study in evaluating this strategy has not been conducted. In patients with AF who receive CRT, it is imperative that ventricular rates are optimally controlled to ensure maximal delivery of BiV pacing. Features available in many contemporary CRT devices, such as "sense assurance", "conducted AF response", "triggered pacing", and "rate regulation" are designed to promote BiV pacing but have yet to be tested for clinical benefit. Holter monitoring studies indicate that device-based pacing counters overestimate the degree of true BiV pacing, probably because of underlying fusion and pseudofusion beats; only patients with very high percentage of complete BiV capture, as confirmed by 12-lead Holter recordings, demonstrated favorable response to CRT.[71]

Whether CRT reduces the incidence of AF among HF patients is debatable. In major CRT trials, such as CARE-HF and COMPANION, patients with AF were excluded and the incidence of new AF during follow-up did not differ between CRT-treated and control patients. In a small comparison study of patients with HF undergoing CRT, the incidence of new-onset AF was lower compared with age- and gender-matched controls with comparable LVEF.[72] The proposed mechanism of the benefit of CRT in reducing AF occurrence includes left atrial reverse remodeling and reduction of MR, but only a small minority of patients with either persistent or permanent AF will show spontaneous conversion to sinus rhythm after CRT.[73] At the present time, the effect of CRT on incidence of either new or recurrent AF remains inconclusive.

Patients with Heart Failure and Narrow QRS Complex

The duration of the QRS complex on 12-lead electrocardiogram (ECG) has been used as the identifying marker of LV dyssynchrony, and consequently, only patients with QRS greater than or equal to 120 ms were enrolled into large clinical trials. Subsequent studies, however, demonstrated that prolonged QRS duration (electrical dyssynchrony) does not completely reflect true LV mechanical dyssynchrony. Significant mechanical LV dyssynchrony may be present in patients with narrow QRS complex (QRS ≤120 ms).[74-78] Although a wide QRS complex is associated with a high prevalence (~70%) of mechanical dyssynchrony, about a third of HF patients with a narrow QRS complex also exhibited mechanical dyssynchrony.[74] This discrepancy between electrical (QRS duration) and mechanical (echocardiographic) dyssynchrony may be due to the fact that the QRS duration primarily reflects total ventricular activation time, but may not reflect regional inhomogeneities of LV contraction (i.e., intra-LV dyssynchrony). Rapid RV depolarization may offset electrical delays in LV, consequently normalizing QRS duration on a surface ECG.[79] Thus, QRS duration may be a convenient but inaccurate surrogate for the ventricular dyssynchrony that CRT is designed to correct. Since approximately two-thirds of HF patients have a narrow QRS complex,[80] a large portion of HF patients with mechanical LV dyssynchrony will not be offered CRT.

Initially, several small single-center, nonrandomized studies provided promising results in the efficacy of CRT among patients with a narrow (≤120 ms) QRS complex and echocardiographically-detected mechanical dyssynchrony[81,82] (Table 2). In one study, only those HF patients with echocardiographic dyssynchrony showed reduction in left ventricular end-systolic volume (LVESV), left ventricular end-diastolic volume (LVEDV), and improved LVEF. The degree of LV reverse remodeling was found to be similar between the wide- and narrow-QRS groups, provided the extent of mechanical dyssynchrony was comparable, regardless of the baseline QRS duration, suggesting that mechanical dyssynchrony

Table 2 **Cardiac resynchronization therapy trials in heart failure patients with narrow QRS complex**

Trial, year published, reference	*Echocardiographic criteria for dyssynchrony and other inclusion criteria*	*Study arms*	*Study follow-up duration (months)*	*Studied outcome*	*Findings*
Achilli et al. 2003[81]	Posterolateral LV wall activation delay greater than the interval between QRS onset and transmitral filling, difference between RV and LV electromechanical delay >20 ms, incomplete LBBB, NYHA III or IV, LVEF ≤0.35	Narrow QRS (n = 14), wide QRS (n = 38)	6	NYHA Class, LVEF, LVESD, LVEDD, MR, and 6MWD	Improvement in 6MWD was greater in wide-QRS group than in narrow-QRS group. Otherwise, similar and significant improvements in clinical and echo parameters seen in both groups
Bleeker et al. 2006[82]	Maximum delay between peak systolic velocities among the four walls in LV ≥65 ms by TDI, NYHA III or IV HF, LVEF ≤0.35	Narrow QRS (n = 33), wide QRS (n = 33)	6	NYHA Class, QoL, 6MWD, LVESV, LVEDV, and LVEF	All clinical and echo parameters improved and the magnitude of improvement was comparable in both groups
Yu et al. 2006[83]	Standard deviation of time to peak systolic velocity in 12 LV segments (asynchrony index) >32.6 ms by TDI, NYHA III or IV, LVEF <0.40	Narrow QRS (n = 51, only 27 with mechanical dyssynchrony), wide QRS (n = 51)	3	NYHA Class, QoL, LVESV, LVEF, MR, 6MWD, and maximal exercise capacity	All clinical and echo parameters improved. Those with narrow QRS and mechanical dyssynchrony showed a greater extent of LV remodeling than those with narrow QRS but without dyssynchrony
Meta-analysis, Jeevanantham et al. 2008[84]	Three trials listed above are included in the analysis	Narrow QRS (n = 98)	At least 3	Change from baseline in NYHA Class, 6MWD, and LVEF	Significant improvements in NYHA class, 6MWD, and LVEF

Contd...

Contd...

RethinQ, Beshai et al. 2007[85]	An opposing wall delay ≥65 ms on TDI or a mechanical dyssynchrony in the septal-to-posterior wall ≥130 ms on M-mode, NYHA class III HF, LVEF ≤0.35%, QRS <130 ms, optimal medical therapy	Randomly assigned to CRT on (n = 87) or CRT off (n = 85)	6	Primary endpoint: increased peak oxygen consumption (VO_2) during cardiopulmonary exercise, secondary end-points: NYHA, QoL, 6MWD, and HF events	No difference in primary end-point
ESTEEM-CRT, Donahue et al. 2008[87]	Standard deviation of time to peak velocity of 12 LV segments >28.7 ms, NYHA class III HF, LVEF ≤0.35%, QRS <120 ms, optimal medical therapy	Single arm (CRT, n = 67)	6 and 12	NYHA class, QoL, LVESV, and LVEDV	NYHA class and QoL improved. No difference in LVESV or LVEDV

LV, left ventricular; RV, right ventricular; LBBB, left bundle branch block; NYHA class, New York Heart Association Functional Classification; LVEF, left ventricular ejection fraction; LVESD, left ventricular end-systolic diameter; LVEDD, left ventricular end-diastolic diameter; MR, mitral regurgitation; 6MWD, six-minute walk distance; TDI, tissue Doppler imaging; HF, heart failure; QoL, quality of life; LVEDV, left ventricular end-diastolic volume; LVESV, left ventricular end-systolic volume; CRT, cardiac resynchronization therapy; ESTEEM-CRT, Evaluation of Screening Techniques in Electrically-Normal, Mechanically-Dyssynchronous Heart Failure Patients in Cardiac Resynchronization Therapy Study.

may be a more reliable determinant of CRT response.[83] A meta-analysis concluded that CRT improved clinical parameters (NYHA Class, 6MWD) and LV reverse remodeling (improved LVEF and smaller LV volume) in patients with narrow QRS and echocardiographically-detected dyssynchrony.[84]

This initial enthusiasm was tempered by the results of two randomized studies that have failed to provide definitive evidence of CRT benefit in patients with narrow QRS complex. The resynchronization therapy in narrow QRS (RethinQ) study was a double-blind randomized clinical trial evaluating the efficacy of CRT in patients with NYHA Class III HF, LVEF less than or equal to 35%, narrow QRS (<130 ms) and prespecified echocardiographic dyssynchrony [opposing wall delays on tissue Doppler imaging (TDI)].[85] All patients received a CRT device, and were randomly assigned to CRT on or CRT off. At 6 months, there was no significant difference in primary end-point (the proportion of patients who had an increase of at least 1.0 mL/kg/min in peak VO_2 during cardiopulmonary exercise) between the two groups: QoL scores, 6MWD, or echocardiographic measures were also similar. Improvements in peak VO_2 with CRT were seen only with QRS duration between 120 and 130 ms. Limitations of the RethinQ study include the concern that TDI may be unreliable in detecting mechanical dyssynchrony,[86] a relatively short follow-up period of 6 months (the benefits of CRT may become manifest after 6 months), and that the study may have been underpowered.

The Evaluation of Screening Techniques in Electrically-Normal, Mechanically-Dyssynchronous Heart Failure Patients in Cardiac Resynchronization Therapy (ESTEEM-CRT) was a multicenter, single-arm, unblinded study that evaluated the acute and chronic effects of CRT in narrow QRS (<120 ms) HF patients with mechanical dyssynchrony (as defined by more robust echocardiographic parameter—the standard deviation of time to peak velocity in 12 LV segments). At 6-month follow-up, despite significant improvements in patient's symptoms (NYHA functional class, QoL), there was no difference in peak VO_2 or echocardiographic parameters (LVEF, LV mass, and mechanical dyssynchrony).[87]

The question arises as to whether the apparent lack of CRT benefit in patients with narrow QRS is due to a true lack of efficacy in this population or due to unavailability of an accurate method to detect those with truly dyssynchronous ventricles. It is generally agreed upon that QRS duration alone is a modest predictor of clinical and echocardiographic response to CRT.[88] Although it is currently the only accepted criteria for assessing dyssynchrony in potential CRT candidates. Conventional echocardiographic indices in identifying mechanical dyssynchrony are unlikely to accurately represent the highly complex longitudinal, radial, and rotational LV motion.[86] Promising techniques in detecting clinically relevant mechanical dyssynchrony include two-dimensional (2D) strain imaging with speckle tracking,[89-91] three-dimensional (3D) echocardiography,[92] and cardiac magnetic resonance imaging (MRI).[93,94] One small study, Resynchronization in Patients with Heart Failure and a Normal QRS Duration ("RESPOND"), used cardiac MRI to avoid placement of the LV lead over scarred regions in HF patients with NYHA Class III or IV HF, LVEF less than 35% and a narrow QRS, and showed improvement in 6MWD with CRT.[95]

The Echocardiography Guided Cardiac Resynchronization Therapy (EchoCRT) is a randomized, double-blind, multicenter trial currently underway to investigate the efficacy of CRT-D (BiV pacing with a defibrillator back-up) in patients with NYHA Class III or IV HF, narrow QRS (<130 ms), LVEF less than or equal to 35%, LVEDD greater than or equal to 55 mm, and echocardiography-based ventricular dyssynchrony (based on one of two stringent, prespecified criteria).[96] The EchoCRT may definitively clarify the role of CRT in HF patients with narrow QRS and mechanical dyssynchrony.

Patients with Heart Failure and Intermediate QRS Complex Duration

The mean duration of QRS complex of patients enrolled in major CRT trials has consistently been greater than 150 ms which is far greater than the enrollment threshold of greater than 120 ms.[25,26] Across the spectrum of patients with different QRS durations (narrow ≤120 ms, intermediate 120–150 ms, wide >150 ms), there is an incremental increase in a mean septal-to-lateral delay and dyssynchrony (27%, 60%, and 70%, respectively).[74] In prespecified subgroup analyses of COMPANION and CARE-HF trials, the benefits of CRT in patients with intermediate QRS durations were diminished or absent, as compared to patients with a wider QRS duration.[25,26]

At the present time, there is no single gold standard imaging modality for measuring mechanical dyssynchrony. Given the variables of complex ventricular contraction patterns, V-V interaction, and other varying myocardial substrates. It seems unlikely that we will find a single parameter that defines mechanical dyssynchrony and consistently predicts response to CRT. A more comprehensive "dyssynchrony score" consisting of clinical factors, a QRS duration, and multiple imaging parameters may be necessary to predict an individual patient's response to CRT.[79]

Heart Failure Patients with Standard Pacing Indication for Bradycardia

Current guidelines recommend CRT for patients with NYHA Class III or IV HF, LVEF less than or equal to 35% on optimal medical therapy who have frequent dependence on RV pacing (Class IIA indication, level of evidence C).[1] For many years, dual chamber (right atrial and RV) pacing was the standard treatment for patients with HF in need of pacing due to either sinus node dysfunction or AV block. The deleterious effects of conventional RV pacing on LV function and the development of HF have been recognized in the last decade as a result of large pacing mode selection trials.[14,15] It is now generally accepted that, especially in patients with a narrow QRS complex, RV pacing should be minimized in patients with pacemakers or defibrillators, if necessary, even at the expense of AV synchrony.

Recent preliminary data raise the question of whether the benefits of CRT extend beyond patients with Class III or IV HF and low LVEF, to all patients who require frequent RV pacing for standard bradycardia indications. Small randomized crossover trials comparing the benefit of CRT over RV pacing in patients with mild cardiomyopathy (LVEF <40%) and dependence on RV pacing showed improved functional class, LV function and LV remodeling during the period of CRT.[97,98] Evidence for the benefit of upgrading from RV pacing to CRT among patients with mild cardiomyopathy is still scarce and larger prospective controlled studies are warranted.[99]

The Pacing to Avoid Cardiac Enlargement (PACE) study was a prospective, double-blind, randomized multicenter trial investigating the beneficial effects of CRT versus RV apical pacing in 177 patients with "preserved" LVEF (≥45%) and standard indications for pacing including sinus node dysfunction and AV block. At 12 months, both LVEF and LVESV were significantly improved in the CRT group.[100] Continued benefits of CRT on LV function and LV remodeling were observed at 2-year follow-up in the same cohort of patients.[101]

The site in the RV where the pacing electrode is placed may also influence outcomes. It is probable that the RV apex, the site where the pacing lead is conventionally placed, may impose the greatest degree of dyssynchrony on the LV and that mid-RV septal pacing may be superior. Two ongoing trials [Right Ventricular Apical and High Septal Pacing to Preserve Left Ventricular Function (Protect Pace) and Right Ventricular Apical versus Septal Pacing (RASP)] will hopefully provide clear direction as to the optimal RV pacing site.[102]

At the present time, there is no convincing evidence that CRT should be recommended uniformly to patients in need of chronic RV pacing, especially in those with preserved LVEF. Progressive Ventricular Dysfunction Prevention in Pacemaker Patients (Prevent-HF) is a multicenter, prospective, and randomized study, designed to address whether BiV pacing is superior to RV pacing in patients with no or minimal HF who are expected to have a high amount of ventricular pacing for bradycardia. This small pilot study (n = 108) showed that there was no significant LV volume difference between the two pacing modes after 12 months.[103]

CARDIAC RESYNCHRONIZATION THERAPY NONRESPONDERS AND METHODS TO IMPROVE RESPONSE

Despite the impressive results of major clinical trials in CRT, it is clear that the benefits of CRT are not uniform within this patient's population. As many as a third of patients receiving CRT are considered "nonresponders". Long-term clinical benefits of CRT are greatly influenced by patient selection, lead placement, and device programming. Table 3 lists potential variables that may contribute to CRT nonresponse.

The definition of a "nonresponder" has not been uniform in CRT trials which adds to the confusion regarding what end-points ought to be considered appropriate measures of CRT response. There are three categories of indices commonly used to determine CRT response: (1) clinical (QoL scores, 6MWD, and NYHA functional class); (2) hemodynamic (dP/dT_{max}, cardiac index); and (3) volumetric (LVEF, LVEDV, and LVESV measured by echocardiography).[104] "Clinical response" is the most subjective index of CRT response with poor interobserver reliability, yet undoubtedly the most important target of treatment from the patient's perspective.[105] Furthermore, CRT has a significant placebo effect seen in the large clinical studies such as MIRACLE, with 39% of patients reporting symptomatic improvement (change in the NYHA Class) even when CRT is not turned on.[23] Interestingly, "hemodynamic measures" do not necessarily correlate with patients' symptoms or NYHA functional class.[106] However, "echocardiographic response" correlates relatively well with clinical response and concordant clinical and echocardiographic responses are seen approximately in 70% of the patients receiving CRT.[107-109] In a large cohort

Table 3 Causes for cardiac resynchronization therapy nonresponse

Factors related to patient selection
• Absence of mechanical dyssynchrony
• Ischemic etiology
• Isolated RBBB or IVCD
• Lateral or posterolateral wall scar
• Short PR interval (probable)
Factors related to individual patient
• Atrial anatomic distortion leading to nonengageable coronary sinus
• Lack of suitable venous branch in lateral or posterolateral walls
• High LV pacing threshold leading to loss of consistent capture
• High burden of AF with rapid ventricular response and/or frequent ventricular arrhythmias
• Conduction delay from LV pacing site (scar, hibernating myocardium)
Factors related to device programming
• Failure to adjust AV delay to optimize AV blood flow
• Failure to adjust V-V timing
• Failure to adjust LV output to accommodate high LV capture threshold

RBBB, right bundle branch block; IVCD, intraventricular conduction delay; LV, left ventricular; AF, atrial fibrillation; AV, atrioventricular; V-V, interventricular.

of HF patients with CRT (n = 440), 28% of the population experienced clinical response without LV reverse remodeling; such discrepant responses were more likely in patients with ischemic dilated cardiomyopathy (ICM), relatively narrow QRS complexes, or less LV dyssynchrony.[109] The magnitude of echocardiographic volumetric LV reverse remodeling can predict the subsequent outcome of patients with CRT.[110,111] In a subanalysis of MADIT-CRT, improvement in LVEDV at 1 year predicted subsequent death or HF and each 10% decrease in end-diastolic volume was associated with a 40% reduction in the primary outcome of death or HF event.[112] It appears that volumetric response may be the most robust and practical predictor of long-term CRT success.

Several patient factors for nonresponse to CRT deserve mention:

- As discussed previously in the section about CRT in patients with a narrow or intermediate QRS duration, CRT is the most effective in HF patients with the widest QRS duration (>150 ms)
- Subanalysis of major CRT trials has demonstrated that there is a significantly diminished benefit of CRT among patients with isolated RBBB, or nonspecific IVCD as compared to LBBB.[53,113-117] The lack of response in patients with RBBB may seem intuitively obvious as a delay in RV activation by itself would be unlikely to benefit from the addition of LV pacing. However, the presence of RBBB pattern does not always imply healthy left-sided conduction; it simply means that the right bundle branch is the more diseased branch. There may be subsets of patients with RBBB, for example with concomitant left hemiblock, that respond well to CRT. It is likely that these patients have a significant mechanical LV dyssynchrony despite an apparent lack of major left-sided conduction disease on the surface ECG.[118-121] Therefore, at the present time, it may be premature to exclude patients with RBBB from receiving CRT
- The importance of presence and location of a scar tissue within the LV, and the relationship of scar location to LV lead location, has been increasingly recognized. The presence of lateral or posterolateral LV scar, especially when it is transmural, is associated with a low-CRT response and increased morbidity and mortality among HF patients receiving CRT.[122] Some studies have found global LV scar burden to be crucial,[123,124] whereas others found the lateral or posterolateral location of the scar to be more influential.[125,126] Importance of a lateral wall scar was also seen in patients with NICM.[126] Viability of the paced LV segment, which ideally should correspond to the latest site of LV activation, seems to be an important determinant of response to CRT. The higher prevalence of a scar in patients with ICM may partially explain a relatively unfavorable response to CRT among patients with ICM compared with idiopathic dilated cardiomyopathies[127-130]
- As previously discussed, a high burden of atrial and ventricular arrhythmias [rapid ventricular rates in AF, frequent premature ventricular contractions

(PVCs), and/or nonsustained ventricular tachycardia (VT)], prevent effective delivery of BiV pacing and compromises benefits of CRT[59]

- Finally, some patients with wide QRS complexes do not appear to have any mechanical dyssynchrony and these patients have a lower probability of response to CRT and a poor prognosis after initiation of CRT.[131] Other contributing factors for CRT nonresponse include NYHA Class IV, severe MR, and severely dilated LV cavity (LVEDD ≥75 mm)[37] and concomitant RV failure/dysfunction[132-134]
- Surface ECG correlates: Some "surface ECG findings" have been associated with improved CRT response. The development of increasing R amplitude in leads V1 through V2 after CRT, along with a left-to-right frontal axis shift, were positive predictors of LV reverse remodeling.[135] In some studies, QRS narrowing after CRT (indexed to baseline QRS duration) was significantly associated with improved LV reverse remodeling after adjusting for multiple confounders.[136] A recent Predictors of Response to Cardiac Re-Synchronization Therapy (PROSPECT)-ECG substudy has also demonstrated a predictive value of QRS narrowing in clinical outcomes among patients implanted with a CRT device.[137] A prolonged PR interval or first-degree AV block is often viewed as a relatively benign finding, but may have important implications in CRT. Very prolonged AV conduction times result in delayed ventricular activation, leading to a delayed diastole, which results in superimposed or fused E and A waves during mitral inflow, as seen on pulsed wave Doppler echocardiography. This induces "diastolic" MR, decreasing LV preload, and consequently leading to a low-cardiac output.[138] Programming of physiologic AV delays during CRT for patients with underlying PR prolongation restores a physiologic left-sided AV contraction sequence. Conversely, in patients with short baseline PR intervals, CRT requires programming of even shorter AV delays which result in truncation of transmitral flow due to early LV pacing. Such short AV delays cause reduced LV preload and eventually low-cardiac output. In such cases, the A wave on transmitral Doppler signal is truncated by early mitral valve closure.[139] Therefore, at least in theory, a sufficiently prolonged baseline PR interval may be an important contributor to maximum CRT response. In a subanalysis of the COMPANION trial, CRT benefits were more pronounced in the subset of patients with PR prolongation.[140] Similarly, in a substudy of the RethinQ trial, a significant increase in peak VO_2 at 6 months was seen only among patients with PR interval greater than or equal to 180 ms.[141] The evidence that CRT provides better outcomes in those with a longer PR interval is still not established and needs to be explored in larger controlled trials.
- Echocardiographic correlates: Currently, there is no single echocardiographic dyssynchrony parameter or index that has demonstrated an accurate predictive value in selecting CRT responders.[86,142] Novel echocardiographic techniques including 2D strain imaging (speckle tracking approach), 3D echocardiography,

and cardiac MRI seem promising, but randomized trials need to be conducted before echocardiographic dyssynchrony assessment can be incorporated into the current CRT guidelines

- Recently, "LV lead positioning" has been shown to be important in improving CRT response. Whether placing a LV lead either surgically or transvenously, targeting the lateral or posterolateral wall has been generally recommended.[143,144] By utilizing 2D speckle-tracking radial strain analysis to assess LV dyssynchrony, it has been demonstrated that the lateral, posterior, and inferior LV segments are the most common sites of the latest mechanical activation in HF patients eligible for CRT.[8] In a substudy of MADIT-CRT, similar CRT benefits were seen for LV leads in the anterior, lateral, or posterior position, but "apical lead locations were associated with a significantly increased risk for HF event or death" (HR = 1.72, P = 0.019) after adjustment for the other clinical covariates.[145] Left ventricular leads placed at sites different from the site of the latest mechanical activation may worsen adverse LV remodeling and clinical outcomes, whereas LV lead placement guided by real-time intraprocedural imaging may lead to better clinical outcomes and LV reverse remodeling.[146-149] Limitations of transvenous LV lead placement include inability to cannulate the coronary sinus, absence of suitable veins, suboptimal performance, and instability of the lead and phrenic nerve stimulation. Failure to place a transvenous LV lead placement ranges from 5–10%; in these patients, surgical epicardial LV lead implantation via left anterior or lateral minithoracotomy, video-assisted thoracoscopy, or robotically-enhanced telemanipulation systems is recommended.[150-152]

Coordinated multidisciplinary care of HF patients with a CRT device is of paramount importance and the cardiac electrophysiologist responsible for CRT optimization plays a crucial role. A comprehensive protocol-driven CRT optimization clinic is feasible and leads to fewer adverse events.[153] Each inpatient and outpatient encounter offers an opportunity to optimize CRT device programming including adjustment of AV delay, ensuring a high percentage of BiV pacing, and adequate LV capture. However, the Frequent Optimization Study Using the QuickOpt Method (FREEDOM) trial compared intracardiac electrogram (IEGM)-based frequent AV and V-V delay optimization to conventional management (empiric programming or one-time non-IEGM-based optimization), and failed to demonstrate improved outcomes with frequent IEGM-based optimization.[154] Some data suggest individualized echocardiographic V-V optimization of CRT improved hemodynamic and echocardiographic parameters in the short-term.[155-157] Preliminary data from the response of cardiac Resynchronization Therapy Optimization with V-V timing in Heart Failure Patients (RESPONSE-HF) trial showed the promising results of V-V optimization among CRT nonresponders, as compared to simultaneous BiV pacing alone.[158] Two well-designed randomized studies (RHYTHM II ICD, DECREASE-HF) have shown no benefits for clinical or echocardiographic improvements with V-V optimized sequential BiV pacing compared with simultaneous BiV stimulation.[159,160]

In summary, it may be recommended that "patient selection" should favor LBBB morphology, wider QRS complexes, nonischemic etiology, low-scar burden, and possibly longer PR intervals. "Procedural recommendations" include avoidance of RV and LV apical lead locations, and if possible, selection of late activating LV sites. "Programming considerations" should include attempts at obtaining a QRS duration that is narrower than baseline, a leftward shift in frontal axis, and positive QRS deflections in V1 and V2; these are often attained by programming LV pacing before RV pacing. In the face of clinical nonresponse, patients should be referred for echocardiographically-guided optimization of AV and V-V delays. Close coordination between the HF physician and the electrophysiologist is associated with improved outcomes.

COMPLICATIONS OF CARDIAC RESYNCHRONIZATION THERAPY

A systematic review of seven randomized clinical trials of CRT revealed the following major complication rates: in-hospital mortality 0.3%, pneumothorax 0.9%, coronary sinus complication 2.0%, and lead dislodgment 5.7%.[161] Cardiac resynchronization therapy device implantation in patients without interruption of warfarin therapy in patients at high-risk of thromboembolic events appears to be safe and associated with a reduced risk of pocket hematoma and shorter length of hospital stay.[162]

There have been numerous case reports and small observational studies of increased incidence of life-threatening ventricular tachyarrhythmias (VTA) following a CRT device implantation.[163-165] Reversal of the normal endocardium-to-epicardium ventricular activation due to epicardial LV pacing may be associated with increased transmural dispersion of repolarization and consequently prolongs QT and JT intervals.[166] Conversely, some studies have shown that CRT is associated with a decrease in the incidence of VTA, likely due to improved hemodynamic effects, diminished myocardial ischemia, and a more favorable neurohumoral state.[167] Subanalysis of major CRT trials has reported neutral impact of CRT on the incidence of VTA.[168,169] A significant reduction in the risk of life-threatening VTA in CRT responders as compared to implantable cardioverter defibrillator (ICD)-only patients and low-CRT responders is an encouraging finding.[170]

FUTURE DIRECTIONS

The future is likely to see continued broadening of the eligible patients for CRT. The current dyssynchrony criteria based on QRS duration may be replaced by a more comprehensive set of parameters for dyssynchrony incorporating QRS duration, emerging echocardiographic indices of dyssynchrony, and clinical factors. Hopefully, such criteria will translate into reduced CRT nonresponse rates. More sensitive and specific dyssynchrony indices may identify narrow QRS complex patients who may benefit from CRT, and help to minimize wide QRS complex nonresponders.

Left ventricular endocardial or epicardial multisite pacing may enhance the response rate and benefits of CRT.[151] Improved LV reverse remodeling has been demonstrated in a small study utilizing multisite ventricular stimulation (1 RV and 2 LV leads).[171] In contrast to nonphysiological epicardial pacing which reverses the direction of myocardial depolarization and repolarization, endocardial LV pacing is considered more physiologic and less arrhythmogenic. The endocardial LV lead may be advanced across the interatrial septum into the LV cavity, allowing optimal LV lead positioning unconstrained by coronary venous anatomy. Risk of systemic thromboembolism, need for anticoagulation, and infection are the major safety concerns associated with LV endocardial lead placement.[172-174] Another emerging pacing strategy is LV-only pacing (as opposed to BiV pacing). Preliminary data suggest that LV-only pacing is noninferior to BiV pacing in a 6-month follow-up with regard to clinical and echocardiographic responses.[175] A meta-analysis of randomized controlled trials comparing LV-only and BiV pacing demonstrated similar improvements in 6MWD, QoL, peak VO_2, and NYHA functional class between the two pacing groups.[176] Further studies are warranted to define the clinical role and safety of these emerging pacing strategies.

ACCF/AHA/HRS GUIDELINES: WHAT IS NEW?

The following discussion summarizes the new CRT recommendations from 2012 ACCF/AHA/HRS focused update incorporated into the ACCF/AHA/HRS 2008 guidelines for device-based therapy of cardiac rhythm abnormalities.[177] It should be noted that the Class I indication is limited to patients with LBBB, with a QRS duration greater than or equal to 150 ms. In contrast, CRT for patients with a QRS duration greater than 120 ms but with a non-LBBB pattern (RBBB and IVCD) are downgraded to Class II recommendations in these guidelines. Recently published appropriate use criteria for CRT can also facilitate individual decision making in CRT implantation in various clinical settings.[178]

- **Class I: CRT is indicated for:**
  - Patients who have LVEF less than or equal to 35%, sinus rhythm, LBBB with a QRS duration greater than or equal to 150 ms, and NYHA Class II, III, or ambulatory IV symptoms on guideline-directed medical therapy (GDMT) (Level of Evidence: A for NYHA Class III/IV; Level of Evidence: B for NYHA Class II)
- **Class IIa: CRT can be useful for:**
  - Patients who have LVEF less than or equal to 35%, sinus rhythm, LBBB with a QRS duration 120–149 ms, and NYHA Class II, III, or ambulatory IV symptoms on GDMT (Level of Evidence: B)

- Patients who have LVEF less than or equal to 35%, sinus rhythm, a non-LBBB pattern with a QRS duration greater than or equal to 150 ms, and NYHA Class III/ambulatory Class IV symptoms on GDMT (Level of Evidence: A)
- Patients with AF and LVEF less than or equal to 35% on GDMT if a) the patient requires ventricular pacing or otherwise meets CRT criteria, or b) AV nodal ablation or pharmacologic rate control will allow near 100% ventricular pacing with CRT (Level of Evidence: B)
- Patients on GDMT who have LVEF less than or equal to 35% and are undergoing new or replacement device placement with anticipated requirement for significant (>40%) ventricular pacing (Level of Evidence: C)

- **Class IIb: CRT may be considered for:**
  - Patients who have LVEF less than or equal to 30%, ischemic etiology of HF, sinus rhythm, LBBB with a QRS duration of greater than or equal to 150 ms, and NYHA Class I symptoms on GDMT (Level of Evidence: C)
  - Patients who have LVEF less than or equal to 35%, sinus rhythm, a non-LBBB pattern with QRS duration 120 to 149 ms, and NYHA Class III/ambulatory Class IV on GDMT (Level of Evidence: B)
  - Patients who have LVEF less than or equal to 35%, sinus rhythm, a non-LBBB pattern with a QRS duration greater than or equal to 150 ms, and NYHA Class II symptoms on GDMT (Level of Evidence: B)
- **Class III: CRT is NOT recommended for:**
  - Patients with NYHA Class I or II symptoms and non-LBBB pattern with QRS duration less than 150 ms (Level of Evidence: B)
  - Patients whose co-morbidities and/or frailty limit survival with good functional capacity to less than 1 year (Level of Evidence: C).

REFERENCES

1. Epstein AE, DiMarco JP, Ellenbogen KA, et al. ACC/AHA/HRS 2008 Guidelines for Device-Based Therapy of Cardiac Rhythm Abnormalities: a report of the American College of Cardiology/American Heart Association Task Force on Practice Guidelines (Writing Committee to Revise the ACC/AHA/NASPE 2002 Guideline Update for Implantation of Cardiac Pacemakers and Antiarrhythmia Devices): developed in collaboration with the American Association for Thoracic Surgery and Society of Thoracic Surgeons. Circulation. 2008;117(21):e350-408.
2. McAlister F, Ezekowitz J, Wiebe N, et al. (2004). Cardiac resynchronization therapy for congestive heart failure. [online] Available from: archive.ahrq.gov/downloads/pub/evidence/pdf/resynchf/resynchf.pdf [Accessed April, 2013].
3. Baldasseroni S, Opasich C, Gorini M, et al. Left bundle-branch block is associated with increased 1-year sudden and total mortality rate in 5517 outpatients with congestive heart failure: a report from the Italian network on congestive heart failure. Am Heart J. 2002;143(3):398-405.
4. Aaronson KD, Schwartz JS, Chen TM, et al. Development and prospective validation of a clinical index to predict survival in ambulatory patients referred for cardiac transplant evaluation. Circulation. 1997;95(12):2660-7.

5. Dhingra R, Pencina MJ, Wang TJ, et al. Electrocardiographic QRS duration and the risk of congestive heart failure: the Framingham Heart Study. Hypertension. 2006;47(5):861-7.
6. Blanc JJ, Etienne Y, Gilard M, et al. Evaluation of different ventricular pacing sites in patients with severe heart failure: results of an acute hemodynamic study. Circulation. 1997;96(10):3273-7.
7. Huvelle E, Fay R, Alla F, et al. Left bundle branch block and mortality in patients with acute heart failure syndrome: a substudy of the EFICA cohort. Eur J Heart Fail. 2010;12(2):156-63.
8. van Bommel RJ, Ypenburg C, Mollema SA, et al. Site of latest activation in patients eligible for cardiac resynchronization therapy: patterns of dyssynchrony among different QRS configurations and impact of heart failure etiology. Am Heart J. 2011;161(6):1060-6.
9. Tse HF, Lau CP. Long-term effect of right ventricular pacing on myocardial perfusion and function. J Am Coll Cardiol. 1997;29(4):744-9.
10. Vernooy K, Verbeek XA, Peschar M, et al. Left bundle branch block induces ventricular remodelling and functional septal hypoperfusion. Eur Heart J. 2005;26(1):91-8.
11. Prinzen FW, Hunter WC, Wyman BT, et al. Mapping of regional myocardial strain and work during ventricular pacing: experimental study using magnetic resonance imaging tagging. J Am Coll Cardiol. 1999;33(6):1735-42.
12. Spragg DD, Akar FG, Helm RH, et al. Abnormal conduction and repolarization in late-activated myocardium of dyssynchronously contracting hearts. Cardiovasc Res. 2005;67(1):77-86.
13. de Teresa E, Chamorro JL, Pulpon A, et al. An even more physiological pacing: changing the sequence of ventricular activation. In: Steinbach K (Ed). Cardiac Pacing: Proceedings of the 7th World Symposium on Cardiac Pacing, Vienna. Darmstadt, Germany: Dr Dietrich Steinkopff Verlag, GmbH & Co. KG; 1983. pp. 395-401.
14. Wilkoff BL, Cook JR, Epstein AE, et al. Dual-chamber pacing or ventricular backup pacing in patients with an implantable defibrillator: the Dual Chamber and VVI Implantable Defibrillator (DAVID) Trial. JAMA. 2002;288(24):3115-23.
15. Sweeney MO, Hellkamp AS, Ellenbogen KA, et al. Adverse effect of ventricular pacing on heart failure and atrial fibrillation among patients with normal baseline QRS duration in a clinical trial of pacemaker therapy for sinus node dysfunction. Circulation. 2003;107(23):2932-7.
16. Cazeau S, Ritter P, Bakdach S, et al. Four chamber pacing in dilated cardiomyopathy. Pacing Clin Electrophysiol. 1994;17(11 Pt 2):1974-9.
17. Foster AH, Gold MR, McLaughlin JS. Acute hemodynamic effects of atrio-biventricular pacing in humans. Ann Thorac Surg. 1995;59(2):294-300.
18. Leclercq C, Cazeau S, Le Breton H, et al. Acute hemodynamic effects of biventricular DDD pacing in patients with end-stage heart failure. J Am Coll Cardiol. 1998;32(7):1825-31.
19. Daubert JC, Ritter P, Le Breton H, et al. Permanent left ventricular pacing with transvenous leads inserted into the coronary veins. Pacing Clin Electrophysiol. 1998;21(1 Pt 2):239-45.
20. Higgins SL, Hummel JD, Niazi IK, et al. Cardiac resynchronization therapy for the treatment of heart failure in patients with intraventricular conduction delay and malignant ventricular tachyarrhythmias. J Am Coll Cardiol. 2003;42(8):1454-9.
21. Abraham WT, Young JB, León AR, et al. Effects of cardiac resynchronization on disease progression in patients with left ventricular systolic dysfunction, an indication for an implantable cardioverter-defibrillator, and mildly symptomatic chronic heart failure. Circulation. 2004;110(18):2864-8.
22. Cazeau S, Leclercq C, Lavergne T, et al. Effects of multisite biventricular pacing in patients with heart failure and intraventricular conduction delay. N Engl J Med. 2001;344(12):873-80.

23. Abraham WT, Fisher WG, Smith AL, et al. Cardiac resynchronization in chronic heart failure. N Engl J Med. 2002;346(24):1845-53.
24. Bradley DJ, Bradley EA, Baughman KL, et al. Cardiac resynchronization and death from progressive heart failure: a meta-analysis of randomized controlled trials. JAMA. 2003;289(6):730-40.
25. Bristow MR, Saxon LA, Boehmer J, et al. Cardiac-resynchronization therapy with or without an implantable defibrillator in advanced chronic heart failure. N Engl J Med. 2004;350(21):2140-50.
26. Cleland JG, Daubert JC, Erdmann E, et al. The effect of cardiac resynchronization on morbidity and mortality in heart failure. N Engl J Med. 2005;352(15):1539-49.
27. Abraham WT, Young JB, Leon AR. (2002). Medtronic InSync® ICD Cardiac Resynchronization System (DRAFT - Sponsor Presentation - Medtronic Corporation ppt/htm). [online]. Available from: www.fda.gov/ohrms/dockets/ac/02/briefing/3843b2.htm. [Accessed April, 2013].
28. Kass DA, Chen CH, Curry C, et al. Improved left ventricular mechanics from acute VDD pacing in patients with dilated cardiomyopathy and ventricular conduction delay. Circulation. 1999;99(12):1567-73.
29. Bleeker GB, Schalij MJ, Nihoyannopoulos P, et al. Left ventricular dyssynchrony predicts right ventricular remodeling after cardiac resynchronization therapy. J Am Coll Cardiol. 2005;46(12):2264-9.
30. Healey JS, Davies RA, Tang AS. Improvement of apparently fixed pulmonary hypertension with cardiac resynchronization therapy. J Heart Lung Transplant. 2004;23(5):650-2.
31. Nelson GS, Berger RD, Fetics BJ, et al. Left ventricular or biventricular pacing improves cardiac function at diminished energy cost in patients with dilated cardiomyopathy and left bundle-branch block. Circulation. 2000;102(25):3053-9.
32. Young JB, Abraham WT, Smith AL, et al. Combined cardiac resynchronization and implantable cardioversion defibrillation in advanced chronic heart failure: the MIRACLE ICD Trial. JAMA. 2003;289(20):2685-94.
33. Vinereanu D. Mitral regurgitation and cardiac resynchronization therapy. Echocardiography. 2008;25(10):1155-66.
34. Breithardt OA, Sinha AM, Schwammenthal E, et al. Acute effects of cardiac resynchronization therapy on functional mitral regurgitation in advanced systolic heart failure. J Am Coll Cardiol. 2003;41(5):765-70.
35. Kanzaki H, Bazaz R, Schwartzman D, et al. A mechanism for immediate reduction in mitral regurgitation after cardiac resynchronization therapy: insights from mechanical activation strain mapping. J Am Coll Cardiol. 2004;44(8):1619-25.
36. Lancellotti P, Mélon P, Sakalihasan N, et al. Effect of cardiac resynchronization therapy on functional mitral regurgitation in heart failure. Am J Cardiol. 2004;94(11):1462-5.
37. Diaz-Infante E, Mont L, Leal J, et al. Predictors of lack of response to resynchronization therapy. Am J Cardiol. 2005;95(12):1436-40.
38. Cabrera-Bueno F, García-Pinilla JM, Peña-Hernández J, et al. Repercussion of functional mitral regurgitation on reverse remodelling in cardiac resynchronization therapy. Europace. 2007;9(9):757-61.
39. Yu CM, Fang F, Zhang Q, et al. Improvement of atrial function and atrial reverse remodeling after cardiac resynchronization therapy for heart failure. J Am Coll Cardiol. 2007;50(8):778-85.
40. Grassi G, Vincenti A, Brambilla R, et al. Sustained sympathoinhibitory effects of cardiac resynchronization therapy in severe heart failure. Hypertension. 2004;44(5):727-31.
41. Gould PA, Kong G, Kalff V, et al. Improvement in cardiac adrenergic function post biventricular pacing for heart failure. Europace. 2007;9(9):751-6.

42. Fantoni C, Raffa S, Regoli F, et al. Cardiac resynchronization therapy improves heart rate profile and heart rate variability of patients with moderate to severe heart failure. J Am Coll Cardiol. 2005;46(10):1875-82.
43. Sinha AM, Skobel EC, Breithardt OA, et al. Cardiac resynchronization therapy improves central sleep apnea and Cheyne-Stokes respiration in patients with chronic heart failure. J Am Coll Cardiol. 2004;44(1):68-71.
44. Janousek J, Tomek V, Chaloupecký VA, et al. Cardiac resynchronization therapy: a novel adjunct to the treatment and prevention of systemic right ventricular failure. J Am Coll Cardiol. 2004;44(9):1927-31.
45. Valzania C, Gadler F, Winter R, et al. Effects of cardiac resynchronization therapy on coronary blood flow: evaluation by transthoracic Doppler echocardiography. Eur J Heart Fail. 2008;10(5):514-20.
46. Henrikson CA, Spragg DD, Cheng A, et al. Evidence for electrical remodeling of the native conduction system with cardiac resynchronization therapy. Pacing Clin Electrophysiol. 2007;30(5):591-5.
47. Linde C, Abraham WT, Gold MR, et al. Randomized trial of cardiac resynchronization in mildly symptomatic heart failure patients and in asymptomatic patients with left ventricular dysfunction and previous heart failure symptoms. J Am Coll Cardiol. 2008;52(23):1834-43.
48. Moss AJ. QRS duration in the selection of patients for cardiac resynchronization therapy. Ann Noninvasive Electrocardiol. 2009;14(4):317-8.
49. Tang AS, Wells GA, Talajic M, et al. Cardiac-resynchronization therapy for mild-to-moderate heart failure. N Engl J Med. 2010;363(25):2385-95.
50. Al-Majed NS, McAlister FA, Bakal JA, et al. Meta-analysis: cardiac resynchronization therapy for patients with less symptomatic heart failure. Ann Intern Med. 2011;154(6): 401-12.
51. Linde C, Abraham WT, Gold MR, et al. Cardiac resynchronization therapy in asymptomatic or mildly symptomatic heart failure patients in relation to etiology: results from the REVERSE (REsynchronization reVErses Remodeling in Systolic Left vEntricular Dysfunction) study. J Am Coll Cardiol. 2010;56(22):1826-31.
52. Moss AJ, Hall WJ, Cannom DS, et al. Cardiac-resynchronization therapy for the prevention of heart-failure events. N Engl J Med. 2009;361(14):1329-38.
53. Zareba W, Klein H, Cygankiewicz I, et al. Effectiveness of Cardiac Resynchronization Therapy by QRS Morphology in the Multicenter Automatic Defibrillator Implantation Trial-Cardiac Resynchronization Therapy (MADIT-CRT). Circulation. 2011;123(10):1061-72.
54. Versteeg H, van den Broek KC, Theuns DA, et al. Effect of cardiac resynchronization therapy-defibrillator implantation on health status in patients with mild versus moderate symptoms of heart failure. Am J Cardiol. 2011;108(8):1155-9.
55. Dickstein K, Vardas PE, Auricchio A, et al. 2010 focused update of ESC Guidelines on device therapy in heart failure: an update of the 2008 ESC Guidelines for the diagnosis and treatment of acute and chronic heart failure and the 2007 ESC Guidelines for cardiac and resynchronization therapy. Developed with the special contribution of the Heart Failure Association and the European Heart Rhythm Association. Eur J Heart Fail. 2010;12(11):1143-53.
56. US Food and Drug Administration. (2012). FDA approves pump for heart failure patients awaiting heart transplant. [online]. Available from www.fda.gov/NewsEvents/Newsroom/PressAnnouncements/ucm328818.htm. [Accessed April, 2013].
57. Maisel WH, Stevenson LW. Atrial fibrillation in heart failure: epidemiology, pathophysiology, and rationale for therapy. Am J Cardiol. 2003;91(6A):2D-8D.

58. Ehrlich JR, Nattel S, Hohnloser SH. Atrial fibrillation and congestive heart failure: specific considerations at the intersection of two common and important cardiac disease sets. J Cardiovasc Electrophysiol. 2002;13(4):399-405.
59. Hayes DL, Boehmer JP, Day JD, et al. Cardiac resynchronization therapy and the relationship of percent biventricular pacing to symptoms and survival. Heart Rhythm. 2011;8(9):1469-75.
60. Leclercq C, Walker S, Linde C, et al. Comparative effects of permanent biventricular and right-univentricular pacing in heart failure patients with chronic atrial fibrillation. Eur Heart J. 2002;23(22):1780-7.
61. Leon AR, Greenberg JM, Kanuru N, et al. Cardiac resynchronization in patients with congestive heart failure and chronic atrial fibrillation: effect of upgrading to biventricular pacing after chronic right ventricular pacing. J Am Coll Cardiol. 2002;39(8):1258-63.
62. Hay I, Melenovsky V, Fetics BJ, et al. Short-term effects of right-left heart sequential cardiac resynchronization in patients with heart failure, chronic atrial fibrillation, and atrioventricular nodal block. Circulation. 2004;110(22):3404-10.
63. Valls-Bertault V, Fatemi M, Gilard M, et al. Assessment of upgrading to biventricular pacing in patients with right ventricular pacing and congestive heart failure after atrioventricular junctional ablation for chronic atrial fibrillation. Europace. 2004;6(5):438-43.
64. Doshi RN, Daoud EG, Fellows C, et al. Left ventricular-based cardiac stimulation post AV nodal ablation evaluation (the PAVE study). J Cardiovasc Electrophysiol. 2005;16(11):1160-5.
65. Brignole M, Botto G, Mont L, et al. Cardiac resynchronization therapy in patients undergoing atrioventricular junction ablation for permanent atrial fibrillation: a randomized trial. Eur Heart J. 2011;32(19):2420-9.
66. Delnoy PP, Ottervanger JP, Luttikhuis HO, et al. Comparison of usefulness of cardiac resynchronization therapy in patients with atrial fibrillation and heart failure versus patients with sinus rhythm and heart failure. Am J Cardiol. 2007;99(9):1252-7.
67. Khadjooi K, Foley PW, Chalil S, et al. Long-term effects of cardiac resynchronisation therapy in patients with atrial fibrillation. Heart. 2008;94(7):879-83.
68. Tolosana JM, Hernandez Madrid A, Brugada J, et al. Comparison of benefits and mortality in cardiac resynchronization therapy in patients with atrial fibrillation versus patients in sinus rhythm (Results of the Spanish Atrial Fibrillation and Resynchronization [SPARE] Study). Am J Cardiol. 2008;102(4):444-9.
69. Gasparini M, Auricchio A, Metra M, et al. Long-term survival in patients undergoing cardiac resynchronization therapy: the importance of performing atrio-ventricular junction ablation in patients with permanent atrial fibrillation. Eur Heart J. 2008;29(13):1644-52.
70. Wilton SB, Leung AA, Ghali WA, et al. Outcomes of cardiac resynchronization therapy in patients with versus those without atrial fibrillation: a systematic review and meta-analysis. Heart Rhythm. 2011;8(7):1088-94.
71. Kamath GS, Cotiga D, Koneru JN, et al. The utility of 12-lead Holter monitoring in patients with permanent atrial fibrillation for the identification of nonresponders after cardiac resynchronization therapy. J Am Coll Cardiol. 2009;53(12):1050-5.
72. Fung JW, Yu CM, Chan JY, et al. Effects of cardiac resynchronization therapy on incidence of atrial fibrillation in patients with poor left ventricular systolic function. Am J Cardiol. 2005;96(5):728-31.
73. Kiès P, Leclercq C, Bleeker GB, et al. Cardiac resynchronisation therapy in chronic atrial fibrillation: impact on left atrial size and reversal to sinus rhythm. Heart. 2006;92(4):490-4.

74. Bleeker GB, Schalij MJ, Molhoek SG, et al. Relationship between QRS duration and left ventricular dyssynchrony in patients with end-stage heart failure. J Cardiovasc Electrophysiol. 2004;15(5):544-9.
75. Yu CM, Lin H, Zhang Q, et al. High prevalence of left ventricular systolic and diastolic asynchrony in patients with congestive heart failure and normal QRS duration. Heart. 2003;89(1):54-60.
76. Bleeker GB, Schalij MJ, Molhoek SG, et al. Frequency of left ventricular dyssynchrony in patients with heart failure and a narrow QRS complex. Am J Cardiol. 2005;95(1):140-2.
77. Rouleau F, Merheb M, Geffroy S, et al. Echocardiographic assessment of the interventricular delay of activation and correlation to the QRS width in dilated cardiomyopathy. Pacing Clin Electrophysiol. 2001;24(10):1500-6.
78. Ghio S, Constantin C, Klersy C, et al. Interventricular and intraventricular dyssynchrony are common in heart failure patients, regardless of QRS duration. Eur Heart J. 2004;25(7):571-8.
79. Abraham J, Abraham TP. Is echocardiographic assessment of dyssynchrony useful to select candidates for cardiac resynchronization therapy? Echocardiography is useful before cardiac resynchronization therapy if QRS duration is available. Circ Cardiovasc Imaging. 2008;1(1):79-84.
80. Kashani A, Barold SS. Significance of QRS complex duration in patients with heart failure. J Am Coll Cardiol. 2005;46(12):2183-92.
81. Achilli A, Sassara M, Ficili S, et al. Long-term effectiveness of cardiac resynchronization therapy in patients with refractory heart failure and "narrow" QRS. J Am Coll Cardiol. 2003;42(12):2117-24.
82. Bleeker GB, Holman ER, Steendijk P, et al. Cardiac resynchronization therapy in patients with a narrow QRS complex. J Am Coll Cardiol. 2006;48(11):2243-50.
83. Yu CM, Chan YS, Zhang Q, et al. Benefits of cardiac resynchronization therapy for heart failure patients with narrow QRS complexes and coexisting systolic asynchrony by echocardiography. J Am Coll Cardiol. 2006;48(11):2251-7.
84. Jeevanantham V, Zareba W, Navaneethan S, et al. Meta-analysis on effects of cardiac resynchronization therapy in heart failure patients with narrow QRS complex. Cardiol J. 2008;15(3):230-6.
85. Beshai JF, Grimm RA, Nagueh SF, et al. Cardiac-resynchronization therapy in heart failure with narrow QRS complexes. N Engl J Med. 2007;357(24):2461-71.
86. Chung ES, Leon AR, Tavazzi L, et al. Results of the Predictors of Response to CRT (PROSPECT) trial. Circulation. 2008;117(20):2608-16.
87. Donahue T, Niazi I, Leon A, et al. One year follow-up of CRT in narrow QRS patients with mechanical dyssynchrony: ESTEEM-CRT. Circulation. 2008;118:S-949.
88. Mollema SA, Bleeker GB, van der Wall EE, et al. Usefulness of QRS duration to predict response to cardiac resynchronization therapy in patients with end-stage heart failure. Am J Cardiol. 2007;100(11):1665-70.
89. Suffoletto MS, Dohi K, Cannesson M, et al. Novel speckle-tracking radial strain from routine black-and-white echocardiographic images to quantify dyssynchrony and predict response to cardiac resynchronization therapy. Circulation. 2006;113(7):960-8.
90. Gorcsan J, Tanabe M, Bleeker GB, et al. Combined longitudinal and radial dyssynchrony predicts ventricular response after resynchronization therapy. J Am Coll Cardiol. 2007;50(15):1476-83.
91. Tatsumi K, Tanaka H, Yamawaki K, et al. Utility of comprehensive assessment of strain dyssynchrony index by speckle tracking imaging for predicting response to cardiac resynchronization therapy. Am J Cardiol. 2011;107(3):439-46.

92. van Dijk J, Knaapen P, Russel IK, et al. Mechanical dyssynchrony by 3D echo correlates with acute haemodynamic response to biventricular pacing in heart failure patients. Europace. 2008;10(1):63-8.
93. Westenberg JJ, Lamb HJ, van der Geest RJ, et al. Assessment of left ventricular dyssynchrony in patients with conduction delay and idiopathic dilated cardiomyopathy: head-to-head comparison between tissue Doppler imaging and velocity-encoded magnetic resonance imaging. J Am Coll Cardiol. 2006;47(10):2042-8.
94. Bilchick KC, Dimaano V, Wu KC, et al. Cardiac magnetic resonance assessment of dyssynchrony and myocardial scar predicts function class improvement following cardiac resynchronization therapy. JACC Cardiovasc Imaging. 2008;1(5):561-8.
95. Foley PW, Patel K, Irwin N, et al. Cardiac resynchronisation therapy in patients with heart failure and a normal QRS duration: the RESPOND study. Heart. 2011;97(13):1041-7.
96. ClinicalTrials.gov. (2013). Echocardiography Guided Cardiac Resynchronization Therapy (EchoCRT). [online] Available from: www.clinicaltrials.gov/ct2/show/NCT00683696?term=echocrt&rank=1. [Accessed April, 2013].
97. Kindermann M, Hennen B, Jung J, et al. Biventricular versus conventional right ventricular stimulation for patients with standard pacing indication and left ventricular dysfunction: the Homburg Biventricular Pacing Evaluation (HOBIPACE). J Am Coll Cardiol. 2006;47(10):1927-37.
98. van Geldorp IE, Vernooy K, Delhaas T, et al. Beneficial effects of biventricular pacing in chronically right ventricular paced patients with mild cardiomyopathy. Europace. 2010;12(2):223-9.
99. Leclercq C. Upgrading from right ventricular pacing to biventricular pacing in pacemaker patients with chronic heart failure: Heart failure. Heart. 2008;94(1):102-7.
100. Yu CM, Chan JY, Zhang Q, et al. Biventricular pacing in patients with bradycardia and normal ejection fraction. N Engl J Med. 2009;361(22):2123-34.
101. Chan JY, Fang F, Zhang Q, et al. Biventricular pacing is superior to right ventricular pacing in bradycardia patients with preserved systolic function: 2-year results of the PACE trial. Eur Heart J. 2011;32(20):2533-40.
102. Kaye G, Stambler BS, Yee R. Search for the optimal right ventricular pacing site: design and implementation of three randomized multicenter clinical trials. Pacing Clin Electrophysiol. 2009;32(4):426-33.
103. Stockburger M, Gómez-Doblas JJ, Lamas G, et al. Preventing ventricular dysfunction in pacemaker patients without advanced heart failure: results from a multicentre international randomized trial (PREVENT-HF). Eur J Heart Fail. 2011;13(6):633-41.
104. Versteeg H, Schiffer AA, Widdershoven JW, et al. Response to cardiac resynchronization therapy: is it time to expand the criteria? Pacing Clin Electrophysiol. 2009;32(10):1247-56.
105. Raphael C, Briscoe C, Davies J, et al. Limitations of the New York Heart Association functional classification system and self-reported walking distances in chronic heart failure. Heart. 2007;93(4):476-82.
106. Shah MR, Hasselblad V, Stinnett SS, et al. Dissociation between hemodynamic changes and symptom improvement in patients with advanced congestive heart failure. Eur J Heart Fail. 2002;4(3):297-304.
107. Bleeker GB, Bax JJ, Fung JW, et al. Clinical versus echocardiographic parameters to assess response to cardiac resynchronization therapy. Am J Cardiol. 2006;97(2):260-3.
108. Abdelhadi R, Adelstein E, Voigt A, et al. Measures of left ventricular dyssynchrony and the correlation to clinical and echocardiographic response after cardiac resynchronization therapy. Am J Cardiol. 2008;102(5):598-601.
109. Auger D, van Bommel RJ, Bertini M, et al. Prevalence and characteristics of patients with clinical improvement but not significant left ventricular reverse remodeling after cardiac resynchronization therapy. Am Heart J. 2010;160(4):737-43.

110. Yu CM, Bleeker GB, Fung JW, et al. Left ventricular reverse remodeling but not clinical improvement predicts long-term survival after cardiac resynchronization therapy. Circulation. 2005;112(11):1580-6.
111. Ypenburg C, van Bommel RJ, Borleffs CJ, et al. Long-term prognosis after cardiac resynchronization therapy is related to the extent of left ventricular reverse remodeling at midterm follow-up. J Am Coll Cardiol. 2009;53(6):483-90.
112. Solomon SD, Foster E, Bourgoun M, et al. Effect of cardiac resynchronization therapy on reverse remodeling and relation to outcome: multicenter automatic defibrillator implantation trial: cardiac resynchronization therapy. Circulation. 2010;122(10):985-92.
113. Egoavil CA, Ho RT, Greenspon AJ, et al. Cardiac resynchronization therapy in patients with right bundle branch block: analysis of pooled data from the MIRACLE and Contak CD trials. Heart Rhythm. 2005;2(6):611-5.
114. Gervais R, Leclercq C, Shankar A, et al. Surface electrocardiogram to predict outcome in candidates for cardiac resynchronization therapy: a sub-analysis of the CARE-HF trial. Eur J Heart Fail. 2009;11(7):699-705.
115. Adelstein EC, Saba S. Usefulness of baseline electrocardiographic QRS complex pattern to predict response to cardiac resynchronization. Am J Cardiol. 2009;103(2):238-42.
116. Bilchick KC, Kamath S, DiMarco JP, et al. Bundle-branch block morphology and other predictors of outcome after cardiac resynchronization therapy in Medicare patients. Circulation. 2010;122(20):2022-30.
117. Nery PB, Ha AC, Keren A, et al. Cardiac resynchronization therapy in patients with left ventricular systolic dysfunction and right bundle branch block: a systematic review. Heart Rhythm. 2011;8(7):1083-7.
118. Garrigue S, Reuter S, Labeque JN, et al. Usefulness of biventricular pacing in patients with congestive heart failure and right bundle branch block. Am J Cardiol. 2001;88(12): 1436-41.
119. Aranda JM, Conti JB, Johnson JW, et al. Cardiac resynchronization therapy in patients with heart failure and conduction abnormalities other than left bundle-branch block: analysis of the Multicenter InSync Randomized Clinical Evaluation (MIRACLE). Clin Cardiol. 2004;27(12):678-82.
120. Kronborg MB, Nielsen JC, Mortensen PT. Electrocardiographic patterns and long-term clinical outcome in cardiac resynchronization therapy. Europace. 2010;12(2):216-22.
121. Chandra R, Zolty R, Palma E. A left hemiblock improves cardiac resynchronization therapy outcomes in patients with a right bundle branch block. Clin Cardiol. 2010; 33(2):89-93.
122. Chalil S, Stegemann B, Muhyaldeen SA, et al. Effect of posterolateral left ventricular scar on mortality and morbidity following cardiac resynchronization therapy. Pacing Clin Electrophysiol. 2007;30(10):1201-9.
123. Adelstein EC, Saba S. Scar burden by myocardial perfusion imaging predicts echocardiographic response to cardiac resynchronization therapy in ischemic cardiomyopathy. Am Heart J. 2007;153(1):105-12.
124. Hummel JP, Lindner JR, Belcik JT, et al. Extent of myocardial viability predicts response to biventricular pacing in ischemic cardiomyopathy. Heart Rhythm. 2005;2(11):1211-7.
125. Jansen AH, Bracke F, van Dantzig JM, et al. The influence of myocardial scar and dyssynchrony on reverse remodeling in cardiac resynchronization therapy. Eur J Echocardiogr. 2008;9(4):483-8.
126. Birnie D, DeKemp RA, Ruddy TD, et al. Effect of lateral wall scar on reverse remodeling with cardiac resynchronization therapy. Heart Rhythm. 2009;6(12):1721-6.
127. Molhoek SG, Bax JJ, van Erven L, et al. Comparison of benefits from cardiac resynchronization therapy in patients with ischemic cardiomyopathy versus idiopathic dilated cardiomyopathy. Am J Cardiol. 2004;93(7):860-3.

128. Sutton MG, Plappert T, Hilpisch KE, et al. Sustained reverse left ventricular structural remodeling with cardiac resynchronization at one year is a function of etiology: quantitative Doppler echocardiographic evidence from the Multicenter InSync Randomized Clinical Evaluation (MIRACLE). Circulation. 2006;113(2):266-72.
129. D'Andrea A, Salerno G, Scarafile R, et al. Right ventricular myocardial function in patients with either idiopathic or ischemic dilated cardiomyopathy without clinical sign of right heart failure: effects of cardiac resynchronization therapy. Pacing Clin Electrophysiol. 2009;32(8):1017-29.
130. McLeod CJ, Shen WK, Rea RF, et al. Differential outcome of cardiac resynchronization therapy in ischemic cardiomyopathy and idiopathic dilated cardiomyopathy. Heart Rhythm. 2011;8(3):377-82.
131. Bax JJ, Bleeker GB, Marwick TH, et al. Left ventricular dyssynchrony predicts response and prognosis after cardiac resynchronization therapy. J Am Coll Cardiol. 2004;44(9): 1834-40.
132. Scuteri L, Rordorf R, Marsan NA, et al. Relevance of echocardiographic evaluation of right ventricular function in patients undergoing cardiac resynchronization therapy. Pacing Clin Electrophysiol. 2009;32(8):1040-9.
133. Burri H, Domenichini G, Sunthorn H, et al. Right ventricular systolic function and cardiac resynchronization therapy. Europace. 2010;12(3):389-94.
134. Alpendurada F, Guha K, Sharma R, et al. Right ventricular dysfunction is a predictor of non-response and clinical outcome following cardiac resynchronization therapy. J Cardiovasc Magn Reson. 2011;13:68.
135. Sweeney MO, van Bommel RJ, Schalij MJ, et al. Analysis of ventricular activation using surface electrocardiography to predict left ventricular reverse volumetric remodeling during cardiac resynchronization therapy. Circulation. 2010;121(5):626-34.
136. Rickard J, Popovic Z, Verhaert D, et al. The QRS narrowing index predicts reverse left ventricular remodeling following cardiac resynchronization therapy. Pacing Clin Electrophysiol. 2011;34(5):604-11.
137. Hsing JM, Selzman KA, Leclercq C, et al. Paced left ventricular QRS width and ECG parameters predict outcomes after cardiac resynchronization therapy: PROSPECT-ECG substudy. Circ Arrhythm Electrophysiol. 2011;4(6):851-7.
138. Barold SS, Ilercil A, Leonelli F, et al. First-degree atrioventricular block. Clinical manifestations, indications for pacing, pacemaker management & consequences during cardiac resynchronization. J Interv Card Electrophysiol. 2006;17(2):139-52.
139. Barold SS, Ilercil A, Herweg B. Echocardiographic optimization of the atrioventricular and interventricular intervals during cardiac resynchronization. Europace. 2008;10(Suppl 3): iii88-95.
140. Olshansky B, Day JD, Sullivan RM, et al. Does cardiac resynchronization therapy provide unrecognized benefit in patients with prolonged PR intervals? The impact of restoring atrioventricular synchrony: an analysis from the COMPANION Trial. Heart Rhythm. 2012;9(1):34-9.
141. Stopper MM, Li J, Beshai JF, et al. The impact of baseline PR interval on response to CRT in heart failure with narrow QRS complexes: A Sub-study of the ReThinQ Trial. Circulation. 2011;124:A17944.
142. Anderson LJ, Miyazaki C, Sutherland GR, et al. Patient selection and echocardiographic assessment of dyssynchrony in cardiac resynchronization therapy. Circulation. 2008; 117(15):2009-23.
143. Butter C, Auricchio A, Stellbrink C, et al. Effect of resynchronization therapy stimulation site on the systolic function of heart failure patients. Circulation. 2001; 104(25):3026-9.

144. Dekker AL, Phelps B, Dijkman B, et al. Epicardial left ventricular lead placement for cardiac resynchronization therapy: optimal pace site selection with pressure-volume loops. J Thorac Cardiovasc Surg. 2004;127(6):1641-7.
145. Singh JP, Klein HU, Huang DT, et al. Left ventricular lead position and clinical outcome in the multicenter automatic defibrillator implantation trial-cardiac resynchronization therapy (MADIT-CRT) trial. Circulation. 2011;123(11):1159-66.
146. Becker M, Kramann R, Franke A, et al. Impact of left ventricular lead position in cardiac resynchronization therapy on left ventricular remodelling. A circumferential strain analysis based on 2D echocardiography. Eur Heart J. 2007;28(10):1211-20.
147. Ypenburg C, van Bommel RJ, Delgado V, et al. Optimal left ventricular lead position predicts reverse remodeling and survival after cardiac resynchronization therapy. J Am Coll Cardiol. 2008;52(17):1402-9.
148. Becker M, Altiok E, Ocklenburg C, et al. Analysis of LV lead position in cardiac resynchronization therapy using different imaging modalities. JACC Cardiovasc Imaging. 2010;3(5):472-81.
149. Bai R, Di Biase L, Mohanty P, et al. Positioning of left ventricular pacing lead guided by intracardiac echocardiography with vector velocity imaging during cardiac resynchronization therapy procedure. J Cardiovasc Electrophysiol. 2011;22(9):1034-41.
150. Ailawadi G, Lapar DJ, Swenson BR, et al. Surgically placed left ventricular leads provide similar outcomes to percutaneous leads in patients with failed coronary sinus lead placement. Heart Rhythm. 2010;7(5):619-25.
151. Blendea D, Singh JP. Lead positioning strategies to enhance response to cardiac resynchronization therapy. Heart Fail Rev. 2011;16(3):291-303.
152. Rivero-Ayerza M, Jessurun E, Ramcharitar S, et al. Magnetically guided left ventricular lead implantation based on a virtual three-dimensional reconstructed image of the coronary sinus. Europace. 2008;10(9):1042-7.
153. Mullens W, Grimm RA, Verga T, et al. Insights from a cardiac resynchronization optimization clinic as part of a heart failure disease management program. J Am Coll Cardiol. 2009;53(9):765-73.
154. Abraham WT, Gras D, Yu CM, et al. Rationale and design of a randomized clinical trial to assess the safety and efficacy of frequent optimization of cardiac resynchronization therapy: the Frequent Optimization Study Using the QuickOpt Method (FREEDOM) trial. Am Heart J. 2010;159(6):944-8.
155. Sogaard P, Egeblad H, Pedersen AK, et al. Sequential versus simultaneous biventricular resynchronization for severe heart failure: evaluation by tissue Doppler imaging. Circulation. 2002;106(16):2078-84.
156. Vanderheyden M, De Backer T, Rivero-Ayerza M, et al. Tailored echocardiographic interventricular delay programming further optimizes left ventricular performance after cardiac resynchronization therapy. Heart Rhythm. 2005;2(10):1066-72.
157. Duvall WL, Hansalia R, Wijetunga MN, et al. Advantage of optimizing V-V timing in cardiac resynchronization therapy devices. Pacing Clin Electrophysiol. 2010;33(10):1161-8.
158. Weiss R. V-V Optimization in Cardiac Resynchronization Therapy Non-Responders: RESPONSE-HF trial results. Abstract AB12-5, HRS 2010, Denver, Colorado. 2010.
159. Boriani G, Müller CP, Seidl KH, et al. Randomized comparison of simultaneous biventricular stimulation versus optimized interventricular delay in cardiac resynchronization therapy. The Resynchronization for the HemodYnamic Treatment for Heart Failure Management II implantable cardioverter defibrillator (RHYTHM II ICD) study. Am Heart J. 2006;151(5):1050-8.
160. Rao RK, Kumar UN, Schafer J, et al. Reduced ventricular volumes and improved systolic function with cardiac resynchronization therapy: a randomized trial comparing

simultaneous biventricular pacing, sequential biventricular pacing, and left ventricular pacing. Circulation. 2007;115(16):2136-44.

161. van Rees JB, de Bie MK, Thijssen J, et al. Implantation-related complications of implantable cardioverter-defibrillators and cardiac resynchronization therapy devices: a systematic review of randomized clinical trials. J Am Coll Cardiol. 2011;58(10):995-1000.
162. Ghanbari H, Feldman D, Schmidt M, et al. Cardiac resynchronization therapy device implantation in patients with therapeutic international normalized ratios. Pacing Clin Electrophysiol. 2010;33(4):400-6.
163. Guerra JM, Wu J, Miller JM, et al. Increase in ventricular tachycardia frequency after biventricular implantable cardioverter defibrillator upgrade. J Cardiovasc Electrophysiol. 2003;14(11):1245-7.
164. Mykytsey A, Maheshwari P, Dhar G, et al. Ventricular tachycardia induced by biventricular pacing in patient with severe ischemic cardiomyopathy. J Cardiovasc Electrophysiol. 2005;16(6):655-8.
165. Shukla G, Chaudhry GM, Orlov M, et al. Potential proarrhythmic effect of biventricular pacing: fact or myth? Heart Rhythm. 2005;2(9):951-6.
166. Medina-Ravell VA, Lankipalli RS, Yan GX, et al. Effect of epicardial or biventricular pacing to prolong QT interval and increase transmural dispersion of repolarization: does resynchronization therapy pose a risk for patients predisposed to long QT or torsade de pointes? Circulation. 2003;107(5):740-6.
167. Ermis C, Seutter R, Zhu AX, et al. Impact of upgrade to cardiac resynchronization therapy on ventricular arrhythmia frequency in patients with implantable cardioverter-defibrillators. J Am Coll Cardiol. 2005;46(12):2258-63.
168. McSwain RL, Schwartz RA, DeLurgio DB, et al. The impact of cardiac resynchronization therapy on ventricular tachycardia/fibrillation: an analysis from the combined Contak-CD and InSync-ICD studies. J Cardiovasc Electrophysiol. 2005;16(11):1168-71.
169. Gold MR, Linde C, Abraham WT, et al. The impact of cardiac resynchronization therapy on the incidence of ventricular arrhythmias in mild heart failure. Heart Rhythm. 2011;8(5):679-84.
170. Barsheshet A, Wang PJ, Moss AJ, et al. Reverse remodeling and the risk of ventricular tachyarrhythmias in the MADIT-CRT (Multicenter Automatic Defibrillator Implantation Trial-Cardiac Resynchronization Therapy). J Am Coll Cardiol. 2011; 57(24):2416-23.
171. Leclercq C, Gadler F, Kranig W, et al. A randomized comparison of triple-site versus dual-site ventricular stimulation in patients with congestive heart failure. J Am Coll Cardiol. 2008;51(15):1455-62.
172. Jaïs P, Takahashi A, Garrigue S, et al. Mid-term follow-up of endocardial biventricular pacing. Pacing Clin Electrophysiol. 2000;23(11 Pt 2):1744-7.
173. van Gelder BM, Scheffer MG, Meijer A, et al. Transseptal endocardial left ventricular pacing: an alternative technique for coronary sinus lead placement in cardiac resynchronization therapy. Heart Rhythm. 2007;4(4):454-60.
174. Whinnett Z, Bordachar P. The risks and benefits of transseptal endocardial pacing. Curr Opin Cardiol. 2012;27(1):19-23.
175. Boriani G, Kranig W, Donal E, et al. A randomized double-blind comparison of biventricular versus left ventricular stimulation for cardiac resynchronization therapy: the Biventricular versus Left Univentricular Pacing with ICD Back-up in Heart Failure Patients (B-LEFT HF) trial. Am Heart J. 2010;159(6):1052-8.
176. Liang Y, Pan W, Su Y, et al. Meta-analysis of randomized controlled trials comparing isolated left ventricular and biventricular pacing in patients with chronic heart failure. Am J Cardiol. 2011;108(8):1160-5.

177. Epstein AE, DiMarco JP, Ellenbogen KA, et al. 2012 ACCF/AHA/HRS focused update incorporated into the ACCF/AHA/HRS 2008 guidelines for device-based therapy of cardiac rhythm abnormalities: a report of the American College of Cardiology Foundation/American Heart Association Task Force on Practice Guidelines and the Heart Rhythm Society. J Am Coll Cardiol. 2013;61:e6-75.

178. Russo AM, Stainback RF, Bailey SR, et al. ACCF/HRS/AHA/ASE/HFSA/SCAI/SCCT/SCMR 2013 appropriate use criteria for implantable cardioverter-defibrillators and cardiac resynchronization therapy: a report of the American College of Cardiology Foundation appropriate use criteria task force, Heart Rhythm Society, American Heart Association, American Society of Echocardiography, Heart Failure Society of America, Society for Cardiovascular Angiography and Interventions, Society of Cardiovascular Computed Tomography, and Society for Cardiovascular Magnetic Resonance. J Am Coll Cardiol. 2013;61:1318-68.

CHAPTER 10

Sudden Cardiac Death and Implantable Cardioverter-Defibrillator

Toshimasa Okabe, Behzad B Pavri

INTRODUCTION

Sudden cardiac death (SCD) continues to be a leading cause of death in the United States and the estimated annual incidence is between 300,000 and 350,000.[1,2] According to American College of Cardiology/American Heart Association/European Society of Cardiology (ACC/AHA/ESC) 2006 Guidelines, SCD is defined as "death from an unexpected circulatory arrest, usually due to a cardiac arrhythmia occurring within an hour of the onset of symptoms." Ventricular tachycardia (VT) and ventricular fibrillation (VF) are the most commonly encountered arrhythmias in SCD.[3] Patients that suffer from acute myocardial infarction (MI), left ventricular (LV) dysfunction and congestive heart failure (CHF) are particularly prone to a fatal ventricular tachyarrhythmia (VTA) episode.

More than three decades have passed since the first human implantable cardioverter-defibrillator (ICD) was implanted at Johns Hopkins Hospital in 1980.[4,5] The ICD has now become the treatment of choice for SCD prevention by providing rapid defibrillation during episodes of fatal VTA to restore viable cardiac rhythms. At present, active areas of ICD research include improvement in candidate selection, arrhythmia recognition, and hardware technology (lead, battery, and implantation technology).

The purpose of this chapter is to discuss:

1. Major clinical trials in ICD and overview of current guidelines.
2. Some controversial issues in ICD (selection criteria, patient subgroups with limited data, disparity in ICD use).
3. Complications of ICD.
4. Psychological and ethical issues in ICD.
5. Emerging technology and future directions in ICD.

IMPLANTABLE CARDIOVERTER-DEFIBRILLATOR TRIALS AND GUIDELINES IN SECONDARY SUDDEN CARDIAC DEATH PREVENTION

The earliest ICDs required patients to undergo surgical implantation of epicardial pacing leads and defibrillator patches via thoracotomy with the ICD generator inserted into the abdomen. Because of significant procedural mortality and morbidity with this approach, patients qualified for an ICD only after they had survived sudden cardiac arrest. In the late 1980s, transvenous insertion of endovascular leads with defibrillation coils was introduced and subsequent miniaturization of pulse generators enabled nonsurgeons to safely implant ICDs in the pectoral region in early 1990s.

As clinicians and scientists were able to better understand the mechanisms of VTA and SCD, and pivotal clinical trials in empirical antiarrhythmic drugs (AAD) for high-risk patients, such as the Cardiac Arrhythmia Suppression Trial (CAST) failed to improve mortality, the focus of SCD prevention shifted from empiric antiarrhythmic drugs to ICD implantation in early 1990s. In 1985, the FDA approved the ICD device for patients who were either cardiac arrest survivors or with recurrent VTA; however, at that time, there were no randomized clinical trials that proved mortality benefit of ICD therapy. Three landmark prospective randomized trials were undertaken in secondary SCD prevention:

- Antiarrhythmics versus Implantable Defibrillators (AVID) in the United States[6]
- Canadian Implantable Defibrillator Study (CIDS) in Canada[7]
- Cardiac Arrest Study Hamburg (CASH) in Europe (Table 1).[8]

Cardiac Arrest Study Hamburg enrolled cardiac arrest survivors due to VTA from 1987 to 1996, and randomized them to ICD or one of the three AAD groups (ICD/amiodarone/metoprolol/propafenone in a 1:1:1:1 design). The propafenone arm was discontinued in 1992 after an interim analysis revealed an increased all-cause mortality rate compared to the ICD. Eventually, 288 patients were recruited to the three remaining groups. During a mean follow-up of 57 months, the difference in survival rate between ICD group and AAD groups (amiodarone/metoprolol) did not reach statistical difference (ICD: AAD, HR 0.766, P = 0.081), although survival-free of sudden death was significantly higher in ICD group than in AAD group (HR 0.423, P = 0.005). Notably, perioperative mortality was as high as 5.1% (5.4% in epicardial implantation and 4.5% in endocardial implantation), which may have mitigated the benefit of ICD therapy.

Canadian Implantable Defibrillator Study randomly assigned 659 patients who had been resuscitated from VT/VF or had syncope due to VT to either ICD therapy or amiodarone between the years of 1990 and 1997. During the 3-year follow-up, there was a statistically nonsignificant decrease in arrhythmic death (3.0% vs. 4.5% per year; P = 0.094) and mortality reduction in ICD group compared to amiodarone group (8.3% vs. 10.2% per year; P = 0.142); a higher use of beta-blockers in ICD group (34% in ICD vs. 21% in amiodarone) clouded the results.

Table 1 **Summary of primary prevention implantable cardioverter-defbrillator trials**

Trials (reference number)	*Year published*	*Inclusion criteria*	*Exclusion criteria*	*Study arms*	*Number of patients in ICD arm/ control arm*	*Mean EF in each arm*	*Index arrhythmia*	*ICM (%)*	*Beta-blocker use*	*RAAS inhibition with ACEI or ARB*	*Measured outcomes*
AVID[6]	1997	Resuscitated VF, VT + syncope, symptomatic VT + EF ≤0.4	High risk (life expectancy < 1 year, NYHA IV CHF, awaiting transplant, on mechanical or inotropic support), low risk (event within 5 days of CABG, angioplasty or MI), previous ICD implant	ICD vs. Class III AAD	n = 1,016, ICD: 507, AAD: 509 (amiodarone 95.8%, sotalol 2.8%)	ICD: 0.32, AAD: 0.31	ICD: VF 226 vs. VT 281, AAD: VF 229 vs VT 280	ICD: 81%, AAD: 81%	ICD: 42%, AAD: 17%	ICD: 69%, AAD: 68%	Overall mortality
CIDS[7]	2000	Resuscitated VF/VT or unmonitored syncope likely due to VT	Events within 72 hours post-MI, or electrolyte abnormalities, ICD or amiodarone not considered appropriate, excessive preoperative risk for ICD, previous amiodarone therapy for	ICD vs. amiodarone	n = 659, ICD: 328, amiodarone: 331	ICD: 0.34, amiodarone: 0.33	ICD: VF or cardiac arrest 45%, VT 40%, amiodarone: VF or cardiac arrest 50%, VT 38%	ICD: 83%, amiodarone: 82%	ICD: 34%, amiodarone: 21%	NA	Overall mortality

Contd...

Contd...

			>6 weeks, life expectancy <1 year, LQTS								
CASH[8]	2000	SCD survivors	Cardiac arrest within 72 hours post-MI, cardiac surgery, electrolyte abnormalities, or proarrhythmic drug effect	ICD vs. 3 AAD groups (amiodarone, propafenone, metoprolol). Assignment to propafenone was discontinued early	n=288; ICD: 99, amiodarone: 92, metoprolol: 97	ICD: 0.46, amiodarone: 0.44, metoprolol: 0.47	VF: 84%, VT: 16%	ICD: 73%, amiodarone: 77%, metoprolol: 70%	ICD: 0%, and amiodanone group: 0%	ICD: 45%, amiodarone: 40%, metoprolol: 40%	Overall mortality

EF, ejection fraction; ICD, implantable cardioverter-defibrillator; ICM, ischemic cardiomyopathy; RAAS, renin angiotensin aldosterone sytem; ACEI, angiotensin-converting enzyme inhibitor; ARB, aldosterone receptor blocker; SCD, sudden cardiac death; VF, ventricular fibrillation;VT, ventricular tachycardia; NYHA, New York Heart Association; CHF, congestive heart failure; CABG, coronary artery bypass graft; MI, myocardial infarction; AAD, antiarrhythmic drug.

Antiarrhythmics versus Implantable Defibrillators, the largest trial but with the shortest patient enrollment duration of the three trials, randomly assigned 1,016 patients presenting with a history of resuscitated VT/VF and symptomatic VT (syncope, near-syncope, CHF, or angina) to either ICD therapy or Class III AAD (95.8% amiodarone) between the years of 1993 and 1997. The study was terminated early due to an observed mortality reduction in favor of ICD therapy. Over a mean follow-up of 18.2 months, the crude death rates in ICD group and AAD group were 15.8% and 24%, respectively ($P < 0.02$). Similar to CIDS, a shortcoming of the study was a consistently higher use of beta-blockers in the ICD group throughout the trial period (ICD: AAD, 42.3% vs. 16.5% at discharge, and 39.4% vs. 10.1% at 24 months), although multivariate analysis demonstrated persistent beneficial effect of ICD therapy. In subgroup analysis, survival benefit was limited to patients whose left ventricular ejection fraction (EF) was 35% or less.

A meta-analysis of the above-mentioned three trials was published in 2000.[9] This compared 934 patients treated with ICD therapy against 932 patients treated with amiodarone. In this study, ICD therapy was associated with significant reductions in all-cause mortality (HR 0.72, $P = 0.0006$) and in arrhythmic death (HR 0.50, $P < 0.0001$). As was seen in AVID trial, patients with EF less than or equal to 35% derived significantly more benefit than those with EF more than 35%. This possible lack of ICD benefit in sudden cardiac arrest survivors with preserved EF has not been translated into current ICD guidelines.

The occurrence of VTA prompts investigation for potentially reversible causes, such as recent or recurrent myocardial ischemia, electrolyte abnormalities, and drug effects. Subsequently, it becomes essential to determine whether an ICD is necessary. Below are the current Class I recommendation for ICD implantation for secondary SCD prevention:[10]

- Survivors of cardiac arrest due to VF or hemodynamically unstable VT (Level of Evidence: A)
- Structural heart disease with spontaneous VT (Level of Evidence: B).

IMPLANTABLE CARDIOVERTER-DEFIBRILLATOR TRIALS AND GUIDELINES IN PRIMARY SUDDEN CARDIAC DEATH PREVENTION

The majority of SCD events occur among those who never had a cardiac arrest. Therefore, there has been great interest in identifying high-risk patients in the general population who could benefit from prophylactic ICD implantation.[11] In general, trials that identify high-risk patients for ICD therapy integrate noninvasive and invasive testing for risk assessment. Furthermore, much attention has been paid to define the role of ICD therapy for patients with ischemic cardiomyopathy (ICM) and nonischemic cardiomyopathy (NICM). To date, there have been 10 major clinical trials evaluating the role of ICD in primary prevention of SCD in various pathophysiologic states (Table 2).

Table 2 Summary of primary prevention ICD trials

ICM vs. NICM			
ICM			
Trials [reference number]	MUSTT[14]	MADIT I[12]	MADIT II[15]
Year published	1999	1996	2002
EF cutoff	0.4	0.35	0.3
Other inclusion criteria	NSVT 4 or more days post-MI	MI 3 weeks or more before entry, NYHA I to III CHF, NSVT and inducible and nonsuppresible VT/VF, age 25-80 yrs	Age >21 (no upper age limit), more than 1 month post-MI
Study arms	EPG Rx (AAD or ICD if AAD failed) vs. No Rx	ICD (98 transthoracic and 98 transvenous implants) vs. control	ICD (single chamber or dual chamber) vs. control
Number of patients in ICD arm/control arm	n=704, EPG Rx: 351 (ICD: 161), No Rx: 353	n=196, ICD: 95, control: 101	n=1,232, ICD: 742, control: 490
Mean EF in each arm	EPG Rx: 0.30, No Rx: 0.29	ICD: 0.25, control: 0.27	ICD: 0.23, control: 0.23
ICM (%)	100	100	100
Measured outcomes	Primary: cardiac arrest or arrhythmic death, Secondary: overall mortality, cardiac death, spontaneous sustained VT	Overall mortality	Overall mortality
Beta-blocker use	EPG Rx: 29%, No Rx: 51%	At 1 month, ICD: 28%, control: 9%	ICD: 70%, control: 70%
RAAS inhibition with ACEI or ARB	EPG Rx: 72%, No Rx: 51%	At 1 month, ICD: 65%, control: 60%	ICD: 68%, control: 72%
Result	Median f/u 39 mo, cardiac arrest or arrhythmic death at 5 yrs in EPG: 25%, in No Rx: 32% (RR 0.73, P= 0.04), overall mortality at 5 yrs in EPG: 42%, in No Rx: 48% (RR 1.80, P= 0.06)	Mean f/u 27 mo, death in ICD: 15, in control: 39 (HR 0.46, P=0.009)	Mean f/u 20 mo, death in ICD: 14.2%, in control: 19.8% (HR 0.69, P=0.016)
Comments	In EPG group, 5-yr rate of cardiac arrest or arrhythmic death was 9% in ICD group and 37% in AAD group (P=0.001). No significant difference in spontaneous VT between EPG and No Rx group	More nonarrhythmic deaths in control group	Statistically nonsignificant increase in new or worsened HF in ICD group. NYHA IV CHF excluded

Contd...

Contd...

ICM vs NICM			
	ICM	Implant early after MI	
Trials [reference number]	CABG-PATCH[16]	DINAMIT[22]	IRIS[23]
Year published	1997	2004	2009
EF cutoff	0.36	0.35	0.4
Other inclusion criteria	Elective CABG, abnormal SAECG, age <80 yrs	6-40 days post-MI, low HRV or elevated HR on Holter monitoring at least 3 days post-MI, age 18-80 yrs	5–31 days post-MI, heart rate ≥90 bpm on first ECG or NSVT ≥150 bpm on Holter, age 18–80 yrs
Study arms	Epicardial ICD vs. control	Single-chamber ICD (VVI 40) vs. control	ICD (81% single chamber VVI 40) vs. control
Number of patients in ICD arm/control arm	n=900, ICD: 446, control: 454	n=674, ICD: 332, control: 342	n=898, ICD: 445, control: 453
Mean EF in each arm	ICD: 0.27, control: 0.27	ICD: 0.28, control: 0.28	ICD: 0.35, control: 0.35
ICM (%)	100	100	100
Measured outcomes	Overall mortality	Overall mortality	Overall mortality
Beta-blocker use	At hospital discharge, ICD: 18%, control: 24%	ICD: 87%, control: 87%	ICD: 89%, control: 86%
RAAS inhibition with ACEI or ARB	ICD: 55%, control: 54%	ICD: 95%, control: 94%	ICD: 82%, control: 82%
Result	Mean f/u 32 mo, death in ICD: 101, in control: 95 (HR 1.07, P=0.64)	Mean f/u 30 mo, death in ICD: 62, in control: 58 (HR 1.08, P=0.66)	Mean f/u 37 mo, death in ICD: 116, in control: 117 (HR 1.04, P=0.78)
Comments	More postoperative infections in ICD group	Statistically significant increase in non-arrhythmic death in ICD group (HR 1.75, P=0.02). NYHA IV CHF excluded	Statistically significant increase in non-SCD (HR 1.92, P=0.001). NYHA IV CHF excluded

Contd...

Contd...

ICM vs NICM				
	NICM			Both (ICM and NICM)
Trials [reference number]	AMIOVIRT[19]	CAT[18]	DEFINITE[20]	SCD-HeFT[21]
Year published	2003	2002	2004	2005
EF cutoff	0.35	0.3	0.36	0.35
Other inclusion criteria	Asymptomatic NSVT lasting <30 s, NYHA I to III CHF, age >18 yrs	Recent onset NICM ≤9 mo, NYHA II or III CHF, age 18–70 yrs	Ambient arrhythmias (NSVT or 10 PVCs /hr on Holter), NYHA I to III CHF	NYHA II or III CHF, age >18 yrs
Study arms	ICD vs. amiodarone	ICD (VVI 40) vs. control	Single-chamber ICD (VVI 40) vs. control	Conventional + placebo vs. conventional + amiodarone vs conventional + shock-only, single-lead ICD (VVI 34)
Number of patients in ICD arm/control arm	n=103, ICD: 51, smiodarone: 52	n=104, ICD: 50, Control: 54	n=458, ICD: 229, control: 229	n=2,521, placebo: 847, amiodarone: 845, ICD: 829
Mean EF in each arm	ICD: 0.22, amiodarone: 0.23	ICD: 0.24, Control: 0.25	ICD: 0.21, control: 0.22	Placebo: 0.25, amiodarone: 0.25, ICD: 0.24
ICM (%)	0	0	0	52
Measured outcomes	Overall morality	Overall mortality	Overall mortality	Overall mortality
Beta-blocker use	At last follow-up, ICD: 53%, amiodarone: 50%	ICD: 4%, Control: 3.7%	ICD: 86%, control: 84%	Placebo: 69%, amiodarone: 69%, ICD: 69%
RAAS inhibition with ACEI or ARB	At last follow-up, ICD: 90%, amiodarone: 81%	ICD: 94%, Control: 98%	(ACE-I) ICD: 84%, control: 87%, (ARB) ICD: 14%, control: 9%	Placebo: 98%, amiodarone: 97%, ICD: 94%
Result	Mean f/u 24 mo, No difference in survival at 1 yr and 3 yrs. (P=0.8)	Mean f/u 5.5 yrs, at 4 yrs, cumulative survival in ICD: 80% in control: 86%. (P=0.554)	Mean f/u 29 mo, death in ICD: 28, in control :40 (HR 0.65, P=0.08)	Mean f/u 46 mo, death in placebo: 244, in amiodarone: 240, in ICD: 182. ICD but not amiodarone reduced mortality (HR 0.77, P=0.007)
Comments		The only predictor of total mortality was lower EF ≤0.21 compared with EF ≥0.28	Statistically significant reduction in arrhythmic death in ICD (P=0.006). NYHA IV CHF excluded	Decreased mortality with ICD was seen in NYHA II CHF, not in NYHA III CHF. Antitachycardia pacing was not permitted for this study

ICM, ischemic cardiomyopathy; NICM, nonischemic cardiomyopathy; MUSTT, Multicenter Unsustained Tachycardia Trial; DINAMIT, Defibrillator in Acute Myocardial Infarction Trial; IRIS, Immediate Risk Stratification Improves Survival; AMIOVIRT, Amiodarone versus Implantable Defibrillator Trial; CAT, Cardiomyopathy Trial; DEFINITE, Defibrillators in Non-Ischemic Cardiomyopathy Treatment Evaluation; NYHA, New York Heart Association; CHF, congestive heart failure; EF, ejection fraction; RAAS, renin angiotensin aldosterone system; NSVT, nonsustained ventricular tachycardia; ACEI/ARB, angiotensin-converting-enzyme inhibitor/angiotensin receptor blocker; MI, myocardial infarction; SCD-HeFT, Sudden Cardiac Death in Heart Failure Trial; Rx, treatment/therapy; AAD, antiarrhythmic drug; f/u, follow-up; EPG, electrophysiological study guided; RR; relative risk; HR, hazard ratio; SAECG, signal averaged electrocardiography; HRV, heart rate variability; PVC, premature ventricular complex; mo, month; yr, year.

Implantable Cardioverter-Defibrillators in Coronary Artery Disease Cardiomyopathy

The Multicenter Unsustained Tachycardia Trial (MUSTT) and the Multicenter Automatic Defibrillator Trial (MADIT) I targeted patients with ICM and required both nonsustained VT (NSVT) and inducible VT/VF by programmed electrical stimulation (PES). Published in 1996, MADIT I was the first large primary ICD trial, in which 196 patients with prior MI (3 weeks or more before entry), EF less than or equal to 35%, The New York Heart Association (NYHA) I to III CHF, and inducible VT/VF (not suppressed by procainamide) were randomly assigned to either ICD (n = 95) or conventional medical therapy (n = 101).[12] During a mean follow-up of 27 months, there were 15 deaths in the ICD group and 39 deaths in the conventional therapy group (HR 0.46, P = 0.009). Once again, there was a significantly higher rate of beta-blocker use in the ICD group, and a subgroup analysis showed only patients with EF less than or equal to 26% derived survival benefit from ICD.[13]

The MUSTT, published in 1999, further confirmed the benefit of ICDs in patients with ICM.[14] MUSTT tested the hypothesis that electrophysiologically-guided antiarrhythmic therapy (EPG therapy) would reduce the risk of SCD among patients with ICM EF less than or equal to 40% and NSVT. Patients with inducible VT/VF at electrophysiological (EP) study were randomly assigned to either EPG therapy (n = 351) or non-AAD therapy (n = 353). Patients assigned to EPG therapy underwent serial drug testing to identify an effective AAD, and ICD was recommended (in almost half the patients) after one or more unsuccessful drug trials. MUSTT was unique when compared to other primary prevention trials in two aspects:

- MUSTT studied the role of EP study in patient selection for ICD implantation; MUSTT did not directly compare ICD to AAD therapy, since assignment between AAD and ICD (in AAD nonresponders) was not randomized
- The primary end-point was arrhythmic death or cardiac arrest, not total mortality. Nevertheless, the 5-year estimates of incidence of the primary end-point were 25% in EPG therapy and 32% in those not receiving AAD (RR 0.73, P = 0.04). The survival benefit associated with EPG therapy was primarily due to the use of ICD, not to AAD. It is noteworthy that only a minority of patients (16% in EPG therapy group and 18% in those receiving no AAD) was enrolled within 1 month post-MI; the median time between MI and enrollment was 39 months.

Multicenter Automatic Defibrillator Trial II was designed to more directly compare ICD therapy to conventional therapy; the trial had simplified inclusion criteria by eliminating the requirement of NSVT and VT/VF inducibility by PES.[15] A total of 1,232 patients with EF less than or equal to 30% who were at least 1 month post-MI were randomly assigned in a 3:2 ratio to receive either an ICD or conventional medical therapy. During a mean follow-up of 20 months, death occurred in 14.2% in ICD therapy and 19.8% in conventional therapy group (HR 0.69, P = 0.016). In a subgroup analysis, survival benefit was again only seen in those with lower EF group (EF ≤25%). The use of beta-blockers was comparable in both groups. The incidence of either new or worsened CHF was slightly higher in the ICD group than in the conventional therapy group; this association was not initially understood, but eventually led to the recognition of deleterious effects of right ventricular (RV) pacing, as discussed later.

The Coronary Artery Bypass Graft-patch (CABG-PATCH) was a negative ICD trial for primary prevention in patients with ICM.[16] It enrolled 900 patients with EF less than 36% and abnormal signal-average electrocardiogram (SAECG) who were undergoing elective coronary artery bypass grafting (CABG). All the patients received an epicardial ICD patches and were randomly assigned to either ICD group or control group. At a mean follow-up of 32 months, there was no mortality difference between the two groups, but there were more postoperative infections in the ICD group. Favorable effect of revascularization via CABG and poor prognostic performance of SAECG for predicting future fatal VTA were felt to be responsible for the negative results.

Implantable Cardioverter-Defibrillators in Nonischemic Cardiomyopathy

The prevalence of NICM is substantial and SCD or life-threatening arrhythmia affects patients with ICM and NICM.[1,17] The earliest trials including patients with NICM were the Cardiomyopathy Trial (CAT) and the Amiodarone Versus Implantable Defibrillator Trial (AMIOVIRT).

The Cardiomyopathy Trial began enrollment in 1991 in Germany and included patients with a new diagnosis of NICM (<9 months), EF less than or equal to 30% and NYHA II or III CHF.[18] A total of 104 patients were randomized to ICD or control group, but the trial was terminated early due to lack of benefit. Cumulative survival rate was not significantly different between the two groups at 2, 4, and 6 years of follow-up. In this study, the only predictor of mortality was EF less than or equal to 21%.

Similarly, AMIOVIRT also failed to provide evidence in favor of ICD for primary SCD prevention in the NICM population.[19] The trial enrolled a total of 103 patients with NICM, EF less than or equal to 35%, NSVT, and NYHA I to III CHF between 1996 and 2000 and randomized them to either ICD or amiodarone. There was no difference in survival between the ICD versus amiodarone groups at 1 and 3 years. In both these small trials, the mortality rates were significantly lower than expected, which accounted for the apparent lack of ICD benefit.

In the midst of the growing skepticism for ICD benefit in the NICM population, the result of the Defibrillators in Non-ischemic Cardiomyopathy Treatment Evaluation (DEFINITE) became available in 2003 and was published in 2004.[20] The trial randomized 458 patients with NICM, NYHA Class I to III CHF and ambient arrhythmias [defined as NSVT or an average of at least 10 premature ventricular complexes (PVCs) per hour on Holter monitoring] to either ICD or control. The ICDs were all single-chamber devices and programmed to back up VVI pacing at 40 bpm. After a mean follow-up of 29 months, despite a significant reduction in arrhythmic death in the ICD group (HR 0.20, P = 0.006), this trial again failed to demonstrate mortality difference in the two groups (HR 0.65, P = 0.08). The authors speculated that the high compliance with lifesaving evidence-based CHF regimen (including angiotensin converting enzyme inhibitors, angiotensin II receptor blockers, beta-blockers, and aldosterone antagonists) and a lower than expected deaths in the control group due to arrhythmias may have lowered all-cause mortality and diminished potential benefit of ICD in this population. In conclusion, all three trials targeting solely on the NICM population failed to demonstrate mortality benefit of ICD therapy.

Implantable Cardioverter-Defibrillators in Heart Failure of Any Etiology

The largest trial for primary prevention of SCD with ICD is the Sudden Cardiac Death in Heart Failure Trial (SCD-HeFT) published in 2005.[21] The trial was unique in that enrolled both ICM and NICM population with EF less than or equal to 35% and mild-to-moderate CHF (NYHA functional Class II or III). A total of 2,521 patients were randomized to three arms:

- Standard CHF therapy and placebo (n = 847)
- Standard therapy and amiodarone (n = 845), and
- Standard therapy and shock-only, single-lead ICD (n = 829).

After a median follow-up of 45.5 months, there was no mortality difference between the amiodarone and placebo (HR 1.06, P = 0.53), but there was significant reduction in mortality in the ICD arm compared with the placebo arm (HR 0.77, P = 0.007). SCD-HeFT provided some basis for ICD indication for primary prevention in NICM population, although a prespecified subgroup analysis based on etiology of cardiomyopathy failed to reach statistical significance (P = 0.06) in patients with NICM. Interestingly, in the prespecified subgroup analysis, among those patients with NYHA Class III CHF, ICD did not reduce risk of death.

Implantable Cardioverter-Defibrillators in New Onset (within 30 days of Myocardial Infarction) Ischemic Cardiomyopathy

It is recognized that the risk of SCD is greatest in the healing phase (first 30 days) after MI among patients with reduced EF, CHF or both; this prompted investigation as to the optimal timing of ICD placement for the prevention of SCD. Two trials, The Defibrillator in Acute Myocardial Infarction Trial (DINAMIT) published in 2004 and the Immediate Risk Stratification Improves Survival (IRIS) trial published in 2009 targeted such patients.

The DINAMIT enrolled total 674 patients 6–40 days after MI with a reduced EF (≤0.35) and impaired cardiac autonomic function [defined as low-heart-rate variability (HRV) or an elevated HR on Holter recordings], and randomly assigned to ICD or no ICD.[22] Despite significant reduction in arrhythmic death in the ICD group (HR 0.42, P = 0.009), there was no difference in overall mortality between the two groups during the mean follow-up period of 30 months. There was an unexpected (almost two-fold) higher incidence of death from nonarrhythmic causes in the ICD group which negated the beneficial effect of ICD in reducing arrhythmic death. The reason for this increase in nonarrhythmic death in ICD group was not entirely clear, but it was speculated that ICD merely "shifted" deaths from arrhythmic to nonarrhythmic, most notably from systolic heart failure. Majority of DINAMIT patients were in NYHA Class II or III CHF (87% in ICD, 88% in control) and the mean EF was 28%, which did not improve 6 weeks later.

The IRIS included a larger sample size with longer follow-up duration and demonstrated results consistent with DINAMIT.[23] IRIS enrolled total 898 patients 5–31 days after MI and heart rate (HR) more than or equal to 90 bpm on the first ECG or NSVT on Holter monitor, and randomly assigned them to ICD or non-ICD. Overall mortality did not differ between the two groups during the follow-up period of 37 months (HR 1.04, P = 0.78). The same disproportionate trend of reduced SCD and increased non-SCD was observed in this trial. Based on these two trials, the ACC/AHA/Heart Rhythm Society (HRS) 2008 guidelines for device-based therapy do not recommend ICD for primary prevention within the first 40 days after MI.[10]

For primary SCD prevention, current guideline gives ICD Class I indications for the patient groups below:

- Ischemic cardiomyopathy EF less than or equal to 35% at least 40 days post-MI and in NYHA functional Class II or III (Level of Evidence: B)
- Ischemic cardiomyopathy EF less than or equal to 30% at least 40 days post-MI and in NYHA functional Class I (Level of Evidence: A)
- Ischemic cardiomyopathy EF less than or equal to 40%, NSVT, inducible VF, or sustained VT by EP study (Level of Evidence: B)
- Nonischemic cardiomyopathy EF less than or equal to 35% and in NYHA functional Class II and III (Level of Evidence: B)
- Syncope of undetermined origin with hemodynamically significant VT or VF induced by EP study (Level of Evidence: B).

REFINING IMPLANTABLE CARDIOVERTER-DEFIBRILLATORS SELECTION CRITERIA

Critical Appraisal of Left Ventricular Ejection Fraction-Based Patient Selection

Impaired left ventricular systolic function and the presence of CHF, whether caused by ICM or NICM, are the most consistent and powerful predictors of cardiac mortality. Despite this, impaired EF has low sensitivity and specificity in predicting SCD, and a substantial number of such patients with ICDs do not receive appropriate therapy from their devices. ICDs are also associated with myriad device-related complications and adverse psychological effects. Finally, current guidelines for primary SCD prevention with ICD target patients with depressed EF and patients with preserved EF who may be at high-risk of SCD are missed. It is sobering to note that the majority of SCD occurs in general population, and SCD is not an uncommon cause of death in patients with isolated diastolic HF or HF with preserved EF.[24]

Only MUSTT and IRIS adopted an EF threshold of less than or equal to 0.40, while other primary prevention trials selected either less than or equal to 0.30 or less than or equal to 0.35 as the inclusion criteria. Among patients enrolled in these trials, however, the average EFs range much lower than the threshold values. In SCD-HeFT (where the inclusion EF criterion was ≤0.35), median EF was 25% and interquartile range for EF was 20–30%.[21] A prespecified subgroup of patients with EF more than 30% in SCD-HeFT did not confer ICD benefit. A similar finding was seen in a subgroup analysis of MADIT II between patients with EF less than or equal to 0.25 and those with EF more than 0.25. There appears to be an inverse relationship between EF and relative benefit from ICD; however, the true optimal EF threshold for consideration of ICD remains unclear. Issues such as the modality and method of measuring EF, and the timing of EF measurement after an index MI, are still matters of debate.

It has been increasingly recognized that reduced EF alone cannot accurately identify the patient at increased risk of arrhythmic SCD. Arrhythmogenic triggers, such as genetic predisposition, myocardial ischemia, exacerbation of HF, electrolyte abnormalities, drug effects, autonomic nervous system activation, and psychosocial factors have been proven to be risk factors that contribute to VTA/SCD. Therefore, retrospective analyses of major ICD trials have examined patient characteristics to delineate risks for VTA/SCD. A subanalysis of MUSTT showed an increased risk of future SCD in ICM population with a greater NYHA functional class, the presence of NSVT, prolonged/abnormal QRS [namely left bundle branch block (LBBB)], VT inducibility by EP study, and the presence of atrial fibrillation (AF).[25] In this study, patients whose only risk factor was low EF (without any of the above-listed variables) had a remarkably low risk of arrhythmic death (<5% of arrhythmic death in 2 years). The importance of incorporating additional clinical variables into the SCD prediction in improving the net benefit of ICD was also demonstrated in a *post hoc* analysis of MADIT II and SCD-HeFT. Goldberg et al. applied a simple risk stratification score comprising five clinical factors (NYHA functional Class > II, age > 70 years, blood urea nitrogen (BUN) >26 mg/dL, QRS >120 ms, and presence of AF) to the MADIT II cohort and divided the cohort to four subgroups based on the calculated risk (risk 0, 1, 2, ≥3) and very high risk (VHR) due to concomitant severe renal dysfunction.[26]

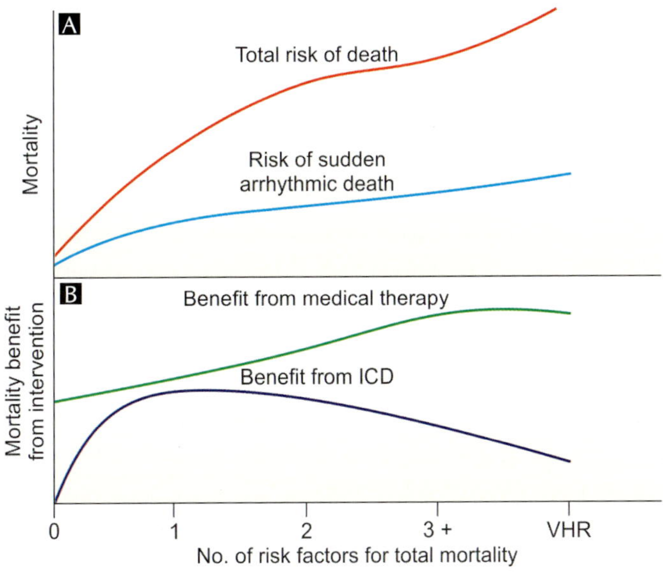

Figure 1: Relationship between total mortality, benefit from ICD implantation, and risk profile in patients with congestive heart failure. **A,** Risk of both overall death and sudden arrhythmic death increase with number of risk factors (NYHA class >II, age >70 years, BUN >26 mg/dL, QRS >120 ms, and AF); however, overall death increases at a greater rate, demonstrating that as the number of risk factors increase, death is more likely to occur from nonarrhythmic causes. **B,** Patients at intermediate risk (1 or 2 risk factors) derive the greatest benefit from ICD implantation; benefit diminishes as more risk factors accrue, related to increasing risk of non-arrhythmic death from competing causes.[26] ICD, implantable cardioverter-defibrillator; BUN, blood urea nitrogen; NYHA, New York Heart Association; VHR, very high risk due to concomitant severe renal disease.

Patients with VHR accounted for 5% of the entire cohort and carried 48% mortality risk during the mean follow-up period of 20 months. In this study, there was no significant survival benefit of primary ICD implant in the lowest-risk subgroup (risk = 0) and in the VHR group; limited efficacy was seen in the high-risk group (risk ≥3). Patients with intermediate risk (risk = 1 or 2) derived the most pronounced benefit. It is particularly noteworthy that patients with severe ICM without other risk factors, accounting for almost one-third of the MADIT II cohort, did not appear to have benefited from primary ICD implant during the follow-up period (mean 20 months) (Fig. 1). This analysis showed, in a compelling manner, the limitation of sole reliance on EF in selecting patients for ICD implantation.

The apparent "U-shaped" curve for ICD efficacy relative to comorbidities was not reproduced in the SCD-HeFT cohort using an externally validated Seattle Heart Failure Model (SHFM) as a risk assessment tool. The SHFM is a simple risk prediction model for HF prognosis, based on age, gender, NYHA functional class, EF, medications, and laboratory values.[27] Levy et al. applied the SHFM to the

SCD-HeFT cohort and showed the benefit of ICD therapy diminishes as predicted mortality increases, but levels off when the predicted annual mortality approaches approximately 20–25%. Unlike MADIT II, there was no subgroup of patients in SCD-HeFT who carried such a low risk of SCD that ICD did not provide mortality benefit.[28]

Value of Noninvasive and Invasive Risk Stratification

Currently, there is no single established noninvasive test capable of predicting SCD risk in a variety of patient populations.[29] In the major primary prevention ICD trials, various noninvasive parameters were incorporated into inclusion criteria (in addition to left ventricular EF) in an attempt to select patients at high risk for SCD. These parameters included resting heart rate, HR variability, NSVT, frequent PVCs, and signal-averaged electrocardiography (SAECG).

Signal-averaged electrocardiography, an electrocardiographic risk stratifying method used in the CABG-PATCH trial, requires specialized equipment that processes and computes small variations in high-frequency, low-amplitude signals in the terminal portion of the QRS complex, the so-called "late potentials". An abnormal SAECG is associated with the substrate for VTA after MI, with a prevalence ranging from 15–35%.[30] Owing to a relatively high-negative predictive value in the ICM population, SAECG may be useful in identifying patients at low risk for SCD. The value of SAECG in predicting SCD and mortality among patients with NICM is less well studied and available data is conflicting.[31] Although low-HRV, used in DINAMIT, signifies impaired "autonomic function" and is associated with increased mortality, its role in SCD risk prediction is not established.[32]

Among all the nonestablished noninvasive tests that are available to assess the risk of SCD (including QRS duration, QT interval, QT dispersion, heart rate turbulence, and baroreflex sensitivity), the most promising risk stratifying tool may be microvolt T-wave alternans (MTWA).[33] TWA is a reflection of repolarization alternans at the level of a single cell and is a rate-dependent phenomenon. Measurement of MTWA requires an exercise treadmill test and special software. TWA occurs at a relatively lower HR in patients susceptible to VTA. There is no randomized controlled trial to date examining the role of MTWA in primary ICD trials. In a substudy of SCD-HeFT, consisting of 490 patients, the result of TWA test did not predict an arrhythmic event.[34] A recent meta-analysis of MTWA in patients with reduced EF found an association between a positive MTWA result and the risk of mortality or severe arrhythmic events occurring within 1–2 years.[35] Major limitations of MTWA testing are lack of applicability in patients who are unable to exercise, patients with AF or frequent PVCs, and intrinsic or iatrogenic (drug-induced) chronotropic incompetence. Additionally, the predictive value of MTWA varies considerably depending on the population studied.[36] Despite moderately promising evidence supporting the use of MTWA, clinical utility of MTWA, especially when it is combined with other known invasive and noninvasive risk-stratifying tools, needs to be determined in additional studies.

Monomorphic VT induced by programmed electrical stimulation at the time of EP study in patients with ICM is a strong risk factor for arrhythmic death, but noninducibility does not necessarily indicate a low risk. Value of VT inducibility by PES among patients with NICM is limited.[33] VT inducibility by PES is utilized in MUSTT, and demonstrated a powerful prognostic value in patients with ICM, EF less than or equal to 40% and NSVT.[14]

SPECIAL POPULATIONS WITH LIMITED OR NONESTABLISHED IMPLANTABLE CARDIOVERTER-DEFIBRILLATOR BENEFIT

Ischemic Cardiomyopathy versus Nonischemic Cardiomyopathy

One of the most striking gaps between the current ICD guidelines and available clinical trials is the role of ICD in primary SCD prevention among patients with NICM. Despite the lack of a single trial showing a statistically significant mortality benefit (see above), including a subgroup analysis of SCD-HeFT, a Class I indication of ICD placement for primary prevention is granted to patients with NICM, EF less than or equal to 35% and NYHA functional Class II or III CHF.

A significant mortality reduction with primary prevention ICD therapy was seen only in a meta-analysis (n = 1,854) combining the results of CAT, AMIOVIRT, DEFINITE, SCD-HeFT, and Comparison of Medical Therapy Pacing and Defibrillation in Heart Failure (COMPANION).[37] This meta-analysis has estimated that the number needed to treat with ICD to prevent one death at 2 years (primary prevention) in NICM is 25 patients, in contrast to 18 patients in ICM.[38]

Men versus Women, Race and Ethnicity

Despite continued efforts to recruit more women, they are still generally underrepresented in contemporary cardiovascular clinical trials, and disproportionately fewer women have been enrolled into ICD trials.[39,40] Furthermore, non-White race and female sex are associated with lower utilization of any implantable cardiac device including ICD.[41] Santangeli et al. conducted a meta-analysis including five studies (MADIT-II, MUSTT, SCD-HeFT, DEFINITE, COMPANION) that enrolled total 7,229 patients, of whom 22% were female.[42] This study showed that the benefit of ICD on mortality was significant in men (HR 0.67, $P < 0.001$), but did not reach statistical significance in women (HR 0.78, $P = 0.1$). In this analysis, the number of ICD implantations to prevent one death in women was nearly double than in men (number needed to treat: 20 in men vs. 12 in women). It is also concerning that the overall rate of adverse events, including ICD complications, has been reported to be higher in women.[43]

Implantable Cardioverter-Defibrillator in Patients with Severe Renal Disease

The current ICD guidelines do not recommend withholding ICD implants in patients with any specific comorbidity; however, the benefit of an ICD in patients with reduced EF and severe renal impairment is not clear. SCD is the most common mode of death among patients receiving dialysis, accounting for approximately 27% of all-cause mortality;[44] however, dialysis patients were excluded from all major ICD trials. Dialysis patients may have multiple, unique myocardial substrates that make them particularly susceptible to fatal VTAs, including a high prevalence of underlying ischemic heart disease and structural heart disease, such as left ventricular hypertrophy, different response to coronary revascularization, rapid electrolyte shifts during a hemodialysis session, hyperkalemia especially before the first hemodialysis session of the week due to nonphysiologic thrice-weekly schedules, ectopic calcium deposition, altered myocardial structure at the cellular level, and elevated defibrillation thresholds.[45,46] The use of ICDs among dialysis patients, both for primary and secondary SCD prevention, has been widespread in the United States, but recent studies indicate all-cause mortality in this population remains alarmingly high.[47,48] A high rate of ICD infection and postprocedure bleeding among patients with end-stage renal disease may further attenuate the net benefit of ICD.[49] Given the high mortality rate despite ICD therapy, and a high prevalence of other competing nonarrhythmic causes of death, such as CHF, malignancy, infection, sepsis, and vascular complications, there is a clear need for a better risk stratifying strategy in this rapidly expanding population with reduced EF and kidney failure who have more than 1 year of life expectancy.[50]

Implantable Cardioverter-Defibrillator Paradox in Patients Early After Myocardial Infarction

The current guidelines recommend prophylactic ICD implantation for patients suffering from ICM with reduced EF, assessed at least 40 days after a qualifying MI. Although the risk of arrhythmic events is highest in the days and weeks following an MI, DINAMIT, and IRIS, enrolling patients with ICM within 40 days and 30 days after acute MI, respectively, did not demonstrate the benefit of ICD implantation. Conversely, both studies showed a significant increase in nonarrhythmic death in the ICD group, negating the benefit of ICD therapy. Additionally, a substudy of MADIT II indicated the survival benefit of ICD was greater in patients whose MI was more remote and the mortality benefit sustained up to more than 15 years.[51] The most plausible explanation is that the ICD can abort fatal arrhythmic events but does not prevent nonarrhythmic death, and patients in the healing phase of MI commonly suffer nonarrhythmic death (pump failure, mechanical complications). Another possibility is that risk-stratifying tools used in DINAMIT and IRIS (HRV, resting heart rate, and NSVT) did not appropriately select patients at increased risk for arrhythmic events. In fact, low-HRV, high-heart rate, and NSVT have also been associated with an increased risk of nonarrhythmic death.[52] Possible interactions between ICD shocks and worsening CHF may also play a role. Prognostic importance of ICD shocks was evaluated in a subanalysis of SCD-HeFT, in which both appropriate and inappropriate shocks were shown to be associated with significant increases in mortality.[53] It has been suggested that some patients are vulnerable to electrical injury and myocardial dysfunction from ICD shocks, potentially leading to CHF exacerbation.[54] For healthcare providers taking care of CHF patients who received ICD shocks, a sense of relief from averted SCD should be accompanied by heightened and aggressive CHF surveillance and management.[55] Presence of supraventricular and ventricular arrhythmias leading to ICD shocks are generally considered a marker of deteriorating overall cardiac status.

Some authors have challenged this paradox of a lack of ICD benefit early after MI by targeting particularly high-risk patients with EP study-guided risk stratification.[56,57] Kumar et al. performed an EP study 9 days after ST-elevation MI and recommended ICD implantation if VT with cycle length more than or equal to 200 ms was induced with less than or equal to 4 extrastimuli (EP positive group). An ICD was implanted a median of 21 days post-MI. At 2 years, the rate of primary end-point of sudden death or spontaneous ventricular arrhythmias was lower in the EP positive group than in the EP negative group ($P < 0.001$), although all-cause mortality was not significantly different. The survival benefit of this aggressive targeted approach needs to be confirmed in a larger study with a primary end-point of all-cause mortality.[57]

DISPARITY IN ICD USE AND NONEVIDENCE-BASED ICD IMPLANTATIONS

Data from "Get With The Guidelines—Heart Failure" (GWTG-HF) Registry indicates that there is significant, unexplained hospital variation in the use of ICD among eligible CHF patients in the United States.[58] Only one-fifth of "eligible" patients receive ICD implants nationwide. After adjusting for patient case mix, a larger hospital bed size, and procedural capabilities in percutaneous coronary intervention, coronary artery bypass graft surgery, and heart transplant were independently associated with a higher ICD use.

In sharp contrast, an analysis of the National Cardiovascular Data Registry-ICD Registry between the years of 2006 and 2009 revealed a 22.5% rate of nonevidence-based ICD implantation, including patients early after MI, with NYHA functional Class IV CHF, and recent diagnosis of CHF. An association between nonevidence-based ICD implantation and a significantly higher risk of in-hospital mortality and postprocedure complications was noted. There was no clear decrease in the rate of nonevidence-based ICD during the studied period of 2006–2009.[59] In addition to ongoing efforts to improve ICD candidate selection, dissemination of evidence-based ICD guidelines needs to be achieved.

COMPLICATIONS OF IMPLANTABLE CARDIOVERTER-DEFIBRILLATOR

There are mainly three types of ICD-related complications: procedural complications, lead or pulse generator-related complications, and untoward effects of ICD, such as inappropriate shocks and worsening CHF.

Procedural Complications

Periprocedural complications of ICD implantation include bleeding, infection, pneumothorax, cardiac perforation, lead dislodgment, and rarely death. The procedural complication rate has dramatically fallen since technological innovations transformed a large-sized device implanted surgically in the abdomen to a much smaller device inserted transvenously in the pectoral region. In-hospital mortality related to nonthoracotomy ICDs is 0.2%.[60] Recent trends in multiple centers of not performing defibrillation safety margin testing may also have contributed to lower implant-related complications, although the true safety of this strategy awaits the results of ongoing trials. It has been increasingly recognized that complication rates of ICD generator replacements and upgrade procedures are not as low as previously thought, and these procedures carry a notable risk.[61] Procedural complication rates are lower when ICDs are implanted by trained electrophysiologists rather than cardiologists or surgeons.[62]

Lead or Pulse Generator-Related Complications

Complications related to transvenous leads include lead fracture, insulation defect, lead failure (oversensing and undersensing), and tricuspid regurgitation. Recent highly publicized lead failures have exposed the lead to be the "Achilles' heel" of ICD systems and pose significant problems for patients and physicians.[63] Such "recalled" leads require regular surveillance, and failure rates tend to increase over time.[64] A pulse generator may migrate or cause skin erosion and necrosis. Rarely, ICD component failures have been reported.

Inappropriate Shocks

Implantable cardioverter-defibrillators may inappropriately deliver a therapy (antitachycardia pacing and/or shock) for supraventricular tachyarrhythmias (SVT). Inappropriate shocks, accounting for approximately 20–25% of all shocks, are associated with increased mortality, and may cause a variety of adverse effects including proarrhythmic effects, early battery depletion, and psychosocial morbidities.[65] Common underlying rhythms for inappropriate shocks are sinus tachycardia, AF, and other SVTs. Modern ICDs are equipped with built-in features (so-called "SVT discriminators") to distinguish SVT from VT/VF, but the key to inappropriate shock avoidance is correct programming of these features. Many patients will require intensified drug therapy and/or catheter-based radio-frequency ablation to control SVTs if device programming fails to prevent inappropriate shocks. Although some authors have suggested that dual-chamber ICDs may be better at decreasing AF-related inappropriate shocks,[66,67] the current consensus is that correctly programmed single chamber devices are recommended when there is no bradycardia-related indication for an atrial lead.

The prognostic significance of atrial arrhythmias in subgroup analyses of the major ICD trials has been controversial. Van Gelder et al. showed in a subanalysis of the Primary Prevention Parameters Evaluation (PREPARE) study that primary ICD patients with atrial tachycardia (AT) or AF are more likely to receive inappropriate shock, but mortality was not significantly increased.[68] On the other hand, in a subanalysis of the Inhibition of Unnecessary RV Pacing with AV Search Hysteresis in ICDs (INTRINSIC RV) study, Bunch et al. showed that newly detected AF in ICD patients was associated with significantly increased mortality.[69] It is indisputable that AF is a major cause of inappropriate shocks and the occurrence of shocks is independently associated with reduced quality of life in ICD recipients.[70]

In MADIT II and SCD-HeFT subanalyses, inappropriate shocks from any cause were indeed associated with an increased all-cause mortality; however, Dichtl et al. did not find a similar association in a large cohort (n = 1,117) of mixed primary and secondary ICD preventions. They concluded that only appropriate ICD shocks had a negative impact on overall survival.[71] The reason for this apparent discrepancy is unclear. Interestingly, a subanalysis of SCD-HeFT demonstrated that a beneficial effect of ICD was only seen in patients with sinus rhythm.[72] It is unclear whether the lack of ICD benefits in the non-sinus rhythm patients is due to detrimental hemodynamic effects of inappropriate shocks or simply due to the fact that nonsinus rhythms (most commonly AF) represent more advanced disease status with higher mortality.

Right Ventricular Pacing and Heart Failure

Previously, large pacing mode selection trials discovered detrimental effects of conventional RV apical pacing on cardiac structure and LV function, leading to HF. RV apical pacing results in dyssynchronous electrical and mechanical activation of the LV (similar to LBBB). Atrial-based cardiac pacing is the only treatment for chronotropic incompetence and symptomatic bradycardia caused by sinus node dysfunction and various degrees of atrioventricular block. Pacemakers also allow aggressive uptitration of beta-blockers in CHF patients, and of AV nodal blocking agents in patients with tachy-brady syndrome (AF with rapid ventricular response rate alternating with conversion pauses and sinus bradycardia). Maintaining atrioventricular synchrony by forced dual-chamber pacing was initially believed to be beneficial for CHF patients by controlling the timing of atrial and ventricular contractions and optimizing transmitral flow; however, this was soon replaced by the understanding of the importance of interventricular synchrony, as reflected by a narrow (native) QRS complex.

In the Dual Chamber and VVI Implantable Defibrillator (DAVID) trial, patients with EF less than or equal to 40% and no persistent atrial arrhythmias were randomly assigned to either VVI at backup pacing at 40 bpm (VVI-40) or DDDR at 70 bpm (DDDR-70).[73] One-year survival free of death or HF admissions was 83.9% in VVI-40 compared with 73.3% in DDDR-70 (CI = 1.06–2.44), and the study was terminated early due to potential harm with dual-chamber pacing. Due to the programmed short AV interval (180 ms) in the DDDR-70 group, nearly 60% of all ventricular beats were paced, in contrast to 1% RV pacing in the VVI-40 group. Percent RV pacing was correlated with the primary end-point of death or HF hospitalization.[74] Deleterious effects of RV pacing on ventricular function and HF progression are more pronounced in patients with reduced EF at baseline, but have also been reported in patients with previously preserved EF.[75-77] A subanalysis of the Mode Selection Trial (MOST) in patients with sinus node dysfunction and normal baseline QRS duration showed higher cumulative RV pacing was associated with risk of HF hospitalization and AF, regardless of the pacing mode (DDDR vs. VVIR); in this study the median EF was 55%.[75]

In a MADIT II substudy, cumulative RV pacing more than 50% of the time (high RV pacing group) was associated with a significantly increased risk of new or worsened CHF and appropriate shocks for VT/VF,[76] and long-term follow-up demonstrated that increased mortality and attenuated ICD efficacy in predominantly paced patients. The deleterious effect was most pronounced in non-LBBB patients.[78] However, it should be noted that patients in the high RV pacing group were generally "sicker" and showed advanced age, severe CHF, LBBB, and more frequent use of dual-chamber device.[79]

Regardless of the pacing system chosen, careful programming to minimize RV pacing has become the standard of care in pacemaker programming. In patients in whom RV pacing is likely high in spite of attempts to minimize it, cardiac resynchronization therapy (CRT) should be considered (chapter 9 on CRT).

PSYCHOSOCIAL AND ETHICAL ISSUES IN IMPLANTABLE CARDIOVERTER-DEFIBRILLATOR

A high prevalence of depression among patients with cardiovascular disease is increasingly recognized.[80] ICD therapy, especially shock delivery, poses a significant psychosocial burden on patients. Unfortunately, psychosocial issues related to ICD are often neglected among cardiovascular practitioners and rarely perceived as ICD complications. Psychological morbidity in adult ICD recipients is well documented, with the prevalence of anxiety ranging from 13 to 46% and depression from 24 to 46%.[81] ICD shocks are clearly the most prominent experience among such patients, and heightened arrhythmia and CHF management and comprehensive assessment of patients' psychosocial well-being should be an integral part of the post-shock evaluation. Participation in support groups and appropriate referral to a psychiatrist or a psychologist should be considered.

It is evident that the ICD is meant to avert untimely SCD, but cannot prevent eventual death from a variety of nonarrhythmic causes. Lack of clear communication between practitioners and ICD patients regarding limitations of ICD therapy and appropriateness of device deactivation in end-of-life situations may contribute to unrealistic expectations or anxiety. A survey of ICD patients showed that 70% of ICD recipients wished to keep the ICD turned on while approaching death from cancer. More than half (55%) would keep the ICD active in the face of experiencing daily shocks, and none opted for deactivation even when suffering from constant dyspnea at rest.[82] In a survey of 414 hospice centers nationwide, 97% reported having patients with active ICDs and 58% reported at least one patient who had been shocked in hospice in the past year.[83] HRS consensus statement provides ethical, legal and medical backgrounds, and concise guidelines on how to approach device deactivation in patients nearing end-of-life or requesting withdrawal of therapy.[84]

EMERGING TECHNOLOGY AND FUTURE DIRECTIONS

New or emerging algorithms in single and dual chamber ICDs to recognize SVT and lead-related noise are expected to reduce inappropriate shocks.[85]

Analysis of randomized ICD trials for primary and secondary prevention have shown that the number of "appropriate" shocks consistently exceeds the SCD and overall mortality rates in the control group without ICD. This discrepancy indicates that "appropriate" shocks delivered for VT/VF are not always "necessary" or lifesaving shocks, because many ventricular arrhythmias may be self-terminating, or do not cause sudden death. Antitachycardia pacing (ATP) effectively reduces shocks for VTA by terminating VT, and is most effective for slower, monomorphic VT. ATP has a more than 90% success rate in terminating spontaneous VT slower than 180 bpm, eliminating the need for shock delivery, conserving a device battery, and avoiding pain.[86]

Given the perceived problems with endovascular ICD leads, entirely subcutaneous so-called "leadless" ICDs have been tested in small, nonrandomized studies. These devices have been shown to consistently detect and converted VF induced during EP studies.[87] The major limitations of the subcutaneous ICD are lack of pacing for bradycardia and for delivery of ATP for VT. Initial data suggest that appropriate detection of VTA and SVT discrimination for subcutaneous ICD system are comparable to or better than conventional transvenous ICDs.[88]

REFERENCES

1. Myerburg RJ, Kessler KM, Castellanos A. Sudden cardiac death: epidemiology, transient risk, and intervention assessment. Ann Intern Med. 1993;119(12):1187-97.
2. Zheng ZJ, Croft JB, Giles WH, et al. Sudden cardiac death in the United States, 1989 to 1998. Circulation. 2001;104(18):2158-63.
3. Zipes DP, Camm AJ, Borggrefe M, et al. ACC/AHA/ESC 2006 guidelines for management of patients with ventricular arrhythmias and the prevention of sudden cardiac death: a report of the American College of Cardiology/American Heart Association Task Force and the European Society of Cardiology Committee for Practice Guidelines (Writing Committee to Develop Guidelines for Management of Patients With Ventricular Arrhythmias and the Prevention of Sudden Cardiac Death). J Am Coll Cardiol. 2006;48(5):e247-346.
4. Mirowski M, Reid PR, Mower MM, et al. Termination of malignant ventricular arrhythmias with an implanted automatic defibrillator in human beings. N Engl J Med. 1980; 303(6):322-4.
5. Mirowski M. The automatic implantable cardioverter-defibrillator: an overview. J Am Coll Cardiol. 1985;6(2):461-6.
6. AVID. A comparison of antiarrhythmic-drug therapy with implantable defibrillators in patients resuscitated from near-fatal ventricular arrhythmias. The Antiarrhythmics versus Implantable Defibrillators (AVID) Investigators. N Engl J Med. 1997;337(22): 1576-83.
7. Connolly SJ, Gent M, Roberts RS, et al. Canadian implantable defibrillator study (CIDS): a randomized trial of the implantable cardioverter defibrillator against amiodarone. Circulation. 2000;101(11):1297-302.
8. Kuck KH, Cappato R, Siebels J, et al. Randomized comparison of antiarrhythmic drug therapy with implantable defibrillators in patients resuscitated from cardiac arrest: the Cardiac Arrest Study Hamburg (CASH). Circulation. 2000;102(7):748-54.
9. Connolly SJ, Hallstrom AP, Cappato R, et al. Meta-analysis of the implantable cardioverter defibrillator secondary prevention trials. AVID, CASH and CIDS studies. Antiarrhythmics vs Implantable Defibrillator study. Cardiac Arrest Study Hamburg. Canadian Implantable Defibrillator Study. Eur Heart J. 2000;21(24):2071-8.
10. Epstein AE, DiMarco JP, Ellenbogen KA, et al. ACC/AHA/HRS 2008 Guidelines for Device-Based Therapy of Cardiac Rhythm Abnormalities: a report of the American College of Cardiology/American Heart Association Task Force on Practice Guidelines (Writing Committee to Revise the ACC/AHA/NASPE 2002 Guideline Update for Implantation of Cardiac Pacemakers and Antiarrhythmia Devices): developed in collaboration with the American Association for Thoracic Surgery and Society of Thoracic Surgeons. Circulation. 2008;117(21):e350-408.
11. Myerburg RJ, Kessler KM, Castellanos A. Sudden cardiac death. Structure, function, and time-dependence of risk. Circulation. 1992;85(1 Suppl):I2-10.
12. Moss AJ, Hall WJ, Cannom DS, et al. Improved survival with an implanted defibrillator in patients with coronary disease at high risk for ventricular arrhythmia. Multicenter Automatic Defibrillator Implantation Trial Investigators. N Engl J Med. 1996;335(26):1933-40.
13. Moss AJ, Fadl Y, Zareba W, et al. Survival benefit with an implanted defibrillator in relation to mortality risk in chronic coronary heart disease. Am J Cardiol. 2001;88(5):516-20.

14. Buxton AE, Lee KL, Fisher JD, et al. A randomized study of the prevention of sudden death in patients with coronary artery disease. Multicenter Unsustained Tachycardia Trial Investigators. N Engl J Med. 1999;341(25):1882-90.
15. Moss AJ, Zareba W, Hall WJ, et al. Prophylactic implantation of a defibrillator in patients with myocardial infarction and reduced ejection fraction. N Engl J Med. 2002;346(12):877-83.
16. Bigger JT. Prophylactic use of implanted cardiac defibrillators in patients at high risk for ventricular arrhythmias after coronary-artery bypass graft surgery. Coronary Artery Bypass Graft (CABG) Patch Trial Investigators. N Engl J Med. 1997 Nov 27;337(22):1569-75.
17. Felker GM, Thompson RE, Hare JM, et al. Underlying causes and long-term survival in patients with initially unexplained cardiomyopathy. N Engl J Med. 2000;342(15):1077-84.
18. Bansch D, Antz M, Boczor S, et al. Primary prevention of sudden cardiac death in idiopathic dilated cardiomyopathy: the Cardiomyopathy Trial (CAT). Circulation. 2002;105(12):1453-8.
19. Strickberger SA, Hummel JD, Bartlett TG, et al. Amiodarone versus implantable cardioverter-defibrillator: randomized trial in patients with nonischemic dilated cardiomyopathy and asymptomatic nonsustained ventricular tachycardia--AMIOVIRT. J Am Coll Cardiol. 2003;41(10):1707-12.
20. Kadish A, Dyer A, Daubert JP, et al. Prophylactic defibrillator implantation in patients with nonischemic dilated cardiomyopathy. N Engl J Med. 2004;350(21):2151-8.
21. Bardy GH, Lee KL, Mark DB, et al. Amiodarone or an implantable cardioverter-defibrillator for congestive heart failure. N Engl J Med. 2005;352(3):225-37.
22. Hohnloser SH, Kuck KH, Dorian P, et al. Prophylactic use of an implantable cardioverter-defibrillator after acute myocardial infarction. N Engl J Med. 2004;351(24):2481-8.
23. Steinbeck G, Andresen D, Seidl K, et al. Defibrillator implantation early after myocardial infarction. N Engl J Med. 2009;361(15):1427-36.
24. Al-Khatib SM, Shaw LK, O'Connor C, et al. Incidence and predictors of sudden cardiac death in patients with diastolic heart failure. J Cardiovasc Electrophysiol. 2007;18(12):1231-5.
25. Buxton AE, Lee KL, Hafley GE, et al. Limitations of ejection fraction for prediction of sudden death risk in patients with coronary artery disease: lessons from the MUSTT study. J Am Coll Cardiol. 2007;50(12):1150-7.
26. Goldenberg I, Vyas AK, Hall WJ, et al. Risk stratification for primary implantation of a cardioverter-defibrillator in patients with ischemic left ventricular dysfunction. J Am Coll Cardiol. 2008;51(3):288-96.
27. Levy WC, Mozaffarian D, Linker DT, et al. The Seattle Heart Failure Model: prediction of survival in heart failure. Circulation. 2006;113(11):1424-33.
28. Levy WC, Lee KL, Hellkamp AS, et al. Maximizing survival benefit with primary prevention implantable cardioverter-defibrillator therapy in a heart failure population. Circulation. 2009;120(10):835-42.
29. Goldberger JJ, Cain ME, Hohnloser SH, et al. American Heart Association/American College of Cardiology Foundation/Heart Rhythm Society scientific statement on noninvasive risk stratification techniques for identifying patients at risk for sudden cardiac death: a scientific statement from the American Heart Association Council on Clinical Cardiology Committee on Electrocardiography and Arrhythmias and Council on Epidemiology and Prevention. Circulation. 2008;118(14):1497-518.
30. McClements BM, Adgey AA. Value of signal-averaged electrocardiography, radionuclide ventriculography, Holter monitoring and clinical variables for prediction of arrhythmic events in survivors of acute myocardial infarction in the thrombolytic era. J Am Coll Cardiol. 1993;21(6):1419-27.

31. Grimm W, Hoffmann J, Knop U, et al. Value of time- and frequency-domain analysis of signal-averaged electrocardiography for arrhythmia risk prediction in idiopathic dilated cardiomyopathy. Pacing Clin Electrophysiol. 1996;19(11 Pt 2):1923-7.
32. Gerritsen J, Dekker JM, TenVoorde BJ, et al. Impaired autonomic function is associated with increased mortality, especially in subjects with diabetes, hypertension, or a history of cardiovascular disease: the Hoorn Study. Diabetes Care. 2001;24(10):1793-8.
33. Kusmirek SL, Gold MR. Sudden cardiac death: the role of risk stratification. Am Heart J. 2007;153(4 Suppl):25-33.
34. Gold MR, Ip JH, Costantini O, et al. Role of microvolt T-wave alternans in assessment of arrhythmia vulnerability among patients with heart failure and systolic dysfunction: primary results from the T-wave alternans sudden cardiac death in heart failure trial substudy. Circulation. 2008;118(20):2022-8.
35. van der Avoort CJ, Filion KB, Dendukuri N, et al. Microvolt T-wave alternans as a predictor of mortality and severe arrhythmias in patients with left-ventricular dysfunction: a systematic review and meta-analysis. BMC Cardiovasc Disord. 2009;9:5.
36. Gehi AK, Stein RH, Metz LD, et al. Microvolt T-wave alternans for the risk stratification of ventricular tachyarrhythmic events: a meta-analysis. J Am Coll Cardiol. 2005;46(1):75-82.
37. Bristow MR, Saxon LA, Boehmer J, et al. Cardiac-resynchronization therapy with or without an implantable defibrillator in advanced chronic heart failure. N Engl J Med. 2004;350(21):2140-50.
38. Desai AS, Fang JC, Maisel WH, et al. Implantable defibrillators for the prevention of mortality in patients with nonischemic cardiomyopathy: a meta-analysis of randomized controlled trials. JAMA. 2004;292(23):2874-9.
39. Melloni C, Berger JS, Wang TY, et al. Representation of women in randomized clinical trials of cardiovascular disease prevention. Circ Cardiovasc Qual Outcomes. 2010;3(2):135-42.
40. Maas AH, van der Schouw YT, Regitz-Zagrosek V, et al. Red alert for women's heart: the urgent need for more research and knowledge on cardiovascular disease in women: proceedings of the workshop held in Brussels on gender differences in cardiovascular disease, 29 September 2010. Eur Heart J. 2011;32(11):1362-8.
41. El-Chami MF, Hanna IR, Bush H, et al. Impact of race and gender on cardiac device implantations. Heart Rhythm. 2007;4(11):1420-6.
42. Santangeli P, Pelargonio G, Dello Russo A, et al. Gender differences in clinical outcome and primary prevention defibrillator benefit in patients with severe left ventricular dysfunction: a systematic review and meta-analysis. Heart Rhythm. 2010;7(7):876-82.
43. Russo AM, Day JD, Stolen K, et al. Implantable cardioverter defibrillators: do women fare worse than men? Gender comparison in the INTRINSIC RV trial. J Cardiovasc Electrophysiol. 2009;20(9):973-8.
44. System URD. USRDS 2010 Annual Data Report. National Institutes of Health, National Institute of Diabetes and Digestive and Kidney Diseases, Bethesda, MD. (2010). Accessed on 12/17/2011.
45. Young BA. Prevention of sudden cardiac arrest in dialysis patients: can we do more to improve outcomes? Kidney Int. 2011;79(2):147-9.
46. Wase A, Basit A, Nazir R, et al. Impact of chronic kidney disease upon survival among implantable cardioverter-defibrillator recipients. J Interv Card Electrophysiol. 2004;11(3):199-204.
47. Charytan DM, Patrick AR, Liu J, et al. Trends in the use and outcomes of implantable cardioverter-defibrillators in patients undergoing dialysis in the United States. Am J Kidney Dis. 2011;58(3):409-17.
48. Sakhuja R, Keebler M, Lai TS, et al. Meta-analysis of mortality in dialysis patients with an implantable cardioverter defibrillator. Am J Cardiol. 2009;103(5):735-41.

49. Tompkins C, McLean R, Cheng A, et al. End-stage renal disease predicts complications in pacemaker and ICD implants. J Cardiovasc Electrophysiol. 2011;22(10):1099-104.
50. Korantzopoulos P, Liu T, Li L, et al. Implantable cardioverter defibrillator therapy in chronic kidney disease: a meta-analysis. Europace. 2009;11(11):1469-75.
51. Wilber DJ, Zareba W, Hall WJ, et al. Time dependence of mortality risk and defibrillator benefit after myocardial infarction. Circulation. 2004;109(9):1082-4.
52. Makikallio TH, Barthel P, Schneider R, et al. Prediction of sudden cardiac death after acute myocardial infarction: role of Holter monitoring in the modern treatment era. Eur Heart J. 2005;26(8):762-9.
53. Poole JE, Johnson GW, Hellkamp AS, et al. Prognostic importance of defibrillator shocks in patients with heart failure. N Engl J Med. 2008;359(10):1009-17.
54. Tokano T, Bach D, Chang J, et al. Effect of ventricular shock strength on cardiac hemodynamics. J Cardiovasc Electrophysiol. 1998;9(8):791-7.
55. Mishkin JD, Saxonhouse SJ, Woo GW, et al. Appropriate evaluation and treatment of heart failure patients after implantable cardioverter-defibrillator discharge: time to go beyond the initial shock. J Am Coll Cardiol. 2009;54(22):1993-2000.
56. Zaman S, Sivagangabalan G, Narayan A, et al. Outcomes of early risk stratification and targeted implantable cardioverter-defibrillator implantation after ST-elevation myocardial infarction treated with primary percutaneous coronary intervention. Circulation. 2009;120(3):194-200.
57. Kumar S, Sivagangabalan G, Zaman S, et al. Electrophysiology-guided defibrillator implantation early after ST-elevation myocardial infarction. Heart Rhythm. 2010; 7(11):1589-97.
58. Shah B, Hernandez AF, Liang L, et al. Hospital variation and characteristics of implantable cardioverter-defibrillator use in patients with heart failure: data from the GWTG-HF (Get With The Guidelines-Heart Failure) registry. J Am Coll Cardiol. 2009;53(5):416-22.
59. Al-Khatib SM, Hellkamp A, Curtis J, et al. Non-evidence-based ICD implantations in the United States. JAMA. 2011;305(1):43-9.
60. van Rees JB, de Bie MK, Thijssen J, et al. Implantation-related complications of implantable cardioverter-defibrillators and cardiac resynchronization therapy devices: a systematic review of randomized clinical trials. J Am Coll Cardiol. 2011;58(10):995-1000.
61. Poole JE, Gleva MJ, Mela T, et al. Complication rates associated with pacemaker or implantable cardioverter-defibrillator generator replacements and upgrade procedures: results from the REPLACE registry. Circulation. 2011;122(16):1553-61.
62. Curtis JP, Luebbert JJ, Wang Y, et al. Association of physician certification and outcomes among patients receiving an implantable cardioverter-defibrillator. JAMA. 2009;301(16):1661-70.
63. Hauser RG. Here we go again--failure of postmarketing device surveillance. N Engl J Med. 2012;366(10):873-5.
64. Birnie DH, Parkash R, Exner DV, et al. Clinical predictors of Fidelis lead failure: report from the Canadian Heart Rhythm Society Device Committee. Circulation. 2012;125(10):1217-25.
65. Daubert JP, Zareba W, Cannom DS, et al. Inappropriate implantable cardioverter-defibrillator shocks in MADIT II: frequency, mechanisms, predictors, and survival impact. J Am Coll Cardiol. 2008;51(14):1357-65.
66. Friedman PA, McClelland RL, Bamlet WR, et al. Dual-chamber versus single-chamber detection enhancements for implantable defibrillator rhythm diagnosis: the detect supraventricular tachycardia study. Circulation. 2006;113(25):2871-9.
67. Ricci RP, Quesada A, Almendral J, et al. Dual-chamber implantable cardioverter defibrillators reduce clinical adverse events related to atrial fibrillation when compared

with single-chamber defibrillators: a subanalysis of the DATAS trial. Europace. 2009;11(5):587-93.
68. van Gelder IC, Phan HM, Wilkoff BL, et al. Prognostic significance of atrial arrhythmias in a primary prevention ICD population. Pacing Clin Electrophysiol. 2011;34(9):1070-9.
69. Bunch TJ, Day JD, Olshansky B, et al. Newly detected atrial fibrillation in patients with an implantable cardioverter-defibrillator is a strong risk marker of increased mortality. Heart Rhythm. 2009;6(1):2-8.
70. Schron EB, Exner DV, Yao Q, et al. Quality of life in the antiarrhythmics versus implantable defibrillators trial: impact of therapy and influence of adverse symptoms and defibrillator shocks. Circulation. 2002;105(5):589-94.
71. Dichtl W, Wolber T, Paoli U, et al. Appropriate therapy but not inappropriate shocks predict survival in implantable cardioverter defibrillator patients. Clin Cardiol. 2011;34(7):433-6.
72. Singh SN, Poole J, Anderson J, et al. Role of amiodarone or implantable cardioverter/defibrillator in patients with atrial fibrillation and heart failure. Am Heart J. 2006;152(5):974, e7-11.
73. Wilkoff BL, Cook JR, Epstein AE, et al. Dual-chamber pacing or ventricular backup pacing in patients with an implantable defibrillator: the Dual Chamber and VVI Implantable Defibrillator (DAVID) Trial. JAMA. 2002;288(24):3115-23.
74. Sharma AD, Rizo-Patron C, Hallstrom AP, et al. Percent right ventricular pacing predicts outcomes in the DAVID trial. Heart Rhythm. 2005;2(8):830-4.
75. Sweeney MO, Hellkamp AS, Ellenbogen KA, et al. Adverse effect of ventricular pacing on heart failure and atrial fibrillation among patients with normal baseline QRS duration in a clinical trial of pacemaker therapy for sinus node dysfunction. Circulation. 2003;107(23):2932-7.
76. Steinberg JS, Fischer A, Wang P, et al. The clinical implications of cumulative right ventricular pacing in the multicenter automatic defibrillator trial II. J Cardiovasc Electrophysiol. 2005;16(4):359-65.
77. Tops LF, Schalij MJ, Bax JJ. The effects of right ventricular apical pacing on ventricular function and dyssynchrony implications for therapy. J Am Coll Cardiol. 2009;54(9):764-76.
78. Barsheshet A, Moss AJ, McNitt S, et al. Long-term implications of cumulative right ventricular pacing among patients with an implantable cardioverter-defibrillator. Heart Rhythm. 2011;8(2):212-8.
79. Benditt DG, Sakaguchi S, Jhanjee R. Right ventricular pacing in MADIT-II: a risk factor for increased mortality, or mainly a marker of increased risk. Heart Rhythm. 2011;8(2):219-20.
80. Yeager KR, Binkley PF, Saveanu RV, et al. Screening and identification of depression among patients with coronary heart disease and congestive heart failure. Heart Fail Clin. 2011;7(1):69-74.
81. Sears SF, Matchett M, Conti JB. Effective management of ICD patient psychosocial issues and patient critical events. J Cardiovasc Electrophysiol. 2009;20(11):1297-304.
82. Stewart GC, Weintraub JR, Pratibhu PP, et al. Patient expectations from implantable defibrillators to prevent death in heart failure. J Card Fail. 2010;16(2):106-13.
83. Goldstein N, Carlson M, Livote E, et al. Brief communication: Management of implantable cardioverter-defibrillators in hospice: A nationwide survey. Ann Intern Med. 2010;152(5):296-9.
84. Lampert R, Hayes DL, Annas GJ, et al. HRS Expert Consensus Statement on the Management of Cardiovascular Implantable Electronic Devices (CIEDs) in patients nearing end of life or requesting withdrawal of therapy. Heart Rhythm. 2010;7(7):1008-26.
85. Corbisiero R, Lee MA, Nabert DR, et al. Performance of a new single-chamber ICD algorithm: discrimination of supraventricular and ventricular tachycardia based on vector timing and correlation. Europace. 2006;8(12):1057-61.

86. Saeed M, Neason CG, Razavi M, et al. Programming antitachycardia pacing for primary prevention in patients with implantable cardioverter defibrillators: results from the PROVE trial. J Cardiovasc Electrophysiol. 2010;21(12):1349-54.
87. Bardy GH, Smith WM, Hood MA, et al. An entirely subcutaneous implantable cardioverter-defibrillator. N Engl J Med. 2010;363(1):36-44.
88. Gold MR, Theuns DA, Knight BP, et al. Head-To-Head Comparison of Arrhythmia Discrimination Performance of Subcutaneous and Transvenous ICD Arrhythmia Detection Algorithms: The START Study. J Cardiovasc Electrophysiol. 2012;23(4):359-66.

CHAPTER 11

Atrial Arrhythmias in Heart Failure

Sumeet K Chhabra, Daniel R Frisch

INTRODUCTION

Patients with heart failure (HF) are at increased risk for various supraventricular arrhythmias, and patients with incessant arrhythmias are at risk for development of new or worsening cardiomyopathy.[1] This interplay of tachyarrhythmias begetting cardiomyopathy and *vice versa* remains one of the most challenging aspects of HF management. Of the various forms of supraventricular tachycardia that may exist in patients with HF, atrial fibrillation (AF) remains the most common and challenging arrhythmia faced by clinicians (Fig. 1). AF is a well-recognized etiology of tachycardia-induced cardiomyopathy,[1] and the contribution towards atrial and ventricular dysfunction often corresponds to the duration and rate of the tachycardia.[2] Accordingly, this chapter focuses on AF [and atrial flutter (AFL)] and the unique challenges inherent to this condition.

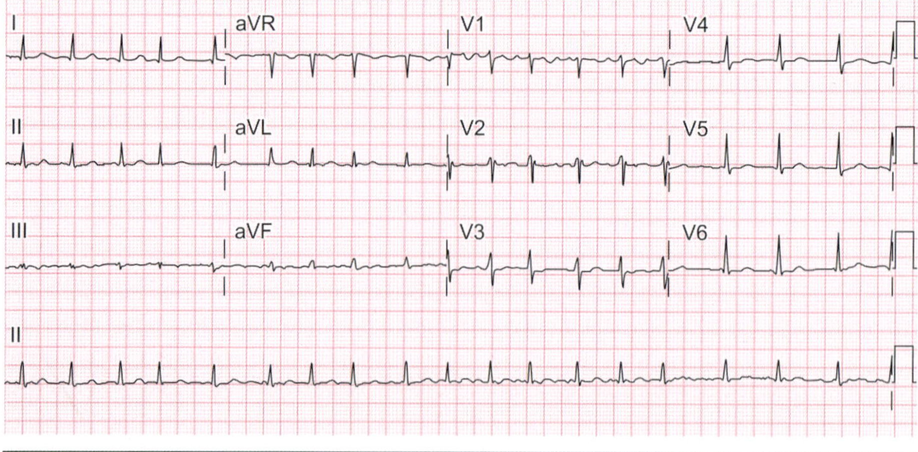

Figure 1: 12-lead electrocardiogram demonstrating atrial fibrillation.

Source: Chhabra SK, Frisch DR.

Dr Eugene Braunwald recognized AF and HF in 1997 as the "two new epidemics of cardiovascular disease".[3] In 2003, a review of data from the Framingham Heart Study confirmed that individuals with either preexisting AF or preexisting HF had a poor prognosis with development of the other condition.[4] Pooled data from 22,651 patients across nine randomized controlled trials[5] has further demonstrated a clear disadvantage to patients with AF and HF, with an odds ratio death of 1.33 (95% CI, 1.12–1.59) for patients in AF compared to sinus rhythm. Accordingly, the management of patients with these concomitant disorders remains a significant clinical, societal, and economic burden to nations and healthcare delivery systems around the world.

EPIDEMIOLOGY

According to 2011 American Heart Association (AHA) Statistics,[6] 5,700,000 people in the United States suffer from HF with nearly 300,000 deaths per year. AF is the most commonly sustained arrhythmia in clinical practice,[7] and the prevalence is projected as over 2.6 million patients in the general population.[6] This prevalence increases with advancing age, and the median age of patients with AF is 75 years.[8] Since the mid-1980s, there has been a 60% increase in hospital admissions for AF, independent of changing patient risk factor profiles.[9] In the United States, the primary indication for hospitalization for AF patients remains HF exacerbation.[6]

Data from the Framingham Heart Study cite an increase in the risk of AF by 4.5-fold in men and 5.9-fold in women in the setting of HF.[10] Other studies have reported that the prevalence of AF in patients with HF increases from less than 10% in those with New York Heart Association (NYHA) Class I symptoms to approximately 50% in patients with NYHA Class IV HF symptoms.[11] The overall prevalence of AF is thought to be similar in both patients with preserved ejection fraction (EF) or reduced EF,[12] but the manifestations may differ in these populations. The indolent nature of this pathologic association is highlighted in the ALPHA (T-wave Alternans in Patients with Heart Failure) registry from Europe, which reports an AF prevalence of over 20% as seen in 3,513 consecutive HF outpatients during regular follow-up.[13] Authors from this registry report the presence of AF is associated with an odds ratio of 2.5 (95% CI, 2.08–3.00, $P < 0.001$) of being in NYHA Class III or Class IV HF as opposed to Class I or Class II symptoms, despite accounting for age, gender, EF, and etiology of HF.[13] Long-term follow-up data from the Olmstead County population which followed patients with lone AF for a mean duration of 25.2 ± 9.5 years reported a hazard ratio of 2.1 (95% CI, 1.11–3.89, $P = 0.022$) for progression to congestive HF for every decade of age at the time of the initial AF diagnosis.[14]

Once AF occurs in a patient with HF, it is thought to promote structural changes that beget worsening AF. Data from Pappone et al. reported on 5-year follow-up on 106 patients following a first episode of AF, and demonstrated an adjusted hazard ratio

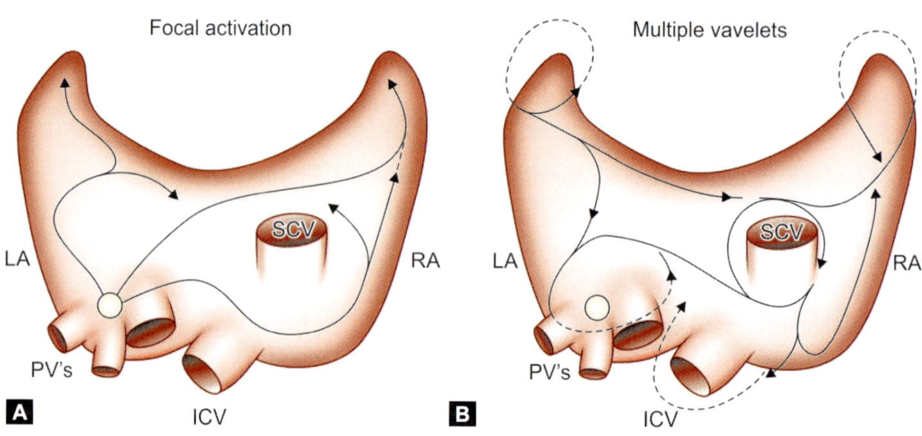

Figure 2: Electrophysiological mechanisms of atrial fibrillation—posterior biatrial view. LA, left atrium; RA right atrium, PV, pulmonary vein; SCV, superior vena cava; ICV, inferior vena cava.

Source: *From* Fuster V, Rydén LE, Cannom DS, et al. 2011 ACCF/AHA/HRS focused updates incorporated into the ACC/AHA/ESC 2006 guidelines for the management of patients with atrial fibrillation: a report of the American College of Cardiology Foundation/American Heart Association Task Force on practice guidelines. Circulation. 2011;123:e269-367, *with permission*.

of 11.2 (95% CI, 3.914–32.059, $P < 0.001$) for progression to permanent AF in patients with concomitant HF.[15] Mortality data reported from the Framingham Heart Study have found that AF is associated with a 1.5- to 1.9-fold mortality risk after adjustment for preexisting cardiac conditions with which AF was related.[16] More recent data in a severe left ventricular dysfunction with implanted cardioverter defibrillator (ICD) population also reports a 1.7-fold increase in mortality in permanent AF (95% CI: 1.0–2.7, $P = 0.033$) despite current and optimal medical therapy in these patients.[17]

PATHOPHYSIOLOGY

Atrial fibrillation is characterized by rapid and chaotic electrical activity with subsequent loss of atrial mechanical function and synchrony with the ventricle. Two major mechanisms thought to play a role are (A) spontaneous depolarizing foci (usually within the pulmonary veins) and (B) multiple reentrant wavelets; these two mechanisms often coexist within the same patient in a complex interaction that is not yet fully understood (Fig. 2).[18,19]

The deleterious relationship between AF and HF is a well-recognized and complex entity with multiple contributing underlying mechanisms[20] (Fig. 3). HF factors including atrial stretch and increased ventricular filling pressures may directly induce the development of AF.[21,22] When AF occurs, the loss of atrial systole (diminished ventricular filling), rapid and irregular ventricular rates

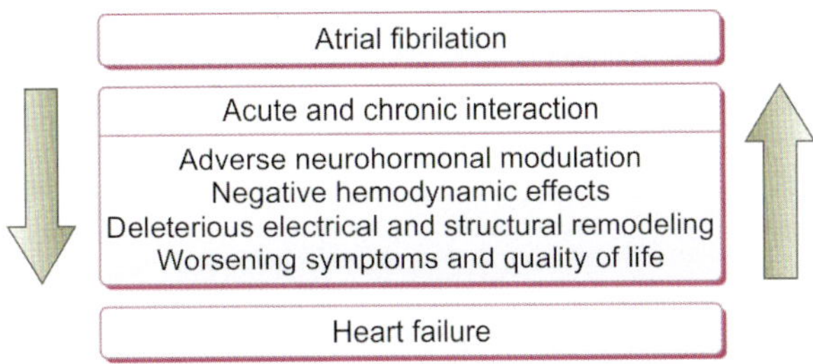

Figure 3: Deleterious patient effects of concomitant atrial fibrillation and heart failure.*

***Source:** Chhabra SK, Frisch DR.

(reduced diastolic filling time), and direct tachycardia-induced cardiomyopathy may all contribute to the development or worsening HF symptoms.[21] Subsequent neurohormonal activation, cellular and extracellular alteration, myocardial fibrosis, and electrophysiological changes have all been implicated in the persistence of AF in HF.[19,21]

It has been clinically demonstrated that persistent AF is associated with a statistically significant decrease in physical activity in patients with advanced HF and low EF.[23] In addition to direct myocardial and hemodynamic effects, AF may also deleteriously affect the efficacy of other known HF treatment strategies, such as cardiac resynchronization therapy (CRT). High AF-induced ventricular rates have been shown to reduce the percentage of resynchronized biventricular pacing from 98% in sinus rhythm to 71% in atrial tachycardia/AF,[24] effectively nullifying any benefit from this therapy.

TREATMENT

In an isolated tachycardia-induced cardiomyopathy, treatment is directed towards abolition of the arrhythmia and management of any HF symptoms until atrial and ventricular dysfunction improves.[2] However, many patients suffer from other preexisting or concomitant etiologies of HF and treatment remains directed at minimizing symptoms and specific risks incurred by AF. Although the goals of treatment in this group are similar to management of AF in a general population, persistent ventricular dysfunction or HF symptoms frequently limit therapeutic options (Fig. 4). Accordingly, stroke risk should be addressed in all patients, and the decision to pursue rate versus rhythm control should be individualized to patient symptoms.[25]

Anticoagulation

Prevention of thromboembolic events is a central therapeutic target for all AF patients, and is especially important in the setting of HF. Data from 5,070 patients

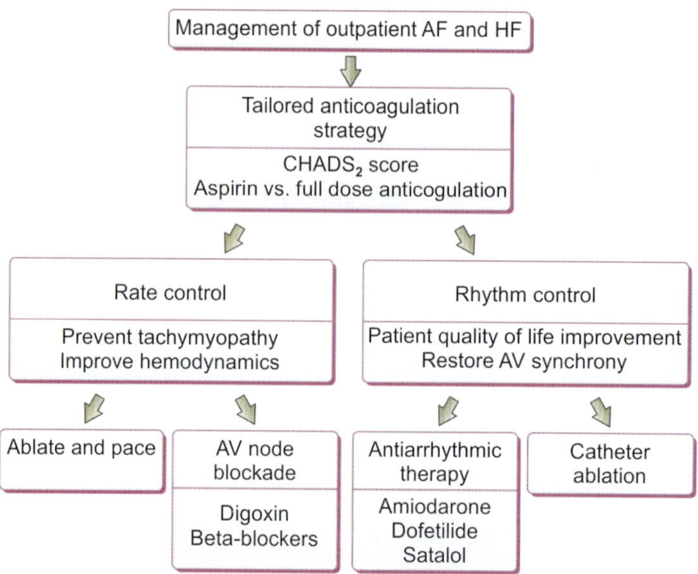

Figure 4: Algorithm for management of outpatient atrial fibrillation (AF) and heart failure (HF).

Source: Chhabra SK, Frisch DR.

in the Framingham Heart Study revealed a 5-fold ($P < 0.001$) age-adjusted incidence of stroke with the presence of AF,[26] yet the exact complement of disease modifying factors (advanced age or specific comorbid conditions) remained elusive until the turn of the century. It was then that data from multiple trials were crystallized into the formation of the $CHADS_2$ scoring system.[27,28] The $CHADS_2$ score assigns one point for each of the following factors: (A) the presence of congestive HF, (B) hypertension, (C) age more than 75 years old, and (D) diabetes. A patient is assigned two points for a history of stroke or transient ischemic attack. Patients with isolated HF ($CHADS_2$ score = 1) have a 2.8% adjusted annual stroke rate, and the choice of full anticoagulation or antiplatelet therapy (commonly with aspirin) is left to the discretion of the treating clinician. Data from the atrial fibrillation clopidogrel trial with irbesartan for prevention of vascular events (ACTIVE A) trial suggest that dual antiplatelet strategy may reduce a composite end-point of vascular events in certain patients with AF and a low $CHADS_2$ score; however, this relationship was not seen upon subgroup analysis in patients with congestive HF.[29] With any $CHADS_2$ score more than 1, current guidelines suggest a full-dose anticoagulation strategy. As many patients with HF have other comorbidities and advanced age, there usually exists an obligate anticoagulation requirement in most situations unless prohibited by clear intolerance (or contraindication) to anticoagulation.

In the United States, the mainstay of oral anticoagulation therapy has historically involved oral vitamin-K antagonism with dose-adjusted warfarin. An international-normalized-ratio (INR) of 2.0–3.0 has been demonstrated to provide sufficient protection against thromboembolic events, without undue risk of major or minor bleeding complications.[30] A 2007 analysis of pooled data from 28,044 patients spanning 29 trials reported that adjusted-dose warfarin reduced stroke by 64% (95% CI, 49–74%) compared to 22% (95% CI, 6–35%) with antiplatelet therapy alone. This increase in efficacy with warfarin was found to result in a relative risk reduction of 39% (CI 22–52%) with less than or equal to 0.3% increase in major extracranial hemorrhage.[31] Accordingly, the 2011 American College of Cardiology Foundation/ American Heart Association/Heart Rhythm Society (ACCF/AHA/HRS) guidelines for the management of patients with AF[19] assign a Class I recommendation to anticoagulate all patients with AF in the absence of contraindications unless the patient is in a low-risk category. These guidelines also report a relative risk of ischemic stroke or systemic embolism of 1.4 in patients with HF, and even recommend anticoagulation in the setting of reduced EF (≤35%) without overt clinical manifestations of HF. Although these particular guidelines recommend oral vitamin-K antagonism, the outpatient oral anticoagulant choices have greatly expanded beyond warfarin since publication. The motivation for alternative agents stems from difficulty maintaining patients in a therapeutic range and from a multitude of pharmacologic and dietary interactions with warfarin.

Dabigatran, an oral direct thrombin inhibitor, was reported on in 2009 in the Randomized Evaluation of Longterm anticoagulation therapY (RE-LY) study, which randomized this agent in comparison to dose-adjusted warfarin in blinded subjects.[32] Of 18,113 patients assigned to one of three study arms (dabigatran 110 mg twice daily, dabigatran 150 mg twice daily, and adjusted-dose warfarin), over 30% of patients in each arm suffered from concomitant HF. At 2-year median follow-up, the authors reported lower rates of stroke and systemic embolism in the group treated with dabigatran 150 mg twice daily, with similar rates of major hemorrhage to adjusted-dose warfarin. In subgroup analysis of patients with HF, no significant difference in the primary end-point between patients receiving 150 mg dabigatran or warfarin was seen (P = 0.33). Dabigatran 150 mg was approved by the USFDA in 2010, with broad commercial availability in 2011. Accordingly, a 2011 update from the ACCF/AHA/HRS guidelines now assigns the use of dabigatran as an alternative to warfarin as a Class I indication in patients with paroxysmal to permanent AF.[33]

In 2011, the results of two randomized trials investigating oral Factor Xa direct inhibitors (rivaroxaban and apixaban) were also reported. Factor Xa is an attractive therapeutic target within the coagulation cascade as it exists at the intersection of the intrinsic and extrinsic coagulation cascade.[34] In the Rivaroxaban Once Daily Oral Direct Factor Xa Inhibition Compared with Vitamin K Antagonism for Prevention of Stroke and Embolism Trial in Atrial Fibrillation (ROCKET-AF) trial published in 2011,[35] rivaroxaban was investigated against warfarin in 14,264 AF patients. At over 1.5-year follow-up, authors found rivaroxaban noninferior to warfarin for the prevention of stroke, with no significant difference between groups in risk of major bleeding. The Apixaban for Reduction in Stroke and other Thromboembolic Events in Atrial Fibrillation (ARISTOTLE) trial[36] compared apixaban to warfarin in 18,201 patients. At nearly 2-year follow-up, apixaban was found to be superior to warfarin in preventing stroke or systemic embolism, with fewer bleeding complications and lower overall mortality. Over 60% of the patients in ROCKET-AF and over 30% of patients in ARISTOTLE (study and control groups) had HF, and future studies are needed to assess efficacy and safety of these new anticoagulants specifically in this population.

Physician attitudes towards new classes of anticoagulants and cost issues for patients remain active areas of research and debate at this time.[37-39] Although initial evidence indicates that these agents are as at least as safe as warfarin, issues of dosage monitoring, cost, and lack of direct reversal agents remain potential problems in wide-spread acceptance and usage (Fig. 5).[40]

Rate Control

According to the 2011 AF Guidelines,[19] rate control goals vary with age but usually involve achieving ventricular rates between 60 and 80 beats per minute at rest and between 90 to 115 beats per minute during exercise. Adherence to this recommendation has long been practiced by clinicians around the world, especially in the setting of HF where poor rate control is thought to further exacerbate already deteriorating hemodynamics.[41-43] With the publication of the rate control efficacy in permanent atrial fibrillation: a comparison between lenient versus strict rate control (RACE-II) trial, however, the strict adherence to tight rate control with aggressive pharmacological therapy has come under question.[44] In this trial, 614 patients with permanent AF were randomized to a lenient rate-control strategy (resting heart rate <110 beats per minute) or a strict rate-control strategy (resting heart rate <80 beats per minute and <110 beats per minute during Moderate exercise). Nearly one-third of the study and control populations had NYHA class II or above symptoms and

Drug	Comment
Warfarin	Monitor interaction with other medicines
Dabigatran	Monitor creatinine clearance
Rivaroxaban	Monitor creatinine clearance
Apixaban	Monitor renal function

Figure 5: Anticoagulation options for atrial fibrillation in heart failure. FDA, Food ad Drug Administration.

Source: Chhabra SK, Frisch DR.

patients were followed for a minimum of 2 years. The authors reported no difference in the incidence of HF at 3 years [3.8% vs. 4.1%, HR 0.97 (90% CI, 0.48–1.96)] and no difference in hospitalization with lenient or strict control (25.1% vs. 27.4%, P = 0.5). These findings may not be applicable to all groups of HF (particularly those patients with NYHA Class IV symptoms or those with preserved EF) and extrapolation of this data remains conditional upon clinical situation.

Beta-blockers remain a mainstay in neurohormonal modification in HF, and are amongst first-line therapies in achieving rate control with concomitant AF.[19] They may be used orally in the outpatient setting, or in intravenous preparation in the inpatient setting, albeit with caution in HF patients (Class I recommendation).[19] They have shown efficacy in reducing hospitalizations and death in HF patients with AF,[45,46] yet need to be administered with caution during acute HF decompensation due to class-wide negative inotropic effects and the potential to worsen acute HF symptoms.[47,48] The benefits of beta-blockers in AF is thought to be a class-effect, and current guidelines[19] recommend nadolol, atenolol, propranolol, esmolol, metoprolol, and carvedilol in oral and intravenous preparations. If a patient is already taking a beta-blocker for HF, a preferable strategy is to up titrate this medication until desired heart rate is achieved or any further increase is limited by hypotension or patient intolerance.

While its efficacy is reduced in states of high sympathetic tone[19] digoxin remains a relevant option in resting heart rate control in AF with HF. Digoxin is a cardiac glycoside and has been in clinical use for over 200 years. Although it is a Class V antiarrhythmic agent, digoxin acts on the atrioventricular (AV) node to increase electrical refractory periods, and is thus useful in the control of atrial arrhythmias.[49] Digoxin has been studied in multiple HF trials and has been proven safe in these patients when part of stable background therapy; however, risks to patients have been reported with withdrawal of this drug in patients already at steady-state.[50-53] Caution must also be exercised in patients with baseline renal dysfunction (or labile renal function), and in patients prescribed other anti-arrhythmic agents (i.e., amiodarone) for possible drug-drug interactions.

Although considered first-line agents in patients with AF and no HF, the use of nondihydropyridine calcium channel antagonists in HF (diltiazem and verapamil) remains a source of concern amongst clinicians. These medications are (at best) infrequently tolerated in the outpatient setting or in patients with preserved EF,[54] and only under close physician supervision. Worsening HF due to negative inotropy is a serious concern with this class of medications,[55,56] and they should be judiciously avoided in the inpatient setting or in patients with labile HF symptoms. Accordingly, the 2011 Guidelines assign this group a Class III contraindication to prevent worsening hemodynamic compromise in patients hospitalized with acute decompensated HF.[19]

Rhythm Control

Several rhythm control agents have been studied in patients with AF and HF, and the mainstay of therapy for those in this group are the Class III antiarrhythmic drugs: amiodarone, dofetilide, and sotalol. Class I antiarrhythmic agents (e.g., quinidine, flecainide, propafenone, procainamide, and disopyramide) should be avoided in HF due to negative inotropic effects and arrhythmogenic side effects.[19,57]

Amiodarone has both sympatholytic and calcium antagonistic properties and acts to slow AV nodal conduction.[19] It is assigned a Class I recommendation in the setting of acute HF exacerbation for rate control and recommended for maintenance of sinus rhythm in patients with HF.[19] Randomized data from 674 patients in the Survival Trial of Antiarrhythmic Therapy in Congestive Heart Failure (CHF-STAT) study demonstrated no increase in mortality in HF patients with amiodarone and safety outcomes comparable to placebo in HF outpatients.[58,59] In the acute setting, bradyarrhythmias are a well-known side effect of amiodarone use, and have even been reported to result in pacemaker placement for HF patients.[60] However, in the chronic setting amiodarone-induced toxicities involving skin, pulmonary, thyroid, hepatic, and ophthalmological complications are well-recognized.[61] Chun et al. examined long-term efficacy of amiodarone in 110 patients and reported a 1-year withdrawal rate of 8% and a 5-year rate of 30% due to adverse effects.[62] No deaths occurred in this study and the most common toxicities reported were skin discoloration (4.5%), pulmonary fibrosis (3.6%), and thyroid toxicity (2.7%). Thus, careful monitoring is required for initiation and outpatient use of amiodarone in all patients.

Dofetilide is also a Class III antiarrhythmic that increases action potential time due to delayed ventricular repolarization. Much of the information of the use of this agent in HF was reported in the Danish Investigations of Arrhythmia and Mortality On Dofetilide in Congestive Heart Failure (DIAMOND-CHF) trial published in 1999.[63] Investigators studied 1,518 patients with severe left ventricular dysfunction randomized to dofetilide or placebo, and found no effect on mortality at a median follow-up of 18 months. Dofetilide is known to block the delayed rectifier potassium current thereby increasing the QT interval, and was the likely cause for the occurrence of torsades de pointes in 3.3% of patients in the DIAMOND-CHF study. The majority of these events (76%) occurred within the first 3 days of initiation of dofetilide, and the authors recommended inpatient initiation and cardiac rhythm monitoring for 72 hours with this agent. Inpatient administration remains an FDA mandate for initiation of this medication. Despite these limitations, dofetilide remains an attractive option in certain patients due to minimal bradycardic effect as compared to other agents.

A third option in AF and HF is the antiarrhythmic sotalol, which demonstrates nonselective beta-adrenergic effects (Class II), and inhibition of the delayed potassium rectifier current, I_k, (Class III) properties.[64] This agent has been shown to be inferior to amiodarone in maintaining sinus rhythm in two large randomized trials—Canadian Trial of Atrial Fibrillation (CTAF)[65] and Sotalol Amiodarone Atrial Fibrillation Efficacy Trial;[66] however, the vast majority of patients in these trials had normal left ventricular function. Given the nonselective beta-blockade effects, one possible limitation to the use of sotalol remains hemodynamic intolerance in patients with HF already on standard-of-care oral vasodilator therapy. Although it is the L-isomer of the drug that accounts for this effect,[64] only the racemic mixture (D, L-sotalol) is available in the United States. Further limiting use of this drug is the Survival with Oral D-Sotalol (SWORD) study, which investigated D-sotalol in 3,121 patients with history of low-EF, HF, or recent myocardial infarction.[67] This trial was stopped early due to increased mortality in the D-sotalol group due to arrhythmogenic effects [relative risk 1.65 (95% CI, 1.15–2.36), P = 0.006)]. Thus, most clinicians advise caution with use of this medication and initiation within a hospital or monitored setting.[68]

Dronedarone, a noniodinated analog of amiodarone, was approved in 2009 in the United States for maintenance of sinus rhythm. Dronedarone is contraindicated in patients with NYHA Class III or above symptoms by the FDA. The exact role of this drug in HF is limited, however, as data suggest that dronedarone also not be used in patients with NYHA Class II or worse symptoms.[69] Additionally, data from the 2011 Permanent Atrial Fibrillation Outcome Study using Dronedarone on Top of Standard Therapy (PALLAS) study has shown increased rates of HF, stroke, and death in patients treated with permanent AF treated with dronedarone.[70] Thus, this agent is best avoided for broad use in a HF population (Fig. 6).

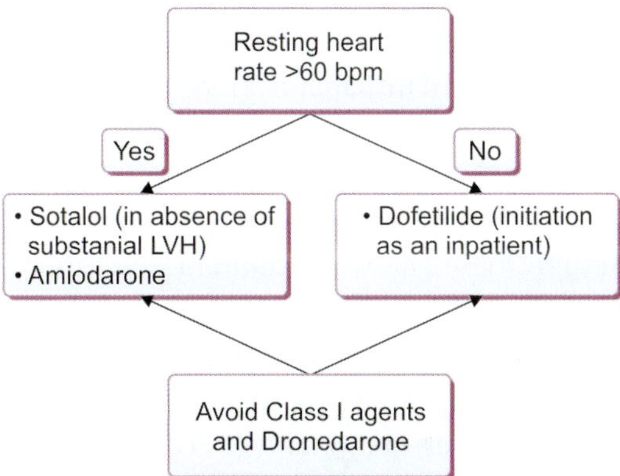

Figure 6: Antiarrhythmic drug therapy in atrial fibrillation in the presence of heart failure. bpm, beats per minute; LVH, left ventricular hypertrophy.

Source: Chhabra SK, Frisch DR.

Rate versus Rhythm Control

The classic rate-control versus rhythm-control study in the general population is the Atrial Fibrillation Follow-up Investigation of Rhythm Management (AFFIRM) trial published in 2002.[71] AFFIRM randomized a total of 4,060 patients to either a rate-control strategy or a rhythm-control strategy. Although roughly 23% of patients in each treatment arm carried a clinical history of HF, actual baseline EF in both groups was preserved. At 5-year follow-up, authors found no survival advantage to a rhythm-control strategy and reported lower adverse drug effects in the rate-control arm. These findings were further reinforced by the RACE trial, also in 2002.[72] RACE randomized 522 patients to pharmacological rate-control (atrioventricular nodal selective agents) or rhythm-control with serial cardioversions and antiarrhythmic therapy. Similar to AFFIRM, rhythm-control in this trial also provided no benefit and may have even resulted in additional adverse events due to antiarrhythmic side effects and intolerance. For several years, these trials remained the mainstay of AF management with findings extended by clinicians to various subpopulations, including patients with HF.

Specific data for rate versus rhythm-control in patients with HF were not available until the publication of the Atrial Fibrillation and Congestive Heart Failure (AF-CHF) trial and the Chronic Atrial Fibrillation and Heart Failure (CAFÉ-II) study.[68] In the AF-CHF multicenter trial, 1,376 patients with an EF less than 35% and NYHA Class II-IV symptoms were randomized to rate-versus rhythm control strategies and followed for a mean of 37 months. At study end, no significant differences were observed in the primary end-point of cardiovascular mortality, or in secondary end-points of all-cause mortality, stroke, worsening HF, or a composite end-point.[73] Although a smaller trial than AFFIRM, these findings confirmed generally held practice guidelines in the choice of pharmacological therapy to patients with HF. A possible signal towards the use of antiarrhythmic therapy emerged with the CAFÉ II study, which randomized 61 patients. Here, the authors found that patients randomized to rhythm control with a Class III agent (amiodarone) had a statistically significant improvement at 1-year follow-up in left ventricular function and quality of life, with greatest improvement in patients where sinus rhythm was maintained once achieved.[74] Despite these gains, the authors noted no difference in repeat 6-minute walk distance or NYHA class between the two groups.

A 2011 meta-analysis from four randomized control trials that included a total of 2,486 patients further addressed the rate versus rhythm control question in HF patients.[75] No difference was seen in mortality (RR 1.03; 95% CI: 0.90–1.17) or CVA/thromboembolic events (RR 1.09; 95% CI: 0.61–1.96) in rate or rhythm control arms.[75] Three out of four studies reported hospitalization data (n = 2,425) and the authors found less frequent hospitalizations with rate-control as compared to rhythm-control (RR 0.92; 95% CI: 0.86–0.98; P = 0.008). Given the relative paucity of data for this population, this area remains fertile ground for further dedicated investigation in definitive treatment strategies.

Ablation of the Atrioventricular Node and Permanent Pacing

In patients who are refractory to pharmacological intervention (rate or rhythm control) and remain symptomatic with AF, especially when there is evidence of tachycardia-induced cardiomyopathy, another possible treatment modality is radiofrequency catheter ablation of the atrioventricular node (AVN) with permanent pacemaker placement.[76] If successful, this approach obviates the need for pharmacological rate- or rhythm-control; however, an obligate anticoagulation requirement remains in patients with a $CHADS_2$ score greater than 1.

An early trial in this modality from 1998 reported on 46 patients with NYHA functional class 2.7 ± 0.6 who underwent AVN ablation with permanent pacemaker placement.[77] The authors reported post-ablation improvement in NYHA class to 1.4 ± 0.8 ($P < 0.001$), improvement in EF from 42% ± 16 to 50% ± 14, and symptomatic improvement in all patients demonstrated by a customized questionnaire. These results led to significant enthusiasm for this treatment strategy, and a meta-analysis published in 2000 spanning 21 studies and 1,181 patients reported "significant improvement" in 18 clinical outcome measures, with 1-year mortality rates comparable with medical therapy.[78]

This enthusiasm, however, has been tempered in recent years with less favorable long-term outcomes, largely due to the deleterious effects of permanent right ventricular apical pacing. Long-term right ventricular pacing may induce left ventricular dyssynchrony in up to 50% of patients, which may herald an increase in HF symptoms.[79] Additionally, right ventricular apical pacing has been identified as a strong independent predictor of worsening left ventricular function,[80] and as a cause of severe mitral regurgitation following AVN ablation.[81] The left ventricular-based cardiac stimulation post-AV nodal ablation evaluation (PAVE) study in 2005 investigated benefits of cardiac resynchronization therapy in such patients, to mitigate any detrimental effects of permanent right ventricular pacing.[82] At 6-month follow-up, the EF in the biventricular paced group was significantly greater than the EF in patients with right ventricular pacing (46% vs. 41%, $P = 0.03$). Subsequent studies have further validated cardiac resynchronization in patients following AVN ablation, and reported favorable outcomes in reducing HF symptoms and hospitalizations.[83]

Pulmonary Vein Isolation

The recognition of the pulmonary veins as a trigger for AF and electrical isolation of all four veins from the left atrium as a therapeutic modality by radiofrequency ablation [(RFA) Fig. 7] was first reported in the early 1990s.[84,85] Since then, thousands of patients around the world have undergone pulmonary vein isolation (PVI) procedures

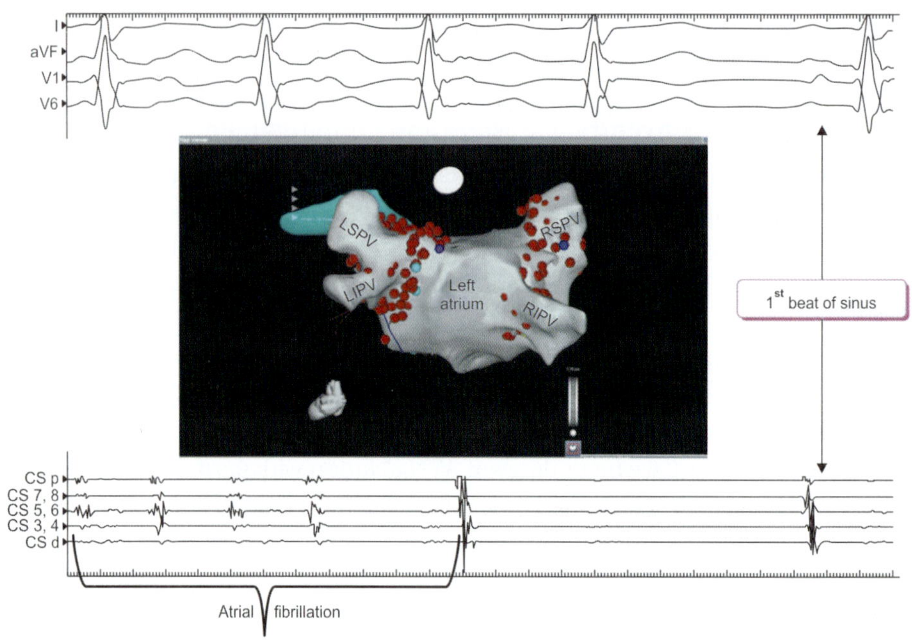

Figure 7: Intracardiac recording of pulmonary vein ablation, (center) electroanatomic map of left atrium. LSPV, left superior pulmonary vein; RSPV, right superior pulmonary vein; LIPV, left inferior pulmonary vein; RIPV, right inferior pulmonary vein.

Source: Chhabra SK, Frisch DR.

with varying degrees of success dependent on the nature of AF, operator/center experience, and the length of follow-up. Most AF ablation studies have traditionally excluded HF patients due to the known deleterious effects of a preexisting poor anatomic substrate. There is also conflicting information in the literature with some centers reporting HF as complication of AF ablation, with an incidence of up to 2.5% of cases.[86] However, as more data and experience has accumulated, the concomitant burden of these diseases has encouraged clinicians to perform PVI procedures on this "sick" population. Initial data was nonrandomized due to procedure volume, and meta-analyses have demonstrated a moderate postablation improvement in EF of 11%.[87,88]

By 2008, randomized studies that specifically investigated PVI in HF patients became available. Pulmonary Vein Antrum Isolation versus AV Node Ablation with Bi-ventricular Pacing for Treatment of Strial Fibrillation in Patients with Congestive Heart Failure (PABA-CHF) was a multicenter trial that randomized 81 patients with symptomatic AF, EF less than 40%, and NYHA Class II or III symptoms to undergo pulmonary vein isolation or atrioventricular-node ablation with biventricular pacing.[89] At 6-months follow-up, the authors reported more favorable outcomes in the group assigned to pulmonary vein isolation, determined by increased scores on the Minnesota Living with HF questionnaire, longer 6-minute-walk distances, and higher EFs (35% vs. 28%, $P < 0.001$). Known periprocedural complications were reported in both arms, and authors concluded that pulmonary vein isolation was superior to atrioventricular-node ablation and biventricular pacing. More recently, however, MacDonald et al.[90] reported on 41 patients in Scotland with NYHA Class II-III HF symptoms and severe left ventricular dysfunction, randomized to medical treatment or pulmonary vein isolation. In this study, the authors found no statistically significant improvement in left ventricular EF, N-terminal pro-B-type natriuretic peptide, or 6-minute walk test with ablation therapy. Furthermore, the authors reported a serious complication rate of 15% with ablation, raising concerns about offering this therapy to patients with HF symptoms.

It is hoped that definitive information regarding pulmonary vein isolation therapy and outcomes will become available with ongoing studies, such as the catheter ablation versus antiarrhythmic drug therapy for atrial fibrillation (CABANA) trial[91] and the catheter ablation versus standard conventional treatment in patients with left ventricular dysfunction and atrial fibrillation trial (CASTLE-AF) trial.[92] Pending results of these trials, catheter ablation remains predominantly an elective procedure and is only rarely performed during a hospitalization for acute HF.[93]

CONCLUSION

Atrial arrhythmias are especially common in HF, either as a cause or as a result of cardiac chamber enlargement and impaired contractile function. AF remains the most common and most challenging arrhythmia faced in HF, with both diseases interacting negatively upon each other when they exist in the same patient. While many proven therapeutic strategies in the general population with AF are applicable to patients with HF, robust randomized data in this patient subset remains limited. Future studies are needed regarding rate versus rhythm control, the applicability of new anticoagulation agents, and the long-term clinical success of atrioventricular node ablation or pulmonary vein isolation. Additionally, as the combined effects of these diseases is better understood, it is possible that new therapeutic targets may be identified to help reverse remodel the electrical, cellular, and structural changes suffered by this population.

REFERENCES

1. Houmsse M, Tyler J, Kalbfleisch S. Supraventricular tachycardia causing heart failure. Curr Opin Cardiol. 2011;26:261-9.
2. Khasnis A, Jongnarangsin K, Abela G, et al. Tachycardia-induced cardiomyopathy: a review of literature. Pacing Clin Electrophysiol. 2005;28:710-21.
3. Braunwald E. Shattuck lecture—cardiovascular medicine at the turn of the millennium: triumphs, concerns, and opportunities. N Engl J Med. 1997;337:1360-9.

4. Wang TJ, Larson MG, Levy D, et al. Temporal relations of atrial fibrillation and congestive heart failure and their joint influence on mortality: the Framingham Heart Study. Circulation. 2003;107:2920-5.
5. Wasywich CA, Pope AJ, Somaratne J, et al. Atrial fibrillation and the risk of death in patients with heart failure: a literature-based meta-analysis. Intern Med J. 2010;40:347-56.
6. Roger VL, Go AS, Lloyd-Jones DM, et al. Heart disease and stroke statistics—2011 update: a report from the American Heart Association. Circulation. 2011;123:e18–e209.
7. Markides V, Peters NS. Mechanisms underlying the development of atrial arrhythmias in Heart Failure. Heart Fail Rev. 2002;7:243-53.
8. Feinberg WM, Blackshear JL, Laupacis A, et al. Prevalence, age distribution, and gender of patients with atrial fibrillation: Analysis and implications. Arch Int Med. 1995;155(5):469-73.
9. Friberg J, Buch P, Scharling H, et al. Rising rates of hospital admissions for atrial fibrillation. Epidemiology. 2003;14:666-72.
10. Benjamin EJ, Levy D, Vaziri SM, et al. Independent risk factors for atrial fibrillation in a population-based cohort. The Framingham Heart Study. JAMA. 1994;271:840-4.
11. Maisel WH, Stevenson LW. Atrial fibrillation in heart failure: epidemiology, pathophysiology, and rationale for therapy. Am J Cardiol. 2003;91:2D-8D.
12. Linssen GC, Rienstra M, Jaarsma T, et al. Clinical and prognostic effects of atrial fibrillation in heart failure patients with reduced and preserved left ventricular ejection fraction. Eur J Heart Fail. 2011;13:1111-20.
13. De Ferrari GM, Klersy C, Ferrero P, et al. Atrial fibrillation in heart failure patients: prevalence in daily practice and effect on the severity of symptoms. Data from the ALPHA study registry. Eur J Heart Fail. 2007;9:502-9.
14. Jahangir A, Lee V, Friedman PA, et al. Long-term progression and outcomes with aging in patients with lone atrial fibrillation: A 30-Year Follow-Up Study. Circulation. 2007;115:3050-6.
15. Pappone C, Radinovic A, Manguso F, et al. Atrial fibrillation progression and management: a 5-year prospective follow-up study. Heart Rhythm. 2008;5:1501-7.
16. Benjamin EJ, Wolf PA, D'Agostino RB, et al. Impact of atrial fibrillation on the risk of death: the Framingham Heart Study. Circulation. 1998;98:946-52.
17. Borleffs CJ, van Rees JB, van Welsenes GH, et al. Prognostic importance of atrial fibrillation in implantable cardioverter-defibrillator patients. J Am Coll Cardiol. 2010;55:879-85.
18. Konings KT, Kirchhof CJ, Smeets JR, et al. High-density mapping of electrically induced atrial fibrillation in humans. Circulation. 1994;89:1665-80.
19. Fuster V, Rydén LE, Cannom DS, et al. 2011 ACCF/AHA/HRS focused updates incorporated into the ACC/AHA/ESC 2006 guidelines for the management of patients with atrial fibrillation: a report of the American College of Cardiology Foundation/ American Heart Association Task Force on practice guidelines. Circulation. 2011;123:e269-367.
20. Anter E, Jessup M, Callans DJ. Atrial fibrillation and heart failure: treatment considerations for a dual epidemic. Circulation. 2009;119:2516-25.
21. Shelton RJ, Clark AL, Kaye GC, et al. The atrial fibrillation paradox of heart failure. Congest Heart Fail. 2010;16:3-9.
22. Kalifa J, Jalife J, Zaitsev AV, et al. Intra-atrial pressure increases rate and organization of waves emanating from the superior pulmonary veins during atrial fibrillation. Circulation. 2003;108(6):668-71.
23. Puglisi A, Gasparini M, Lunati M, et al. Persistent atrial fibrillation worsens heart rate variability, activity, and heart rate, as shown by a continuous monitoring by implantable

biventricular pacemakers in heart failure patients. J Cardiovasc Electrophysiol. 2008;19:693-701.

24. Santini M, Gasparini M, Landolina M, et al. Device-detected atrial tachyarrhythmias predict adverse outcome in real-world patients with implantable biventricular defibrillators. J Am Coll Cardiol. 2011;57:167-72.
25. Darby AE, DiMarco JP. Management of atrial fibrillation in patients with structural heart disease. Circulation. 2012;125:945-57.
26. Wolf PA, Abbott RD, Kannel WB. Atrial fibrillation as an independent risk factor for stroke: the Framingham study. Stroke. 1991;22:983-8.
27. van Walraven C, Hart RG, Wells GA, et al. A clinical prediction rule to identify patients with atrial fibrillation and a low risk for stroke while taking aspirin. Arch Intern Med. 2003;163:936-43.
28. Gage BF, Waterman AD, Shannon W, et al. Validation of clinical classification schemes for predicting stroke: results from the National Registry of Atrial Fibrillation. JAMA. 2001;285:2864-70.
29. Connolly SJ, Pogue J, Hart RG, et al. Effect of clopidogrel added to aspirin in patients with atrial fibrillation. N Engl J Med. 2009;360:2066-78.
30. Singer DE, Chang Y, Fang MC, et al. Should patient characteristics influence target anticoagulation intensity for stroke prevention in nonvalvular atrial fibrillation?: The ATRIA Study. Circ Cardiovasc Qual Outcomes. 2009;2:297-304.
31. Hart RG, Pearce LA, Aguilar MI. Meta-analysis: antithrombotic therapy to prevent stroke in patients who have nonvalvular atrial fibrillation. Ann Intern Med. 2007;146:857-67.
32. Connolly SJ, Ezekowitz MD, Yusuf S, et al. Dabigatran versus warfarin in patients with atrial fibrillation. N Engl J Med. 2009;361:1139-51.
33. Wann SL, Curtis AB, Ellenbogen KA, et al. 2011 ACCF/AHA/HRS Focused Update on the Management of Patients with Atrial Fibrillation (Update on Dabigatran): A Report of the American College of Cardiology Foundation/American Heart Association Task Force on Practice Guidelines. Circulation. 2011;123:1144-50.
34. Ruff CT, Giugliano RP, Antman EM, et al. Evaluation of the novel factor Xa inhibitor edoxaban compared with warfarin in patients with atrial fibrillation: design and rationale for the Effective aNticoaGulation with factor xA next GEneration in Atrial Fibrillation-Thrombolysis In Myocardial Infarction study 48 (ENGAGE AF-TIMI 48). Am Heart J. 2010;160:635-41.
35. Patel MR, Mahaffey KW, Garg J, et al. Rivaroxaban versus warfarin in nonvalvular atrial fibrillation. N Engl J Med. 2011;365:883-91.
36. Granger CB, Alexander JH, McMurray JJ, et al. Apixaban versus warfarin in patients with atrial fibrillation. N Engl J Med. 2011;365:981-92.
37. Freeman JV, Zhu RP, Owens DK, et al. Cost-effectiveness of dabigatran compared with warfarin for stroke prevention in atrial fibrillation. Ann Intern Med. 2011;154:1-11.
38. Del Zopp GJ, Eliasziw M. New options in anticoagulation for atrial fibrillation. N Engl J Med. 2011;365:952-3.
39. Mega JL. A new era for anticoagulation in atrial fibrillation. N Engl J Med. 2011;365:1052-3.
40. Potpara TS, Lip GY. New anticoagulation drugs for atrial fibrillation. Clin Pharmacol Ther. 2011;90(4):502-6.
41. Lazzari JO, Gonzalez J. Reversible high rate atrial fibrillation dilated cardiomyopathy. Heart. 1997;77:486.
42. Nerheim P, Birger-Botkin S, Piracha L, et al. Heart failure and sudden death in patients with tachycardia-induced cardiomyopathy and recurrent tachycardia. Circulation. 2004;110:247-52.

43. Van Gelder IC, Crijns HJ, Blanksma PK, et al. Time course of hemodynamic changes and improvement of exercise tolerance after cardioversion of chronic atrial fibrillation unassociated with cardiac valve disease. Am J Cardiol. 1993;72:560-6.
44. Van Gelder IC, Groenveld HF, Crijns HJ, et al. Lenient versus strict rate control in patients with atrial fibrillation. N Engl J Med. 2010;362:1363-73.
45. Joglar JA, Acusta AP, Shusterman NH, et al. Effect of carvedilol on survival and hemodynamics in patients with atrial fibrillation and left ventricular dysfunction: retrospective analysis of the US Carvedilol Heart Failure Trials Program. Am Heart J. 2001;142:498-501.
46. Swedberg K, Olsson LG, Charlesworth A, et al. Prognostic relevance of atrial fibrillation in patients with chronic heart failure on long-term treatment with beta-blockers: results from COMET. Eur Heart J. 2005;26:1303-8.
47. Packer M, Bristow MR, Cohn JN, et al. US Carvedilol Heart Failure Study Group. The effect of carvedilol on morbidity and mortality in patients with chronic heart failure. N Engl J Med. 1996;334:1349-55.
48. Effect of metoprolol CR/XL in chronic heart failure: metoprolol CR/XL randomized intervention trial in congestive heart failure (MERIT-HF). Lancet. 1999;353:20017.
49. Libby P, Bonow RO, Mann DL, Zipes DP, Braunwald E (Eds). Braunwald's Heart Disease: A Textbook of Cardiovascular Medicine, 8th edition. Philadelphia: Saunders Elsevier: 2007.
50. The Digitalis Investigation Group. The effect of digoxin on mortality and morbidity in patients with heart failure. N Engl J Med. 1997;336:525-33.
51. Packer M, Gheorghiade M, Young JB, et al. Withdrawal of digoxin from patients with chronic heart failure treated with angiotensin-converting-enzyme inhibitors: RADIANCE Study. N Engl J Med. 1993;329:1-7.
52. Uretsky BF, Young JB, Shahidi FE, et al. Randomized study assessing the effect of digoxin withdrawal in patients with mild to moderate chronic congestive heart failure: results of the PROVED trial. PROVED Investigative Group. J Am Coll Cardiol. 1993;22(4):955-62.
53. The effect of digoxin on mortality and morbidity in patients with heart failure. The Digitalis Investigation Group. N Engl J Med. 1997;336(8):525-33.
54. Heart Failure Society of America. Evaluation and management of patients with heart failure and preserved left ventricular ejection fraction. J Card Fail. 2006;12:e80-5.
55. Goldstein RE, Boccuzzi SJ, Cruess D, et al. The Adverse Experience Committee, Multicenter Diltiazem Postinfarction Research Group. Diltiazem increases late-onset congestive heart failure in postinfarction patients with early reduction in ejection fraction. Circulation. 1991;83:52-60.
56. Chew CY, Hecht HS, Collett JT, et al. Influence of severity of ventricular dysfunction on hemodynamic responses to intravenously administered verapamil in ischemic heart disease. Am J Cardiol. 1981;47:917-22.
57. Stevenson WG, Tedrow U. Management of atrial fibrillation in patients with heart failure. Heart Rhythm. 2007;4:S28-30.
58. Deedwania PC, Singh BN, Ellenbogen K, et al. The Department of Veterans Affairs CHF-STAT Investigators. Spontaneous conversion and maintenance of sinus rhythm by amiodarone in patients with heart failure and atrial fibrillation: observations from the veterans affairs congestive heart failure survival trial of antiarrhythmic therapy (CHF-STAT). Circulation. 1998;98:2574-9.
59. Singh SN, Fletcher RD, Fisher SG, et al. Amiodarone in patients with congestive heart failure and asymptomatic ventricular arrhythmia. Survival trial of antiarrhythmic therapy in congestive heart failure. N Engl J Med. 1995;333:77-82.

60. Weinfeld MS, Drazner MH, Stevenson WG, et al. Early outcome of initiating amiodarone for atrial fibrillation in advanced heart failure. J Heart Lung Transplant. 2000;19: 638-43.
61. Papiris SA, Triantafilldou C, Kolilekas L, et al. Amiodarone: review of pulmonary effects and toxicity. Drug Saf. 2010;33 (7):539-58.
62. Chun SH, Sager PT, Stevenson WG, et al. Long-term efficacy of amiodarone for the maintenance of normal sinus rhythm in patients with refractory atrial fibrillation or flutter. Am J Cardiol. 1995;76:47-50.
63. Torp-Pedersen C, Moller M, Bloch-Thomsen PE, et al. Danish Investigations of Arrhythmia and Mortality on Dofetilide Study Group. Dofetilide in patients with congestive heart failure and left ventricular dysfunction. N Engl J Med. 1999;341:857-65.
64. Chaki AL, Caines AE, Miller AB. Sotalol as adjunctive therapy to implantable cardioverter-defibrillators in heart failure patients. Congest Heart Fail. 2009;15:144-7.
65. Roy D, Talajic M, Dorian P, et al. Amiodarone to prevent recurrence of atrial fibrillation. Canadian Trial of Atrial Fibrillation Investigators. N Engl J Med. 2000;342:913-20.
66. Singh BN, Singh SN, Reda DJ, et al. Amiodarone versus sotalol for atrial fibrillation. N Engl J Med. 2005;352:1861-72.
67. Waldo AL, Camm AJ, deRuyter H, et al. Effect of d-sotalol on mortality in patients with left ventricular dysfunction after recent and remote myocardial infarction. The SWORD investigators. Survival with oral d-Sotalol. Lancet. 1996;348:7-12.
68. Seiler J, Stevenson WG. Atrial fibrillation in congestive heart failure. Cardiol Rev. 2010;18:38-50.
69. Hohnloser SH, Crijns HJ, van Eickels M, et al. Dronedarone in patients with congestive heart failure: insights from ATHENA. Eur Heart J. 2010;31:1717-21.
70. Connolly SJ, Camm AJ, Halperin JL, et al. Dronedarone in high-risk permanent atrial fibrillation. N Engl J Med. 2011;365:2268-76.
71. Wyse DG, WaldoAL, DiMarcoJP, et al. A comparison of rate control and rhythm control in patients with atrial fibrillation. N Engl J Med. 2002;347:1825-33.
72. Van Gelder IC, Hagens VE, Bosker HA, et al. A comparison of rate control and rhythm control in patients with recurrent persistent atrial fibrillation. N Engl J Med. 2002;347:1834-40.
73. Roy D, Talajic M, Nattel S, et al. Rhythm control versus rate control for atrial fibrillation and heart failure. N Engl J Med. 2008;358:2667-77.
74. Shelton RJ, Clark AL, Goode K, et al. A randomised, controlled study of rate versus rhythm control in patients with chronic atrial fibrillation and heart failure: (CAFE-II Study). Heart. 2009;95:924-30.
75. Caldeira D, David C, Sampaio C. Rate vs rhythm control in patients with atrial fibrillation and heart failure: A systematic review and meta-analysis of randomized controlled trials. Eur J Intern Med. 2011;22:448-55.
76. Rubenstein JC, Roth JA. Atrioventricular junction ablation and pacemaker implantation for heart failure associated with atrial fibrillation: potential issues and therapies in the setting of acute heart failure syndrome. Heart Fail Rev. 2011;16:457-65.
77. Manolis AG, Katsivas AG, Lazaris EE, et al. Ventricular performance and quality of life in patients who underwent radiofrequency AV junction ablation and permanent pacemaker implantation due to medically refractory atrial tachyarrhythmias. J Interv Card Electrophysiol. 1998;2:71-6.
78. Wood MA, Brown-Mahoney C, Kay GN, et al. Clinical outcomes after ablation and pacing therapy for atrial fibrillation: a meta-analysis. Circulation. 2000;101:1138-44.

79. Tops LF, Schalij MJ, Holman ER, et al. Right ventricular pacing can induce ventricular dyssynchrony in patients with atrial fibrillation after atrioventricular node ablation. J Am Coll Cardiol. 2006;48:1642-8.
80. O'Keefe JH, Abuissa H, Jones PG, et al. Effect of chronic right ventricular apical pacing on left ventricular function. Am J Cardiol. 2005;95:771-3.
81. Twidale N, Manda V, Holliday R, et al. Mitral regurgitation after atrioventricular node catheter ablation for atrial fibrillation and heart failure: acute hemodynamic features. Am Heart J. 1999;138:1166-75.
82. Doshi RN, Daoud EG, Fellows C, et al. Left ventricular-based cardiac stimulation post AV nodal ablation evaluation (the PAVE study). J Cardiovasc Electrophysiol. 2005;16:1160-5.
83. Brignole M, Botto G, Mont L, et al. Cardiac resynchronization therapy in patients undergoing atrioventricular junction ablation for permanent atrial fibrillation: a randomized trial. Eur Heart J. 2011;32:2420-9.
84. Haïssaguerre M, Jaïs P, Shah DC, et al. Spontaneous initiation of atrial fibrillation by ectopic beats originating in the pulmonary veins. N Engl J Med. 1998;339:659-66.
85. Jais P, Haissaguerre M, Shah DC, et al. A focal source of atrial fibrillation treated by discrete radiofrequency ablation. Circulation. 1997;95:572-6.
86. Tan HW, Wang XH, Shi HF, et al. Congestive heart failure after extensive catheter ablation for atrial fibrillation: prevalence, characterization, and outcome. J Cardiovasc Electrophysiol. 2011;22:632-7.
87. Dagres N, Varounis C, Gaspar T, et al. Catheter ablation for atrial fibrillation in patients with left ventricular systolic dysfunction. A systematic review and meta-analysis. J Cardiac Fail. 2011;17:964-70.
88. Wilton SB, Fundytus A, Ghali WA, et al. Meta-analysis of the effectiveness and safety of catheter ablation of atrial fibrillation in patients with versus without left ventricular systolic dysfunction. Am J Cardiol. 2010;106:1284-91.
89. Khan MN, Jaïs P, Cummings J, et al. Pulmonary-vein isolation for atrial fibrillation in patients with heart failure. N Engl J Med. 2008;359:1778-85.
90. MacDonald MR, Connelly DT, Hawkins NM, et al. Radiofrequency ablation for persistent atrial fibrillation in patients with advanced heart failure and severe left ventricular systolic dysfunction: a randomised controlled trial. Heart. 2011;97:740-7.
91. Jais P, Packer DL. Ablation vs. drug use for atrial fibrillation. Eur Heart J. 2007;9:G26-34.
92. Marrouche NF, Brachmann J. Catheter ablation versus standard conventional treatment in patients with left ventricular dysfunction and atrial fibrillation (CASTLE-AF) - study design. Pacing Clin Electrophysiol. 2009;32:987-94.
93. Knight BP, Jacobson JT. Assessing patients for catheter ablation during hospitalization for acute heart failure. Heart Fail Rev. 2011;16:467-6.

CHAPTER

12 Ventricular Tachyarrhythmias in Patients with Congestive Heart Failure

Andrew Yin, Reginald T Ho

INTRODUCTION

Between 300,000 and 450,000 sudden cardiac deaths (SCD) are estimated to occur in the United States each year.[1,2] Ventricular fibrillation (VF) or ventricular tachycardia (VT) deteriorating into VF accounts for approximately 80% of all SCD cases.[2-4] Ventricular tachyarrhythmias frequently occur in patients with left ventricular (LV) dilation and reduced ejection fraction (EF).[5] Coronary artery disease with prior myocardial infarction is the most common cardiovascular disorder associated with VT and it is estimated that 65–70% of all SCD is due to ischemic heart disease.[6] The purpose of this chapter is to discuss the acute and long-term management of ventricular tachyarrhythmias in patients with congestive heart failure (CHF).

INITIAL EVALUATION

Patients having suffered VT or VF require a comprehensive evaluation to identify its cause including an understanding of the underlying cardiac substrate and potential triggers. The 12-lead electrocardiogram provides valuable information including ischemia or infarction, left ventricular hypertrophy, bundle branch block (BBB), and QT prolongation. Transthoracic echocardiography is a quick, safe, and simple means to assess ventricular size and function, valvular abnormalities, and infiltrative myocardial disorders (e.g., amyloidosis). Ventricular tachyarrhythmias can be triggered by myocardial ischemia, electrolyte imbalances, and drugs (proarrhythmia). Patients should undergo evaluation for myocardial ischemia (e.g., cardiac catheterization or stress testing) and a focused history must include a search for proarrhythmic drugs. Electrolyte derangements, especially hypokalemia and hypomagnesemia, should be corrected.

ACUTE THERAPY

The acute management of patients presenting with VT/VF begins with advanced cardiac life support. The first step is to ensure an open and protected airway and assist ventilation. Ventricular tachyarrhythmias causing circulatory arrest should be treated emergently by unsynchronized external defibrillation.[7] For out-of-hospital cardiac arrest, intravenous amiodarone has been shown to increase short-term survival to hospital admission when compared to either placebo or lidocaine but not improve survival to hospital discharge.[7] Hemodynamically stable VT can be treated initially with intravenous (IV) antiarrhythmic drugs (AADs) or low-energy cardioversion (Table 1). Procainamide is often a first-line drug that can both slow and terminate stable monomorphic VT. Lidocaine is a second tier agent that may be effective especially in the setting of myocardial ischemia.[8,9]

Polymorphic Ventricular Tachycardia

Polymorphic VT (PVT) is defined as VT with constantly changing QRS morphologies and axes.[10] In the setting of QT prolongation, it is commonly referred to as "torsade de pointes" (TdP)—a term coined by Dessertenne in 1966.[11] TdP is thought to be initiated by early after-depolarizations which in the setting of heterogenous recovery of activation facilitates reentry.[11] This results in a spiral wave of shifting reentry migrating along the epicardial surface that perpetuates TdP and is responsible for its polymorphic nature. A common cause of rapid PVT is ischemia, infarction, or recurrent infarction which should be treated with aggressive anti-ischemic therapies including revascularization (Fig. 1).[2,12] When PVT occurs in the setting of QT prolongation (TdP), drug toxicity and electrolyte imbalances (particularly, hypokalemia and hypomagnesemia) are often involved (Fig. 2).[13] Acute management of TdP includes intravenous magnesium (2 gm), temporary pacing, or intravenous

Table 1 Intravenous AAD for VT/VF

Agent	*Dose*	*Common side effects*
Amiodarone	150 mg IV over 10 min (300 mg IV for pulseless VT/VF) then 1 mg/min IV x 6 hours followed by 0.5 mg/min IV x 18 hours	Bradycardia, AV block, QT prolongation, torsades de pointes, CHF, hypotension, pulmonary toxicity, hepatotoxicity, hyper- or hypothyroidism
Lidocaine	1–1.5 mg/kg bolus IV Repeat if required at 0.5–0.75 mg/kg bolus IV every 5–10 min to a maximum cumulative dose of 3 mg/kg then 1–4 mg/min IV	Lightheadedness, tremor, confusion, hypotension, blurred vision, tinnitus, anxiety, dizziness, euphoria, drowsiness, lethargy, nausea
Procainamide	15–17 mg/kg IV over 30 min then continue at 1–4 mg/min to a maximum of 1.5 g load and 9 g/day	Hypotension, bradycardia, flushing, pruritus, angioedema, rash, fever, nausea, confusion

AAD, antiarrhythmic drug; VF, ventricular fibrillation; VT, ventricular tachycardia; AV, atrioventricular; CHF, congestive heart failure.

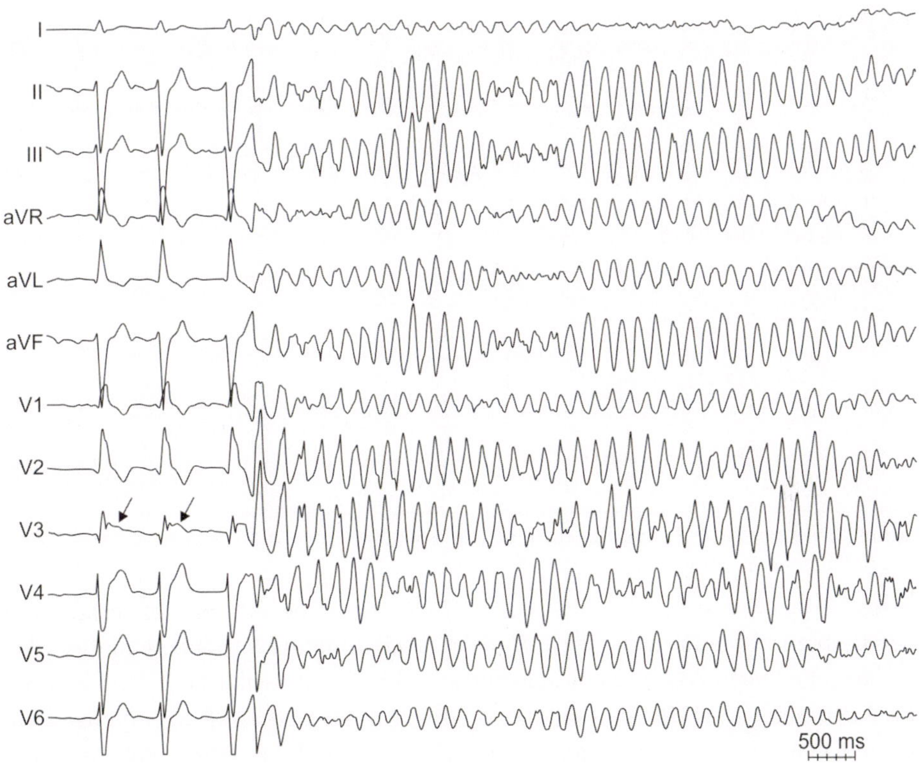

Figure 1: 12-lead electrocardiography of ischemic polymorphic ventricular tachycardia. Note the ST-segment elevation in lead V3 (arrows).

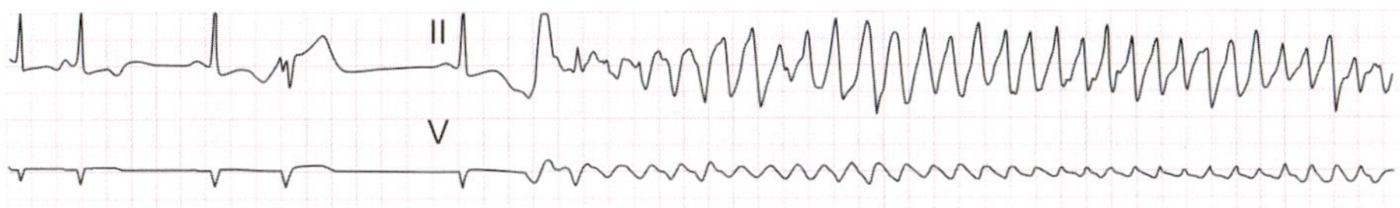

Figure 2: Torsade de Pointe. Note the escalating pause-dependent QT prolongation preceding polymorphic ventricular tachycardia.

isoproterenol to increase the heart rate and shorten the QT interval, correcting electrolyte abnormalities and withdrawing offending medications.

Monomorphic Ventricular Tachycardia

Monomorphic VT in the setting of structural heart disease and CHF are generally due to macroreentry within areas of scar (Fig. 3). Reentry around a fixed anatomical obstacle perpetuates VT and is responsible for its monomorphic nature.[14] Myocardial scar tissue is comprised of isolated tracts of surviving tissue interspersed with inexcitable scar (anatomic obstacle) that provide the substrate for reentry.[15,16]

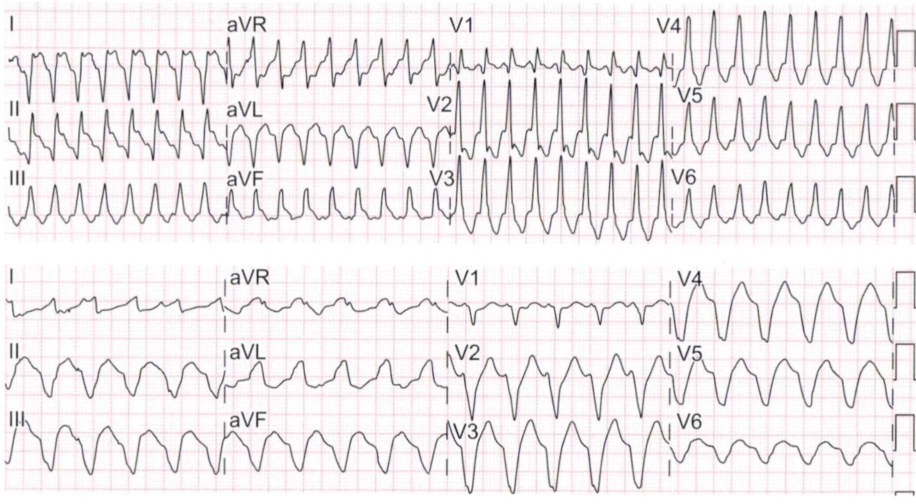

Figure 3: Monomorphic ventricular tachycardia with positive (top) and negative (bottom) precordial concordance.

Bundle branch reentrant tachycardia is a specific macroreentrant monomorphic VT involving the His-Purkinje system and seen in patients with CHF.[10,17] The classic clinical triad is a (1) dilated cardiomyopathy, (2) left BBB, and (3) prolonged HV interval in electrophysiologic study. Catheter ablation of the right bundle branch is curative for this specific VT.

Ventricular Tachycardia Storm

Ventricular tachycardia storm is defined as more than or equal to three episodes of VT within a 24-hour period requiring intervention for termination.[18,14] Patients can present with multiple painful discharges from their implantable cardioverter defibrillator (ICD). Treatment requires (1) acute VT suppression (e.g., IV amiodarone, lidocaine, or procainamide), (2) aggressive treatment of ischemia (e.g., revascularization, beta-blockers), and (3) hemodynamic support as necessary [left ventricular assist devices (LVAD)], extracorporeal membrane oxygenation.[18,19] Emergent catheter ablation and neuraxial modulation can also be effective to suppress VT.[20,21]

Ventricular Tachycardia/Ventricular Fibrillation in Patients with Left Ventricular Assist Devices

Patients with CHF requiring LVAD are a unique population. LVADs are used as a bridge to cardiac transplantation or as destination therapy for end-stage CHF. It has been observed that there is an increased incidence of ventricular arrhythmias in the early period post-LVAD implantation, and new onset monomorphic VT in patient who did not have ventricular arrhythmias before LVAD.[22-25] Between 22 and 52% of LVAD patients have clinically significant ventricular arrhythmias.[22-25] Post-LVAD ventricular arrhythmia is associated with poorer prognosis[24] and often incessant and refractory to AAD therapy.[25] The mechanism of ventricular arrhythmia post-LVAD is thought to be due to myocardial scar, postoperative inotropic and vasopressor use, subendocardial ischemia, and nonusage of beta blocker.[22,24,25]

LONG-TERM THERAPY

Long-term management strategies for VT/VF in patients with CHF focus on sudden death protection with ICD implantation and prevention/treatment of recurrent episodes by AAD therapy and/or VT ablation.[26]

Implantable Cardioverter Defibrillator

The first ICD implantation was performed in 1980 at The Johns Hopkins Hospital in patients who had survived two episodes of cardiac arrest.[27] Since then, the indications for ICD implantation have expanded substantially and supported by multiple clinical trials.[28] By 2009, the National ICD Registry estimates that approximately 120,000 ICDs are implanted annually. The ICD can effectively terminate a ventricular arrhythmia either by antitachycardia pacing or shock therapy (Figs. 4 and 5). Indication for ICD implantation is either for primary or secondary prevention. Primary prevention indication refers to ICD implantation for patients at high risk but who have never experienced a malignant ventricular arrhythmia and including: (1) prior myocardial infarction (MI) and EF less than or equal to 30% (Class

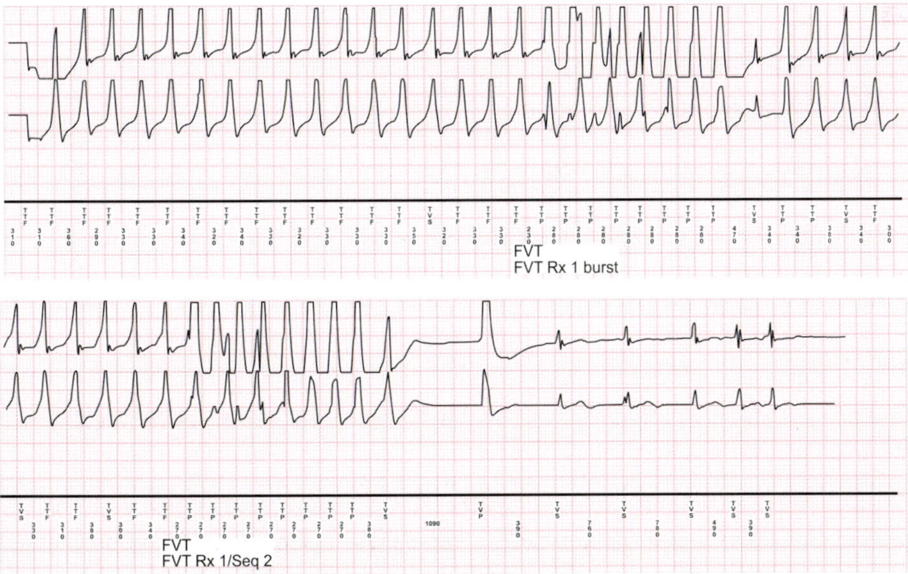

Figure 4: Successful termination of monomorphic ventricular tachycardia by antitachycardia pacing.

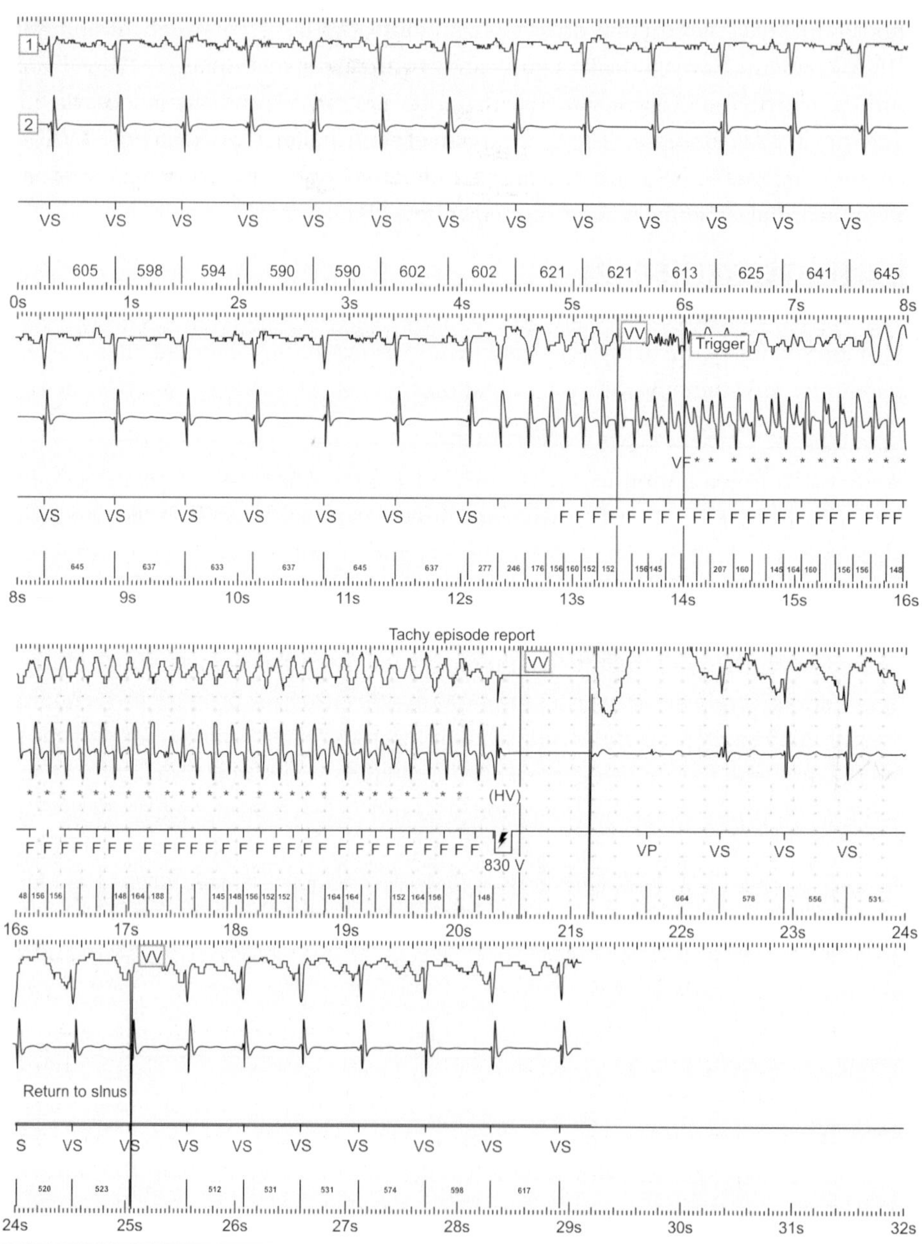

Figure 5: Successful termination of ventricular fibrillation by an implantable cardioverter defibrillator shock.

I indication), (2) NYHA functional Class II or III CHF and EF less than or equal to 35% (Class I indication), and (3) prior MI, EF less than or equal to 40%, nonsustained VT and inducible sustained VT/VF (Class I indication).[28] Secondary prevention indication refers to ICD implantation for patients having survived a malignant ventricular arrhythmia and includes: (1) survivors of SCD due to VT/VF (Class I indication), (2) spontaneous sustained VT in the setting of structural heart disease (Class I indication), (3) spontaneous VT with normal or near-normal ventricular function (Class IIa indication), (4) syncope with inducible sustained VT/VF (Class I indication), and (5) syncope in the setting of a nonischemic cardiomyopathy and significant LV dysfunction (Class IIa indication).[28]

Antiarrhythmic Drug

With the exception of beta-blockers, oral AADs have not been shown to improve survival in patients with VT/VF and CHF, but they are important adjunctive therapies to control VT and reduce ICD shocks.[29-31] In the setting of CHF, AADs is generally limited to Class III agents [(amiodarone, dofetilide, and sotalol) Table 2]. Amiodarone is the most widely used AAD to control VT in CHF patients because of its safety and effectiveness but requires screening for long-term toxicities.[32-35] Alternative AADs include dofetilide and sotalol but dosing is limited by renal impairment. Combination therapy with quinidine/mexiletine is another option when amiodarone fails or is not tolerated. Class Ic AADs (flecainide, and encainide) increase mortality in survivors of myocardial infarction and are generally avoided in patients with CHF.[36] Disopyramide (Class Ia) depresses cardiac contractility and should also be avoided. Procainamide (Class Ia) is generally not used for long-term management of VT because of the concern about long-term side effects.

Amiodarone

Although amiodarone is categorized as a Class III AAD, it is a multichannel blocker, targeting sodium channels, calcium channels, and beta receptors. Multiple trials have evaluated the safety and efficacy of amiodarone in patient with prior myocardial infarction and/or CHF. In CHF-STAT (Survival Trial of Antiarrhythmic Treatment—Congestive Heart Failure), 674 CHF patients were randomized to receive amiodarone or placebo.[34] Amiodarone was effective in suppressing ventricular arrhythmias and improving LV function but did not reduce mortality or SCD. There was a trend towards reduced mortality in patient with nonischemic cardiomyopathy.[34] In Grupo de Estudio de la Sobrevida en la Insuficiencia Cardiaca en Argentina (GESICA), 516 patients with severe CHF (61% nonischemic) and EF less than or equal to 35% were randomized to amiodarone or placebo. Amiodarone was associated with a 28% relative risk reduction in deaths (33.5% vs. 41.4%, $P = 0.024$).[35] Furthermore, fewer patients in the amiodarone group were admitted to the hospital (31% relative risk reduction, $P = 0.0024$).[35] In European Myocardial Infarction Amiodarone Trial (EMIAT) 1,486 survivors of myocardial infarction (EF $\leq$40%) were randomized to amiodarone or placebo.[32] There was no significant difference in all-cause mortality between the two groups but amiodarone reduced arrhythmic deaths (relative risk

Table 2 Oral AAD for VT/VF

Agent	*Dose*	*Common side effects*
Amiodarone	800–1,200 mg daily x 1–3 weeks then 200–400 mg daily	Bradycardia, AV block, QT prolongation, torsades de pointes, pulmonary toxicity, hepatotoxicity, hyper- or hypothyroidism
Dofetilide	125–500 μg every 12 hrs (based upon creatinine clearance) Check QTc 2–3 hours after first dose. If QTc >15% over baseline or >500 ms decrease dose. Check QTc after each subsequent dose x 3 days and discontinue if QTc >500 ms *Must be initiated and monitored in the hospital	QT prolongation, torsades de pointes, headache, chest pain, dizziness, dyspnea, nausea, insomnia, back pain, diarrhea
Sotalol	80 mg–160 mg every 12 hours (based upon creatinine clearance)	QT prolongation, torsades de pointes, CHF, heart block, bradycardia, dyspnea, fatigue, dizziness, chest pain, palpitations, hypotension, headache
Metoprolol XL	12.5–200 mg daily	Fatigue, dizziness, diarrhea, pruritus, rash, depression, dyspnea, bradycardia, CHF
Carvedilol	6.25–25 mg twice daily	Dizziness, fatigue, diarrhea, hyperglycemia, weight gain, hypotension, bradycardia, dyspnea, nausea, headache, CHF

AAD, antiarrhythmic drug; VT, ventricular tachycardia; VF, ventricular fibrillation; AV, atrioventricular; CHF, congestive heart failure.

reduction of 35%, P = 0.05).[32] In Canadian Myocardial Infarction Amiodarone Trial (CAMIAT) 1,202 survivors of myocardial infarction who had at least one run of VT were randomized to amiodarone or placebo.[33] Amiodarone reduced the risk of VF and arrhythmic death (relative risk reduction of 48.5%, P = 0.016) particularly when treated with beta blockers.[33] In Sudden cardiac death in heart failure trial (SCD-HeFT), there was no difference in mortality between amiodarone and placebo in patients with NYHA function Class II–IV and EF less than or equal to 35%.[29] While these trials show that amiodarone is safe in patient with CHF and can reduce arrhythmic death, amiodarone does not improve overall survival.

Dofetilide

Dofetilide, a Class III AAD more commonly used in the management of atrial fibrillation, has not demonstrated an effect on mortality in patients with CHF. In Danish Investigations of Arrhythmia and Mortality on Dofetilide—CHF

(DIAMOND-CHF), 1,518 patients with NYHA function class III–IV CHF and EF less than or equal to 35% were randomized to dofetilide or placebo. There was no difference in mortality compared to placebo (41% vs. 42% P = 0.54).[37] In DIAMOND-MI, 1,510 survivors of MI with severe left ventricular dysfunction (EF $\leq$35%) were randomized to dofetilide versus placebo. Similarly, there was no difference in mortality in the dofetilide group as compared to placebo (31% vs. 32%, P = 0.226). In the subgroup of patients receiving both dofetilide and beta-blockers, there was a borderline significant risk reduction of death (31%, P = 0.05).[38] In both trials, there was a low incidence of TdP observed in the dofetilide group at initiation of therapy.[37,38] These trials show that dofetilide is safe in patients with CHF, but does not improve overall survival.

Beta-Blockers

Beta-blockers are the only AAD demonstrated to reduce mortality in patient with prior MI and CHF. Beta-blockers reduce myocardial ischemia by slowing the heart rate and decreasing myocardial oxygen consumption.[39] In beta-blocker heart attack trial (BHAT), propranolol demonstrated a significant reduction in overall mortality and specifically in SCD in infarct survivors compared to placebo (3.3% vs. 4.6%, $p < 0.05$).[40] The metoprolol CR/XL randomized intervention trial in congestive heart failure (MERIT) trial was the first large, double-blinded, randomized-controlled study to evaluate the mortality benefits of long-acting metoprolol in CHF patients. All-cause mortality was lower in the metoprolol group (7.2% vs. 11.0%, P = 0.00009).[41] There were fewer SCDs and deaths due to worsening heart failure in the metoprolol group.[41] The protective effect of carvedilol in CHF has been studied in several large trials. The US Carvedilol Heart Failure Study Group showed that carvedilol reduced mortality compared to placebo (7.8% vs. 3.2%, P <0.001).[42] Carvedilol also reduced the risk of death as well as hospitalization for cardiovascular causes. The Carvedilol Post Infarct Survival Control in LV Dysfunction (CAPRICORN) study showed survivors of MI with reduced LVEF treated with carvedilol had reduced all-cause and cardiovascular mortality, and lower rates of recurrent nonfatal MIs while Carvedilol Prospective Randomized Cumulative Survival (COPERNICUS) showed that carvedilol in patients with severe CHF improved mortality and reduced length of stay and hospitalization for cardiovascular causes and CHF.[43,44] In Carvedilol or Metoprolol European Trial (COMET), both carvedilol and metoprolol provided similar benefits when patients achieved target doses but patients treated with carvedilol had lower mortality that cannot be explained by the difference in blood pressure or heart rate.[45] Beta-blockers have also been shown to be beneficial in patients with nonischemic cardiomyopathy. In a subgroup analysis of cardiac insufficiency bisoprolol study (CIBIS), 232 patients with idiopathic dilated cardiomyopathy treated with bisoprolol had improved survival compared to placebo.[46]

Non-Antiarrhythmic Drugs

Early data on angiotensin converting enzyme inhibitors (ACEIs) demonstrated that its mortality benefit was reducing progressive HF or recurrent myocardial infarction rather than SCD.[47-49] However, in the second veterans administration cooperative vasodilator-heart failure trial (V-HeFT II), enalapril reduced mortality compared to hydralazine/nitrate (18% vs. 25%, P = 0.016) with the majority of deaths due to SCD.[50] In Trandolapril Cardiac Evaluation (TRACE), trandolapril was associated with reduction in overall mortality (RR = 0.75, P = 0.001) and mortality due to SCD (RR = 0.76, P = 0.03).[51] In Acute Infarction Ramipril Efficacy (AIRE), ramipril reduced overall mortality (RR of 27%, P = 0.002)[52] and deaths due to SCD (RR of 30%, P = 0.011).[53] Data on angiotensin receptor blockers (ARBs) for sudden death protection is limited. In Evaluation of Losartan in the Elderly (ELITE) losartan was associated with a lower all-cause mortality compared to captopril (4.8% vs. 8.7%, P = 0.035) with most deaths attributable to SCD.[54] However, the second ELITE study showed that losartan was not superior to captopril in improving survival.[55] A meta-analysis comparing ACEIs and ARBs did not demonstrate a significant difference in reducing all-cause mortality and HF hospitalizations but ARBs could be regarded as a suitable alternative for ACEIs.[56] Pleotropic effects of statin and omega-3 fatty acids might reduce SCD but data remains inconclusive.

VENTRICULAR TACHYCARDIA ABLATION

In contrast to AAD which electrophysiologically modify the tissue responsible for VT, catheter ablation physically disrupts the VT circuit. It has become an essential tool in the treatment and prevention of recurrent VT that often results in painful ICD discharges (Table 3, Fig. 6). The ideal patient for VT ablation has the following features: (1) easily and reproducibly inducible VT with programmed extrastimulation or burst pacing, (2) VT associated with a discrete scar (MI), (3) VT of a single morphology, and (4) hemodynamically tolerated VT.[57] Such an ideal VT allows for activation, pace- and entrainment mapping to localize and target the ventricular sites critical to the macroreentrant circuit. Three dimensional advanced electroanatomic mapping systems also allow substrate modification involving the border zone of scar when VT is rapid and unmappable.[58] Risks of catheter ablation include local vascular injury (bleeding, infection, pseudoaneurysm, arteriovenous fistula, and thrombosis), cardiac tamponade, air embolism, valve injury, damage to cardiac conduction system or coronary arteries, myocardial ischemia, stroke, and rarely death. Endocardial VT catheter ablation is contraindicated in the presence of a mural LV thrombus. In a multicenter trial, the incidence of major procedural-related complications is approximately 8% with a 3% risk of death.[59]

Table 3 Indications for ventricular tachycardia ablation

- Recurrent symptomatic sustained monomorphic ventricular tachycardia (VT) despite antiarrhythmic drug (AAD) therapy or when antiarrhythmic drugs are not tolerated
- Incessant sustained monomorphic VT or VT storm
- Frequent premature ventricular complexes, nonsustained ventricular tachycardias, or VT causing ventricular dysfunction
- Recurrent sustained polymorphic ventricular tachycardia, and ventricular fibrillation refractory to AAD therapy

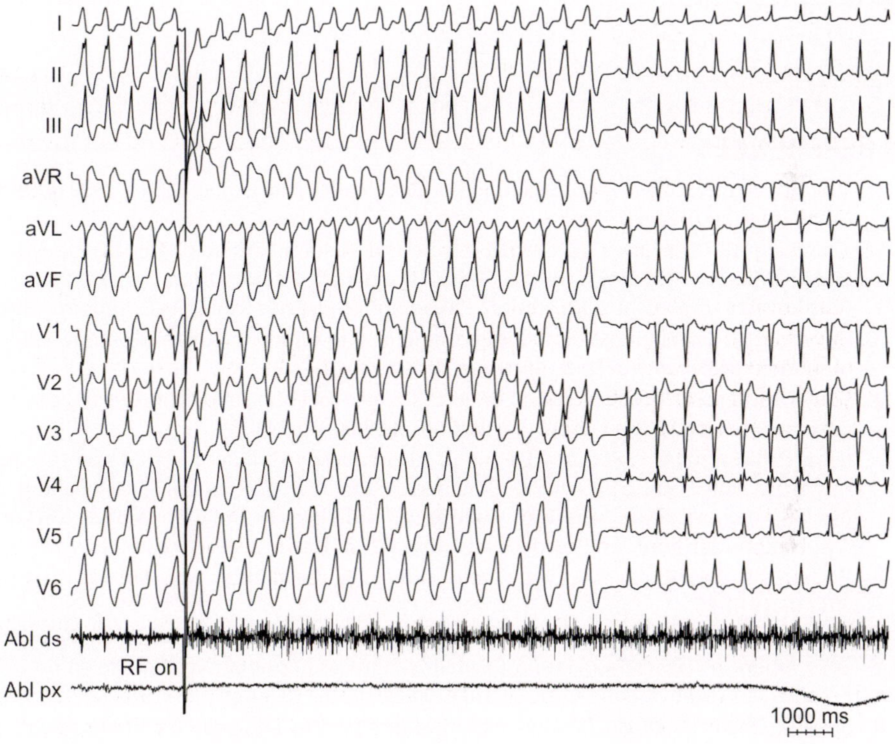

Figure 6: Successful termination of monomorphic ventricular tachycardia (VT) by radiofrequency energy during endocardial VT ablation.

FUTURE DIRECTIONS

The management of VT/VF in patients with CHF continues to evolve. Ranolazine is a promising new AAD being actively investigated for treatment of VT. Thoracic epidural anesthesia and left cardiac sympathetic denervation might be effective to treat VT storm refractory to AAD therapy. Advances in ablation include the use of robotic navigation[60] and incorporation of cardiac MRI into electroanatomic mapping systems to delineate myocardial scar and facilitate target sites for ablation. Advances in ICD therapy include new lead designs for defibrillation and LV pacing and diagnostic capabilities to detect pulmonary edema before development of symptoms. Mechanical circulatory support systems also continue to advance and provide hemodynamic support for the unstable VT/VF patient while awaiting cardiac transplantation.

ACKNOWLEDGMENTS

None.

DISCLOSURES

Reginald T Ho—None.
Andrew Yin—None.

REFERENCES

1. Zheng Z, Croft J, Giles W, et al. Sudden Cardiac Death in the United States, 1989 to 1998. Circulation. 2001;104:2158-63.
2. Myerburg RJ, Castellanos A. Cardiac arrest and sudden cardiac death. In: Zipes DP, Libby P, Bonow RO, Braunwald E (Eds). Braunwald's Heart Disease: A Textbook of Cardiovascular Medicine, 8th edition. Philadelphia: Elsevier Saunders Company; 2007.
3. Myerburg RJ, Castellanos A. Emerging paradigms of the epidemiology and demographics of sudden cardiac arrest. Heart Rhythm. 2006;3:235-39.
4. Luu M, Stevenson WG, Stevenson LW, et al. Diverse mechanisms of unexpected cardiac arrest in advanced heart failure. Circulation. 1989;80:1675-80.
5. Jessup M, Abraham WT, Casey DE, et al. 2009 Focused Update Incorporated Into the ACC/AHA 2005 Guidelines for the Diagnosis and Management of Heart Failure in Adults: A Report of the American College of Cardiology Foundation/American Heart Association Task Force on Practice Guidelines. Circulation. 2009;119:e391-479.
6. Pachón M, Almedral J. Sudden death: managing the patient who survives. Heart. 2011;97:1619-25.
7. Neumar RW, Otto CW, Link MS, et al. Part 8: Adult Advanced Cardiovascular Life Support: 2010 American Heart Association Guidelines for Cardiopulmonary Resuscitation and Emergency Cardiovascular Care. Circulation. 2010;122(18 Suppl 3):S729-67.
8. Nasir N, Taylor A, Doyle TK,. Evaluation of intravenous lidocaine for the termination of sustained monomorphic ventricular tachycardia in patients with coronary artery disease with or without healed myocardial infarction. Am J Cardiol. 1994;74:1183-6.
9. Lie KI, Wellens HJ, van Capelle FJ, et al. Lidocaine in the prevention of primary ventricular fibrillation. A double-blind, randomized study of 212 consecutive patients. N Engl J Med. 1974;291:1324-6.
10. Buxton AE, Calkins H, Callans DJ, et al. ACC/AHA/HRS 2006 key data elements and definitions for electrophysiological studies and procedures: a report of the American College of Cardiology/American Heart Association Task Force on Clinical Data Standards (ACC/AHA/HRS Writing Committee to Develop Data Standards on Electrophysiology). Circulation. 2006;114:2534-70.
11. Dessertenne F. La Tachycardie Ventriculaire a Deux Foyers Opposes Variable. Arch Mal Coeur Vaiss. 1966;59:263-72.
12. Wolfe C, Nibley C, Bhandari A, et al. Polymorphous ventricular tachycardia associated with acute myocardial infarction. Circulation. 1991;84:1543-51.

13. Viskin S, Belhassen B. Polymorphic ventricular tachyarrhythmias in the absence of organic heart disease: classification, differential diagnosis, and implications for therapy. Prog Cardiovasc Dis. 1998;41:17-34.
14. Aliot EM, Stevenson WG, Almendral-Garrote JM, et al. EHRA/HRS expert consensus on catheter ablation of ventricular arrhythmias. Heart Rhythm. 2009;6:886-933.
15. de Bakker JM, Van Capelle F, Janse MJ, et al. Macroreentry in the infarcted human heart: the mechanism of ventricular tachycardias with a "focal" activation pattern. J Am Coll Cardiol. 1991;18:1005-14.
16. Karagueuzian HS, Mandel WJ. Electrophysiologic Mechanisms of Ischemic Ventricular Arrhythmias: Experimental and Clinical Correlations. In: Mandel WJ (Ed). Cardiac Arrhythmias: Their Mechanisms, Diagnosis, and Management, 3rd edition. Philadelphia: JB Lippincott Company; 1995.
17. Blanck Z, Dhala A, Deshpande S, et al. Bundle branch reentrant ventricular tachycardia: cumulative experience in 48 patients. J Cardiovasc Electrophysiol. 1993;4:253-62.
18. Tung R, Boyle NG, Shivkumar K. Catheter ablation of ventricular tachycardia. Circulation. 2011;123:2284-8.
19. Sweeney MO, Sherfesee L, DeGroot PJ, et al. Differences in effects of electrical therapy type for ventricular arrhythmias on mortality in implantable cardioverter-defibrillator patients. Heart Rhythm. 2010;7:353-60.
20. Carbucicchio C, Santamaria M, Trevisi N, et al. Catheter ablation for the treatment of electrical storm in patients with implantable cardioverter-defibrillators: short- and long-term outcomes in a prospective single-center study. Circulation. 2008;117:462-9.
21. Bourke T, Vaseghi M, Michowitz Y, et al. Neuraxial modulation for refractory ventricular arrhythmias: value of thoracic epidural anesthesia and surgical left cardiac sympathetic denervation. Circulation. 2010;121:2255-62.
22. Refaat M, Chemaly E, Lebeche D, et al. Ventricular arrhythmias after left ventricular assist device implantation. Pacing Clin Electrophysiol. 2008;31:1246-52.
23. Anderson M, Videbæk R, Boesgaard S, et al. Incidence of ventricular arrhythmias in patients on long-term support with a continuous-flow assist device (HeartMate II). J Heart Lung Transplant. 2009;28:733-5.
24. Bedi M, Kormos R, Winowich S, et al. Ventricular arrhythmias during left ventricular assist device support. Am J Cardiol. 2007;99:1151-3.
25. Ziv O, Dizon J, Thosani A, et al. Effects of left ventricular assist device therapy on ventricular arrhythmias. J Am Coll Cardiol. 2005;45:1428-34.
26. Zipes DP, Camm AJ, Borggrefe M, et al. ACC/AHA/ESC 2006 Guidelines for Management of Patients With Ventricular Arrhythmias and the Prevention of Sudden Cardiac Death: a report of the American College of Cardiology/American Heart Association Task Force and the European Society of Cardiology Committee for Practice Guidelines (writing committee to develop Guidelines for Management of Patients With Ventricular Arrhythmias and the Prevention of Sudden Cardiac Death): developed in collaboration with the European Heart Rhythm Association and the Heart Rhythm Society. Circulation. 2006;114:e385-484.
27. Mirowski M, Reid PR, Mower MM, et al. Termination of malignant ventricular arrhythmias with an implanted automatic defibrillator in human beings. N Engl J Med. 1980;303:322-4.
28. Epstein AE, DiMarco JP, Ellenbogen KA, et al. ACC/AHA/HRS 2008 Guidelines for Device-Based Therapy of Cardiac Rhythm Abnormalities: a report of the American College of Cardiology/American Heart Association Task Force on Practice Guidelines (Writing Committee to Revise the ACC/AHA/NASPE 2002 Guideline Update for Implantation of Cardiac Pacemakers and Antiarrhythmia Devices): developed in collaboration with

the American Association for Thoracic Surgery and Society of Thoracic Surgeons. Circulation. 2008;117:e350-408.

29. Buxton AE, Lee KL, Fisher JD, et al. A randomized study of the prevention of sudden death in patients with coronary artery disease. N Engl J Med. 1999;341:1882-90.
30. Bardy GH, Lee KL, Mark DB, et al. Amiodarone or an implantable cardioverter-defibrillator for congestive heart failure. N Engl J Med. 2005;352:225-37.
31. Connolly SJ, Dorian P, Roberts RS, et al. Comparison of β-blockers, amiodarone plus β-blockers, or sotalol for prevention of shocks from implantable cardioverter defibrillators: the OPTIC Study: a randomized trial. JAMA. 2006;295:165-71.
32. Julian DG, Camm AJ, Frangin G, et al. Randomised trial of effect of amiodarone on mortality in patients with left-ventricular dysfunction after recent myocardial infarction: EMIAT. Lancet. 1997;349:667-74.
33. Cairns JA, Connolly SJ, Roberts R, et al. Randomised trial of outcome after myocardial infarction in patients with frequent or repetitive ventricular premature depolarizations: CAMIAT. Lancet. 1997;349:675-82.
34. Singh SN, Fletcher RD, Fisher SG, et al. Amiodarone in patients with congestive heart failure and asymptomatic ventricular arrhythmia. Survival Trial of Antiarrhythmic Therapy in Congestive Heart Failure. N Engl J Med. 1995;333:77-82.
35. Doval HC, Nul DR, Grancelli HO, et al. Randomised trial of low-dose amiodarone in severe congestive heart failure. Grupo de Estudio de la Sobrevida en la Insuficiencia Cardiaca en Argentina (GESICA). Lancet. 1994;344:493-8.
36. Echt DS, Liebson PR, Mitchell LB, et al. Mortality and morbidity in patients receiving encainide, flecainide, or placebo. The Cardiac Arrhythmia Suppression Trial. N Engl J Med. 1991;324:781-8.
37. Torp-Pedersen C, Møller M, Bloch-Thomsen P, et al. Dofetilide in patients with congestive heart failure and left ventricular dysfunction. N Engl J Med. 1999;341:857-65.
38. Køber L, Thomsen PEB, Møller M, et al. Effect of dofetilide in patients with recent myocardial infarction and left-ventricular dysfunction: a randomised trial. Lancet. 2000;356:2052-8.
39. Anderson KP. Sympathetic nervous system activity and ventricular tachyarrhythmias: recent advances. Ann Noninvasive Electrocardiol. 2003;8:75-89.
40. β-Blocker Heart Attack Trial Research Group. A randomized trial of propranolol in patients with acute myocardial infarction. I. Mortality results. JAMA. 1982;247:1707-14.
41. MERIT-HF Study Group. Effect of metoprolol CR/XL in chronic heart failure: Metoprolol CR/XL Randomised Intervention Trial in Congestive Heart Failure (MERIT-HF). Lancet. 1999;353:2001-7.
42. Packer M, Bristow MR, Cohn JN, et al. The effect of carvedilol on morbidity and mortality in patients with chronic heart failure. U.S. Carvedilol Heart Failure Study Group. N Engl J Med. 1996;334:1349-55.
43. Dargie HJ. Effect of carvedilol on outcome after myocardial infarction in patients with left-ventricular dysfunction: the CAPRICORN randomised trial. Lancet. 2001;357:1385-90.
44. Packer M, Fowler MB, Roecker EB, et al. Effect of carvedilol on the morbidity and of patients with severe chronic heart failure: results of the carvedilol prospective randomized cumulative survival (COPERNICUS) study. Circulation. 2002;106:2194-9.
45. Metra M, Torp-Pedersen C, Swedberg K, et al. Influence of heart rate, blood pressure, and beta-blocker dose on outcome and the differences in outcome between carvedilol and metoprolol tartrate in patients with chronic heart failure: results from the COMET trial. Eur Heart J. 2005;26:2259-68.
46. CIBIS Investigators and Committees. A randomized trial of beta-blockade in heart failure. The Cardiac Insufficiency Bisoprolol Study (CIBIS). Circulation. 1994;90:1765-73.

47. The CONSENSUS Trial Study Group. Effects of enalapril on mortality in severe congestive heart failure. Results of the Cooperative North Scandinavian Enalapril Survival Study (CONSENSUS). N Engl J Med. 1987;316:1429-35.
48. The SOLVD Investigators. Effect of enalapril on survival in patients with reduced left ventricular ejection fractions and congestive heart failure. N Engl J Med. 1991;325:293-302.
49. Pfeffer MA, Braunwald E, Moyé LA, et al. Effect of captopril on mortality and morbidity in patients with left ventricular dysfunction after myocardial infarction. Results of the survival and ventricular enlargement trial. The SAVE Investigators. N Engl J Med. 1992;327:669-77.
50. Cohn JN, Johnson G, Ziesche S, et al. A comparison of enalapril with hydralazine-isosorbide dinitrate in the treatment of chronic congestive heart failure. N Engl J Med. 1991;325:303-10.
51. Køber L, Torp-Pedersen C, Carlsen JE, et al. A clinical trial of the angiotensin-converting-enzyme inhibitor trandolapril in patients with left ventricular dysfunction after myocardial infarction. Trandolapril Cardiac Evaluation (TRACE) Study Group. N Engl J Med. 1995;333:1670-6.
52. The Acute Infarction Ramipril Efficacy (AIRE) Study Investigators. Effect of ramipril on mortality and morbidity of survivors of acute myocardial infarction with clinical evidence of heart failure. Lancet. 1993;342:821-8.
53. Cleland JG, Erhardt L, Murray G, et al. Effect of ramipril on morbidity and mode of death among survivors of acute myocardial infarction with clinical evidence of heart failure. Eur Heart J. 1997;18:41-51.
54. Pitt B, Segal R, Martinez FA, et al. Randomised trial of losartan versus captopril in patients over 65 with heart failure (Evaluation of Losartan In the Elderly Study, ELITE). Lancet. 1997;349:747-52.
55. Pitt B, Poole-Wilson PA, Segal R, et al. Effect of losartan compared with captopril on mortality in patients with symptomatic heart failure: randomised trial—the Losartan Heart Failure Survival Study ELITE II. Lancet. 2000;355:1582-7
56. Lee VC, Rhew DC, Dylan M, et al. Meta-analysis: angiotensin-receptor blockers in chronic heart failure and high-risk acute myocardial infarction. Ann Intern Med. 2004;141:693-704.
57. Ho RH, Callans DJ. Malignant ventricular arrhythmias. In: Atman EM (Ed). Cardiovascular Therapeutics: A Companion to Braunwald's Heart Disease, 2nd edition. Boston: WB Saunders Co; 2002.
58. Marchlinski FE, Callans DJ, Gottlieb CD, et al. Linear ablation lesions for control of unmappable ventricular tachycardia in patients with ischemic and nonischemic cardiomyopathy. Circulation. 2000;101:1288-96.
59. Calkins H, Epstein A, Packer D, et al. Catheter ablation of ventricular tachycardia in patients with structural heart disease using cooled radiofrequency energy: results of a prospective multicenter study. Cooled RF Multi Center Investigators Group. J Am Coll Cardiol. 2000;35:1905-14.
60. Valderrábano M, Dave AS, Báez-Escudero JL, et al. Robotic catheter ablation of left ventricular tachycardia: initial experience. Heart Rhythm. 2011;8:1837-46.

CHAPTER 13

Heart Transplantation

Gordon R Reeves, Paul J Mather

INTRODUCTION

In appropriately selected patients with advanced heart failure (HF), orthotopic heart transplantation (OHT) can improve long-term survival and quality of life. Heart transplant also brings with it a host of new potential problems including those related to the transplant surgery, graft function, rejection and failure, and the problems associated with long-term immunosuppression therapy. Careful patient selection and meticulous follow-up care are essential to good outcomes and a successful heart transplant program.

The number of heart transplants performed each year has peaked in the mid-1990s and has remained essentially stable for the past decade with current estimates exceeding 5,000 annually worldwide (Fig. 1).[1] The majority of these (> 3,500) are reported to the Registry of the International Society for Heart and Lung Transplantation (ISHLT).[2] Availability of donor organs continues to limit the number of HTs performed. In the Unites States, nearly half of patients awaiting HT spend more than 1 year waiting for a suitable donor organ and nearly 20% die or become too sick to remain eligible before receiving a HT (United States Organ Transplantation annual report 2010).[3]

INDICATIONS

By far the most common indication for OHT is refractory HF, with transplantations for patients with a nonischemic cardiomyopathy (53%) now outnumbering those with ischemic disease (38%) (Fig. 2).[2] Other less common indications for heart transplant (combined <10% of all heart transplants) include congenital heart disease, valvular cardiomyopathy, retransplant, refractory angina, and recurrent life-threatening ventricular arrhythmias.[2,4] See table 1 for a partial list of indications for HT in appropriate patients.

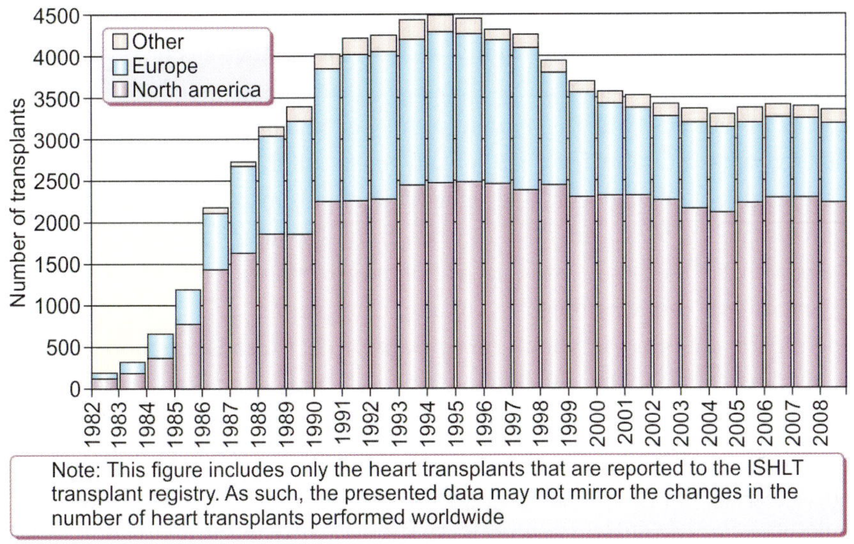

Figure 1: Number of heart transplantations performed annually and stratified by region as reported to the International Society for Heart and Lung Transplantation.[1]

Source: *From* Stehlik J, Edwards LB, Kucheryavaya AY, et al. The Registry of the International Society for Heart and Lung Transplantation: twenty-seventh official adult heart transplant report--2010. J Heart Lung Transplant. 2010;29(10): 1089-103, *with permission.*

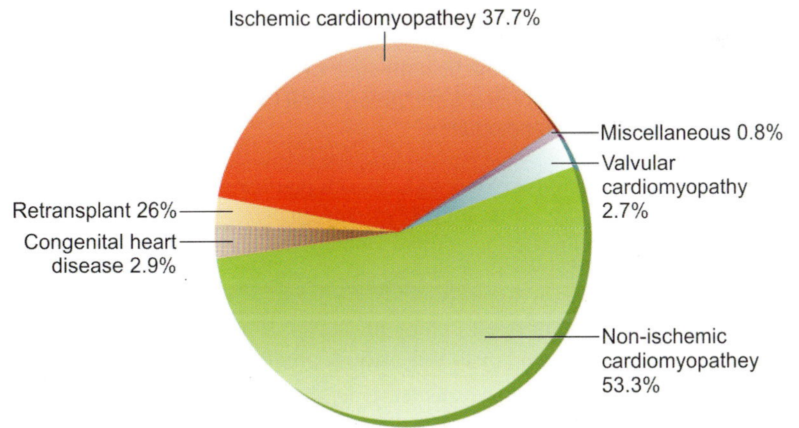

Figure 2: Etiology of heart disease in heart transplantation recipients from June 2005 through June 2010.[2]

Source: *From* Stehlik J, Edwards LB, Kucheryavaya AY, et al. The Registry of the International Society for Heart and Lung Transplantation: Twenty-eighth Adult Heart Transplant Report--2011. J Heart Lung Transplant. 2011;30(10):1078-94, *with permission.*

PATIENT SELECTION

Although improvements in morbidity and mortality have been associated with increased use of neurohormonal blockade and device therapy,[5,6] long-term outcomes in patients with HF remain poor.[7] For patients with HF, HT should be considered once mortality from HF is likely to exceed that of HT. In HT recipients, the highest risk of death occurs in the first year after transplant with 1-year survival of approximately 85%.[2] In subsequent years, mortality rates decrease to about 3–4% per year with median long-term survival of approximately 11 years overall and 14 years for patients surviving the first year after transplant.[2]

Identifying patients for whom their risk from HF exceeds the more immediate risks of transplant can be challenging. Several clinical markers, risk prediction models, and tests have been studied in an effort to identify HF patients at risk for worse outcomes. Patients with advanced HF requiring inotropic support to maintain organ perfusion clearly warrant consideration for transplantation (Table 1). For ambulatory patients with less severe HF, risk scores, such as the heart failure survival

Table 1 Indications for cardiac transplantation

Indications in appropriate patients
- Hemodynamic compromise due to HF
  - Refractory cardiogenic shock
  - Dependence in IV inotropic support to maintain adequate organ perfusion
- Peak VO_2 <10–12 mL/kg/min in an adequate study*
  - Peak VO_2 <14 mL/kg/min if intolerant of beta-blocker therapy*
- Severe symptoms of ischemia that consistently limit routine activity and are not amenable to revascularization, medical therapy, or other therapies
- Recurrent symptomatic ventricular arrhythmias refractory to therapeutic modalities including medical therapy and ablation

Relative indications
- Peak VO_2 12–14 mL/kg/min or Peak VO_2 ≤50% predicted in an adequate study*
- Recurrent unstable ischemia not amenable to therapy
- Recurrent instability of fluid balance/renal function not due to patient adherence

Insufficient indications
- Low left ventricular ejection fraction
- History of NYHA Class III or IV HF symptoms
- Peak VO_2 >15 ml/kg/min and peak VO_2 >50% predicted without other indications*

HF, heart failure; VO_2, oxygen consumption per unit time; NYHA, New York Heart Association

Source: *Adapted from* Hunt SA, Abraham WT, Chin MH, et al. 2009 Focused Update Incorporated Into the ACC/AHA 2005 Guidelines for the Diagnosis and Management of Heart Failure in Adults: a report of the American College of Cardiology Foundation/American Heart Association Task Force on Practice Guidelines: developed in collaboration with the International Society for Heart and Lung Transplantation. *Circulation*. 2009;119:e391-479.

See also Mehra MR, et al. Listing Criteria for Heart Transplantation: International Society for Heart and Lung Transplantation Guidelines for the care of Cardiac Transplant Candidates–2006[24] for further discussion of the role of VO_2 and other criteria for heart transplantation.

*VO_2 should not be used as the sole indication for heart transplantation.

score (HFSS) and the Seattle heart failure model (SHFM), and cardiopulmonary exercise testing (CPET) with measurement of respiratory gas exchange can be helpful in predicting patient prognosis and in risk stratification.

The HFSS was developed as a prognostic tool in ambulatory HF patients to help identify those who may be candidates for HT using seven variables including peak oxygen uptake (VO_2).[8] It has been revalidated more recently in more diverse HF patients, including those receiving contemporary therapies.[9-12] The SHFM was developed later using data from HF patients participating in clinical trials and has the additional feature of estimating the impact of various interventions (medical therapy and device therapy) on survival.[13] It has been validated in ambulatory HF patients referred for HT evaluation, however, may underestimate risk when applied to this population.[14,15] When compared directly in the same cohort of HF patients referred for transplantation, these two tools demonstrated similar ability to discriminate those at high, medium, and low mortality risk and may provide complimentary assessments with improved predictive ability when used in combination.[16]

Peak VO_2 determined by CPET is a long-standing prognostic marker for identifying patients who may warrant HT.[17] CPET is a form of exercise testing that includes the measurement of respiratory gas exchange through the use of a metabolic cart. Peak VO_2 is the highest amount of oxygen uptake achieved during the exercise and lower values are associated with worse outcomes. The original level of less than 14 mL/kg/min used to identify advanced HF patients who may benefit from HT has subsequently been lowered to less than 12 mL/kg/min or less than 10 mL/kg/min due to improved prognosis with advances in chronic HF therapies.[4,18] Several variables obtained from CPET in addition to peak VO_2 provide prognostic information and there are several excellent reviews that provide more detail.[19-22] One variable of particular note is ventilator efficiency, defined as the slope of minute ventilation (VE) to carbon dioxide output (VCO_2). In some studies, this CPET variable has been the strongest predictor of survival.[23] Higher values, thought to reflect increased ventilation-perfusion mismatching and heightened respiratory responses,[21] are associated with worse outcomes and a cut-off of more than or equal to 45 has been proposed to identify those with a particularly poor prognosis.[19]

CONTRAINDICATIONS

Once it has been determined that a patient has an indication for HT, the next step in patient selection is to evaluate absolute and relative contraindications to cardiac transplantation (Table 2). In order to optimize patient outcomes, make appropriate use of the relative shortage of donor organs, and honor the sacrifice of organ donation, it is important to identify patients who are most likely to do well following HT. Contraindications generally fall into one of the following two categories: (a) disease in other organ systems that increase perioperative risk and (b) factors that

Table 2 Potential contraindications to heart transplantation. The distinction between absolute and relative contraindications is variable across transplant centers and continually evolving

Common absolute contraindications

- Systemic illness with life expectancy, <2 years despite HT, including:
  - » Active (other than nonmelanoma skin) or recent malignancy*
  - » AIDS with frequent opportunistic infections
  - » Active, multisystem sarcoid**, amyloidosis**, or systemic lupus erythematosus
  - » Irreversible severe renal, pulmonary, or hepatic dysfunction in patients considered only for HT**
- Fixed pulmonary hypertension**
  - » Pulmonary artery systolic pressure >60 mmHg
  - » Mean transpulmonary gradient >15 mmHg
  - » Pulmonary vascular resistance >5–6 Wood units
- Common relative contraindications
  - » Age >70 years old
  - » Active infection (except for device-related infection in VAD recipients)
  - » Severe or poorly controlled diabetes mellitus with end-organ damage
  - » Severe peripheral vascular or cerebrovascular disease
  - » Morbid obesity (BMI >30 kg/m^2 or >140% ideal body weight)
  - » Pulmonary infarction within 6–8 weeks
  - » Difficult to control hypertension
  - » Irreversible neurological or neuromuscular disorder
  - » Psychological or social (e.g., lack of social support) issue that limit ability to adhere to post-transplantation medication and follow-up regimens
  - » Active or recent (6 months) drug, tobacco, or alcohol abuse
  - » Heparin-induced thrombocytopenia within 3 months or circulating platelet factor 4 antibodies

HT, heart transplantation; AIDS, acquired immune deficiency syndrome; FEV_1, forced expiratory volume in 1 second; VAD, ventricular assist device; BMI, body mass index; INR, international normalized ratio.

Source: *Adapted from* Mancini D, Lietz K. Selection of cardiac transplantation candidates in 2010. Circulation. 2010;122(2):173-83.

See also Mehra MR, et al. Listing Criteria for Heart Transplantation: International Society for Heart and Lung Transplantation Guidelines for the care of Cardiac Transplant Candidates – 200624 for further discussion of contraindication to heart transplantation.

*Time period for cancer remission traditionally more than 5 years but is variable and should be individualized in consultation with oncological expert.

**Sometime considered relative contraindications.

could complicate long-term care of the transplanted heart, including the potentially harmful side-effects of immunosuppression therapy and the ability to adhere with close and careful follow-up. These factors can be highly variable and require a comprehensive evaluation of the prospective recipient by a multidisciplinary team. Early referral to a transplant center not only allows time to complete this evaluation but also can provide the opportunity to intervene on potentially modifiable contraindications to transplantation. The most common reasons transplant may be considered too high risk are listed in table 2 and discussed below.

Age

Although the average age of heart transplant recipients has remained stable, there have been increases in transplants at both ends of the age spectrum.[1] The rising number of successful older transplant recipients may reflect improvements in HF management, so that patients present with end-stage HF at an older age, as well as improvements in the perioperative and long-term management of transplant recipients allowing successful transplantation of older recipients. Although there is no absolute age "cut-off", cardiac transplantation in patients 70 years and older is rare (1–2% of all transplants).[2] Successful transplantation in patients with advanced age requires especially careful selection and may involve using organs from alternative (e.g., older) donors that may not be ideal for younger recipients.

Body Mass Index

Those with a very high or very low BMI may not have good outcomes with transplant and this should be considered in the decision to proceed. Interventions targeting weight loss or improved nutrition as is appropriate can be implemented to improve eligibility.

Pulmonary Disease

Irreversible pulmonary hypertension is a contraindication to transplant, as the donor heart's right ventricle (RV) is likely to fail with the increase in afterload. Pulmonary vascular resistance and transpulmonary gradient (the difference between mean pulmonary artery pressure and pulmonary capillary wedge pressure) are typically used for assessment purposes. These measures help account for pulmonary hypertension that is predominantly due to elevated filling pressures of the left ventricle (LV) that will be corrected with the transplanted heart. The ISHLT guidelines recognize a cut-off of 5 Woods units as a relative contraindication to transplant.[24] Transpulmonary gradients greater than 13 are concerning and the greater than 16–20 is recognized as a relative contraindication.[24] If the pulmonary pressures and pulmonary vascular resistance are elevated, then attempts should be made to show reversibility if possible. Treatment with nesiritide, nitroprusside, milrinione, inhaled nitric oxide, or prostacyclin may acutely reduce the pulmonary pressures to an acceptable range. Short-term treatment with vasoactive agents like those listed above and HF management to optimize LV filling pressures, including inotropic support and diuretic therapy, may reveal reversibility of elevated pulmonary pressures and allow a patient to be listed for transplant. If this is unsuccessful, then longer term support with mechanical devices [e.g., left ventricular assist devices (LVADs)] can be considered. Serial right heart catheterization (RHC) should be performed in patients to ensure ongoing reversibility of the pulmonary hypertension, the frequency of which is likely dependent on how severe and difficult it was to reverse the patient's pulmonary pressures initially.

In addition to fixed pulmonary hypertension, advanced restricted or obstructive lung disease is a contraindication to HT as lung disease increases the perioperative risk and increases immunosuppressive complications. Combined heart-lung transplantation may be an option in a very limited number of these patients.

Diabetes Mellitus

Well-controlled diabetes mellitus without end-organ involvement is generally not a contraindication to HT. However, significant end-organ damage, including neuropathy, nephropathy, or nonhealing diabetic ulcers is a relative contraindication.

Renal Disease

The nephrotoxic effects of immunosuppressive therapy and potential perioperative hemodynamic insult can both negatively affect post-transplant renal function. Heart-kidney transplant can be considered in patients with significant renal impairment (e.g., creatinine clearance less than 40 mL/min).

Hepatic Disease

Advanced hepatic disease increases the perioperative risk and can decrease long-term survival. Heart-liver transplantation is available at some centers for appropriate candidates.

Non-Cardiac Vascular Disease

Significant non-cardiac vascular disease, including peripheral vascular disease and cerebral vascular disease, is a relative contraindication to transplantation.

Infectious Disease

Active infection will generally be worsened by immunosuppression therapy and is typically an absolute contraindication.

Malignancy

With the exceptions of non-melanoma skin cancers, some prostate cancers, and some cardiac tumors, active malignancy is generally an absolute contraindication to transplant. A history of malignancy can be a relative contraindication and detailed records of the cancer diagnosis and management as well as consultation with an oncologist regarding risk of tumor recurrence is warranted.

Substance Abuse

Ongoing use of alcohol, tobacco, or illicit drugs is generally considered a contraindication to transplantation. Abstinent patients with a history of substance abuse may be considered for HT after a thorough assessment of their prior use and risk of relapsing has been undertaken. Laboratory monitoring of ongoing abstinence is also sometimes performed.

Psychosocial

For successful long-term outcomes after HT, patients must be willing and able to adhere to a complex medical regimen and frequent, close follow-up. Adequate social support is also needed. Psychological disease can impact adherence and should be thoroughly evaluated and under good control if transplantation is to be considered.

LISTING AND WAITING FOR TRANSPLANT

Countries have developed different systems for the fair allocation of organs. Generally, the sickest patients listed for transplant are given priority. Policies and procedures related to listing status are updated periodically and vary by country or region. Organ shortages, longer wait periods, and the increasing role of mechanical circulatory support are likely to influence revisions to these systems. It is important to be familiar with and remain adherent to applicable listing regulations to help promote the fair and ethical distribution of donor organs.

DONOR SELECTION

Numerous factors must be considered when evaluating a potential organ donor for a heart transplant recipient, including size, age, clinical course and cause of death, and medical, surgical, and social history. Recipient factors, including urgency of transplantation, age, comorbid disease, extent of preexisting human leukocyte antigens (HLA) antibodies also impact the suitability of a potential organ from a particular donor and must also be considered.

DONOR CARDIAC EVALUATION

Cardiac evaluation will include an electrocardiogram and an echocardiogram in all prospective donors and left heart catheterization in older donors (e.g., >45 years in men and >55 years in women) or other donors where there is increased concern for coronary artery disease (CAD). The procuring surgeon will also conduct a careful direct inspection (through visualization and palpation) of the donor organ for evidence of CAD, contusion, or other abnormalities in function or structure. Both CAD and left ventricular hypertrophy (LVH) (wall thickness >14 mm) are known to increase the risk of early graft failure and can be associated with long-term complications, such as coronary allograft vasculopathy (CAV) and diastolic HF, respectively.[25] Donor hearts with obstructive CAD or significant LVH are generally avoided or only considered for alternative list recipients. The use of donor hearts with abnormalities in LV function is also generally avoided unless considered reversible secondary to the cardiotoxic physiologic environment associated with brain death.

DONOR EXTRA-CARDIAC EVALUATION

Donor age, donor weight, anoxia as cause of death, and allograft ischemic time have all been associated 1-year post-transplant survival in contemporary transplant patients.[2]

Donor Age

The majority of donors for HT are 18–59 years old and the mean age has risen gradually to approximately 33 years old.[1] There is no clear-cut upper age cutoff for donors; however, older donors have been associated with worsened outcomes.[2] Older donor hearts (e.g., >45 or 50 years old) may be more susceptible to prolonged ischemic times (>4 hours) and other factors that could complicate transplantation. Donors of 60 years and older are very rarely used (1–2% of all transplantations)[1] and use of organs from donors more than 55 years should be used very selectively,[25] e.g., in alternative list recipients.

Donor Size

Both oversizing and undersizing of the donor heart can complicate OHT. Oversizing can complicate the ability to close the chest of the recipient after OHT without cardiac compression and associated hemodynamic compromise. An undersized heart may be unable to adequately support the circulatory needs of the larger recipient. It is recommended that generally the donor weight be within 30% of the recipient's weight.[25] Smaller female donor to a larger male recipient and smaller donor to a recipient with elevated pulmonary resistance (>4 Woods units) may carry higher risks.[25,26]

Ischemic Time

An acceptable ischemic time is dependent on both donor and recipient factors. Average ischemic time has risen gradually in recent years to approximately 3 hours[2] and ischemic time of less than 4 hours is generally recommended.[25] However, there are cases, such as with a young adult donor, when longer ischemic time (e.g., >6 hours) can be tolerated with good outcomes. Hypothermia and mechanical arrest of the heart with the use of myocardial preservation solutions helps to preserve the donor organ during the ischemic period.

DONOR HEART IMPLANTATION

The standard biatrial technique for OHT, originally described by Lower and Shumway[27] in 1960, has largely been replaced by the bicaval technique. With the biatrial technique both the donor and the recipient's hearts are excised at the mid-atrial level and the aorta and pulmonary artery are transected above the aortic and pulmonic valves. The bicaval technique leaves the donor atria intact and transects the superior and inferior vena cava to remove the donor heart. This technique allows for improved atrial and ventricular function, improved valvular function (i.e., decreased tricuspid regurgitation), less atrial arrhythmias, and less sinus node dysfunction and heart block after implantation.[28-30]

POSTOPERATIVE MANAGEMENT OF THE HEART TRANSPLANT RECIPIENT

The most common causes of death during for the first 30 days following transplant are graft failure (35–40%), multiorgan failure (20%), infection (11%), and acute rejection (5%).[2] Efforts to optimize graft and other organ function and minimize the risks of infection and rejection are central to the perioperative care of the OHT recipient.

Immediately following OHT, the transplanted heart often requires hemodynamic support. This is especially true for the RV, which has less intrinsic reserve, may be more susceptible to ischemic injury, and may face higher pulmonary pressures in the recipient than it was exposed to in the donor. Pulmonary vasodilators can be used to help reduce RV afterload. Excessive RV preload [i.e., central venous pressure (CVP) >15 mmHg] can cause RV distension and mechanical disadvantage and should be avoided even if aggressive diuresis or hemodialysis are needed to achieve this. LV systolic function is typically preserved initially, but can decline in the early postoperative hours possibly related to ischemic/reperfusion injury and myocardial edema.[31] Even in those with preserved LV systolic function, these factors commonly lead to diastolic dysfunction postoperatively. Hemodynamic monitoring with a pulmonary artery catheter is used to help guide therapy. Transthoracic (TTE) and/or transesophageal (TEE) echocardiography can also be used to evaluate graft performance. Vasoactive and inotropic agents are commonly employed postoperatively and gradually weaned. In cases where these agents are inadequate to support the newly transplanted graft, mechanical support (of the RV, LV, or both) can also be provided.

The atria are also susceptible to ischemic and surgical injury and sinus node dysfunction may result. Typical heart rate (HR) for a denervated heart is 90–110 beats per minute (bpm). Slower heart rates may result from sinus node dysfunction and can compromise cardiac output (CO). This is usually self-limited and temporary epicardial pacing or chronotropic agents, such as isoproterenol, can be used until sinus node function recovers. Permanent pacemaker placement is rarely needed.

Infection of the surgical wound can be minimized with standard aseptic technique and prophylactic perioperative antibiotics targeting usual skin flora. Prophylactic antimicrobial agents to prevent opportunistic infections are also initiated in the early postoperative period.

Induction Therapy

Induction therapy involves the use of polyclonal or monoclonal antibodies to provide intense immunosuppression during the perioperative period. Use is variable with approximately half of transplant receiving some form of induction therapy.[2] Potential benefits include a reduction in early rejection and a delay in the initiation of nephrotoxic immunosuppressive agents (i.e., calcineurin inhibitors). Potential agents include polyclonal antithymocyte globulin (ATG) (derived from equine or rabbit proteins), murine derived monoclonal antibodies targeting the CD3 molecule on T-cells (OKT3), and monoclonal antibodies targeting the IL-2R (CD25) cytokine receptor (basiliximab and daclizumab).[32] Potential adverse effects include allergic reaction, particularly with those agents derived exclusively from animal proteins, increased risk of post-transplant lymphoproliferative disorder (PTLD) (variably observed with ATG and OKT-3) and increased infection risk associated with ATG.[32,33] The potential benefit of induction therapy may be greatest in those with significant preoperative renal impairment and in those at high risk for acute rejection (e.g., those with PRAs >10%).[25,33] The selective use of induction therapy in this later group may explain why these therapies have been associated with increased rates of rejection after the postoperative period.[2] Further prospective research is needed to more clearly define the role of these agents.

IMMUNOSUPPRESSION AND REJECTION

Following transplantation, allografts are susceptible to several different types of rejection. A brief description of each as well as strategies for preventing, identifying, and managing allograft rejection is included in this section.

Hyperacute Rejection

Hyperacute rejection is caused by preformed recipient antibodies binding to donor antigens (HLA, ABO, or endothelial), and occurs within minutes to hours after transplantation.[32] The binding of these alloantibodies to donor antigens leads to compliment fixation causing thrombosis and cell death.[33] Catastrophic graft failure follows and is almost always fatal.

Fortunately, hyperacute rejection is rare thanks to ABO matching and the use of panel reactivity antibody (PRA) tests to help identify and guide the management of recipients at higher risk for rejection from preformed antibodies. The PRA test involves adding the recipient's serum to a sample of lymphocytes from a representative sample of the potential donor pool and measuring what percentage of the sample lymphocytes that undergo lysis.[31] A PRA test threshold of more than or equal to 10% is commonly used to identify a "sensitized" recipient who should undergo prospective cross-matching with a potential donor to determine if any of the recipients existing antibodies target donor antigens.[31,32] The need to perform a prospective cross match further geographically limits the donor pool. Tests to identify to specific HLA antigens to which the recipient has antibodies have been developed and allow a virtual cross match to be performed that does not create additional restrictions to the donor pool.[25,31] This approach has been found to reduce with time for sensitized recipients with similar rates of survival and rejection as performing prospective cross matches.[34] Efforts to desensitize recipients with high levels of HLA antibodies, including intravenous immunoglobulin (IVIG), plasmaphoresis, and monoclonal antibodies targeting immune cells (rituximab) alone or in combination, are also sometimes employed to increase the potential donor pool and decrease rejection risk.[25,31]

Acute Allograft Rejection

Overall, acute allograft rejection occurs in about 30% of heart transplant recipients within the first year after transplant and has been associated with worse long-term survival.[1,2] Younger recipients and female recipients remain at higher risk of rejection[2] and this increase risk appears to remain with various immunosuppression regimens.[1]

Acute rejection is typically initially asymptomatic and when symptoms do develop, they are often nonspecific (e.g., fatigue, malaise, nausea, or fever).[33] Currently, there is no sufficiently reliable clinical or noninvasive method for surveillance and endomyocardial biopsy (EBM) remains the standard of care for detecting acute rejection.[25] Although echocardiographically derived parameters are commonly monitored and can be useful at times, they are neither sensitive nor specific enough to replace EMB.[25,33] Gene expression has shown promise, particularly in patients who are at low risk for rejection and several months post-transplant,[35] but is not applicable to the broader heart transplant population. Routine surveillance EBM is done most frequently in the months immediately following transplant and much less frequently after the first year, reflecting the pattern when acute rejection is most likely to occur.[25]

Acute allograft rejection can be characterized as antibody mediated or cellular and each is described briefly below. These can occur independently or coexist.

Acute Antibody Mediated Rejection

Although less common than acute cellular rejection (ACR), antibody mediated rejection (AMR) occurs in as many as 10–20% of heart transplant recipients with allosensitized patients, female recipients, and certain other subgroups at relatively increased risk.[36] Donor specific antibodies (DSA), which may be preformed or developed de novo, target endothelial antigens causing complement activation, and allograft injury.[33,36] Recommended diagnostic evaluation for AMR includes immunofluorescence testing for immunoglobulin and complement (e.g., C4d) deposition on EBM samples as well as retrospective crossmatching and measurement of DSA levels.[25] Treatment options include the use of high-dose corticosteroids, adjustment to maintenance immunosuppressive regimens, IVIG, plasmapheresis, rituximab, polyclonal antilymphocytic antibodies, bortezomib, and potentially eculizmab.[25,33,36]

Acute Cellular Rejection

The complex pathways leading to this predominantly T-cell mediated immune response have been described in more detail elsewhere[32,33] and a brief summary of these descriptions is presented here. ACR is initiated by the presentation of donor HLA, either by donor antigen presenting cells (APCs) (direct allorecognition) or by recipient APCs (indirect allorecognition), to recipient T cells. This stimulus in the presence of other costimuli activates intracellular pathways, including those mediated by calcineurin, that lead to the production of cytokines, including IL-2. These cytokines stimulate T-cell clonal expansion as well as the expansion of other inflammatory cell lines.[32] An activated form of the enzyme target of rapamycin (TOR) plays a role in the regulation of the cell cycle and lymphocytes proliferation is dependent on de novo synthesis of purines.[32] These steps represent the primary targets of contemporary immunosuppressive agents and regimens,[32] which are reviewed in more detail below.

Immune cell infiltration and associated myocardial damage are the pathological hallmarks of acute cellular rejection.[33] As mentioned previously, EMB remains the standard of care for surveillance and a standard grading system was developed and recently revised[37] (Table 3). This system, along with the presence or absence of graft

Table 3 International Society for Heart and Lung Transplantation standardized grading for presence of rejection in heart biopsies based on cellular rejection

Evidence of rejection (Cellular)	*Grade (1990 system)*	*Grade (2004 system)*
No rejection	0	0 R
Interstitial/perivascular infiltrate without myocyte damage 1 focus of infiltrate with myocyte damage	1A (mild, focal)	1 R (mild)
	1B (mild, diffuse)	
	2 (moderate, focal)	
Two or more foci of mononuclear cell infiltrate with associated myocyte damage	3A (moderate, focal)	2 R (moderate)
Diffuse infiltrate with multifocal myocyte damage with or without edema, hemorrhage, or vasculitis	3B (moderate, diffuse)	3 R (severe)
	4 (severe, extensive)	

Note: "R" indicates revised criteria

Source: *Adapted from* Stewart S, Winters GL, Fishbein MC, et al. Revision of the 1990 working formulation for the standardization of nomenclature in the diagnosis of heart rejection. J Heart Lung Transplant. 2005;24(11):1710-20.

dysfunction (based upon hemodynamic derangement or clinical symptoms) is used to guide the treatment of acute cellular rejection.

Treatment of Acute Cellular Rejection

Mild ACR without any evidence of graft dysfunction is often self-limited and may not require any changes to the immunosuppressive regimen. Severe forms of asymptomatic ACR are typically treated with high-dose intravenous corticosteroids (methylprednisolone 1,000 mg daily for 3 days). Moderate ACR with preserved graft function can be treated in the same manner or with an outpatient regimen of increased oral corticosteroids (1–3 mg/kg/day of prednisone for 3–5 days) based on individual patient risk.[25] In addition, adjustments to the chronic immunosuppressive regimen should be considered for moderate or severe asymptomatic ACR.

Acute cellular rejection with evidence of graft dysfunction requires prompt hospitalization (intensive care setting) and aggressive treatment. Initial therapy consists of high-dose intravenous corticosteroids as described above. Cytolytic therapy with polyclonal [e.g., thymoglobulin or antithymocyte gamma-globulin (ATGAM)] or monoclonal [e.g., muromonoab-CD3 (OKT3) (currently not in production)] may also be required. In addition, augmentation or modification of the maintenance immunosuppressive regimen, either with an adjustment in dose, addition of an agent, or change to an alternative regimen is also recommended.[25] Supportive measures, including hemodynamic support, if needed, prophylaxis against opportunistic infection, and pretreatment with corticosteroids, antihistamines, and antipyretics (acetaminophen) with cytolytic therapy should be provided.[25] Repeat EMB can be performed approximately 2 weeks after completion of therapy to ensure adequate treatment of ACR.

A more extensive discussion of treatment options for acute rejection is available in recently published guidelines.[25,33] It should be noted that the management of immunosuppression and the treatment of acute rejection varies from center to center. The majority of the recommendations on these topics in the guidelines are based upon low levels of evidence reflecting limited amount of high quality studies available in the literature to guide therapy.

Maintenance Immunosuppression

Maintenance immunosuppressive regimens typically involve a combination of three agents, corticosteroids, a calcineurin inhibitor, and antimetabolite. More recently, TOR inhibitors have sometimes been used to replace an antimetabolite or, especially late after transplant, a calcineurin inhibitor. Rejection history and side-effect profiles often dictate changes in chronic immunosuppression regimens.

Corticosteroids

Prednisone therapy remains a standard component of maintenance immunosuppression in heart transplant recipients. They provide potent immunosuppressive and anti-inflammatory effects on all types of leukocytes through the regulation of transcription.[38] Because of the numerous adverse effects associated with long-term use, regimens that wean steroids over the first 6–12 months post-transplantation have been implemented and similar outcomes have been observed as longer steroid regimens.[39] In recent cohorts, approximately 20% of transplant recipients at 1 year and approximately 50% at 5 years after transplant were successfully weaned from prednisone.[2]

Calcineurin Inhibitors

Calcineurin inhibitors (CI), in the form of either cyclosporine or tacrolimus, continue to form the cornerstone of immunosuppression therapy. Both agents inhibit transcription of IL-2 and other cytokines by blocking calcium-activated calcineurin.[38] Although tacrolimus has not been shown to provide a survival benefit over cyclosporine,[38] there is evidence for lower rates of rejection[40] as well as differing side-effect profile (lower rates of hypertension and hyperlipidemia but higher rates of diabetes mellitus) compared to cyclosporine. As a result, tacrolimus is now the dominant CI in clinical use with approximately 75% of heart transplant recipients taking this medication and less than 20% taking cyclosporine.[2] Regardless of the CI used, however, nephrotoxicity remains a major drawback to the use of this class of agents. Regimens where CI use has been reduced or completely eliminated have been investigated with some preliminary success,[41,42] but further research is needed.

Antiproliferatives

Azathioprine (AZA) and mycophenolate mofetil (MMF) both work by blocking lymphocyte proliferation, although MMF is selective for de novo purine synthesis upon which lymphocytes (but not other cells) exclusively depend.[38] Several studies have shown potential benefits of MMF over AZA including a possible survival advantage.[38,43] AZA is now used only rarely in heart transplant recipients where as MMF is taken by approximately 85% of these patients.[2]

Target of Rapamycin Inhibitors

Sirolimus and its analog everolimus inhibit IL-2 mediated proliferation of lymphocytes and smooth muscle cells through cell-cycle arrest in the G1 to S phase.[33] Tolerability of these medications may be more limited due to adverse side effects,[33] however, this class of medications may have a more favorable impact on cardiac allograft vasculopathy and allow for calcineurin-free long-term maintenance therapy.[41,42]

Further research is needed to define the best role for TOR inhibitors, which have been recently found to be used in less than 10% of heart transplant patients.[2]

In summary, the most common maintenance immunosuppression regimen is comprised of prednisone, tacrolimus, and MMF. Efforts to improve regimens to minimize adverse sideeffects and maintain or improve clinical outcomes are ongoing. In addition to the topics discussed here, a thorough understanding of potential drug-drug interactions with immunosuppressive agents[44] is essential for the safe and appropriate management of these medications.

Long-Term Outcomes

Many of the deleterious long-term outcomes in heart transplant recipients are directly related to immunosuppressive therapy, including infection and malignancy, while others are attributable to medication side effects including renal insufficiency, hypertension, hyperlipidemia, and diabetes.

COMPLICATIONS

Infection

Infection remains the major cause of death in the first year after transplant and can come from many sources. Common sources initially are those that arise from the surgical wound, pneumonia, urinary tract infections, indwelling catheters, and involve nosocomial organisms commonly seen in the intensive care unit. After the immediate postoperative period, the infections are more diverse and can be donor acquired as in the case of CMV or toxoplasmosis. The transplant patient is also susceptible to fungi including *Aspergillus, Candida,* and *Pneumocystis* as well as *Mycobacteria, Nocardia,* and *Legionella* species.

Malignancy

Malignancy is common after heart transplant and may develop as a sequela of chronic immunosuppresion. Nonmelanotic cutaneous malignancies are particularly common, as are lymphomas, including post-transplant lymphoproliferative disorder (PTLD).

Hypertension

Although the mechanism is not completely understood, many patients will have post-transplant hypertension. The mechanism may be related to preglomerular vasoconstriction in the kidney.

Diabetes

Chronic steroids often disrupt a patient's ability to handle glucose, and blood sugars elevate. This provides another motivation to get a patient off chronic steroids if possible.

Post-Transplant Vasculopathy

Although the pathogenesis is not fully known, post-transplant vasculopathy or transplant coronary artery disease commonly occurs in the transplanted heart and happens regardless of the patient's original need for transplant. Classically, the disease appears as pruning of the distal vessels on coronary angiography. There is some data to suggest that antiproliferative immunosuppressive agents, such as sirolimus and everolimus may help to prevent or decrease the rate of progression of transplant vasculopathy.[41,45-47]

CONCLUSION

Ongoing efforts to improve candidate selection, maximize the use of available donor organs, optimize immunosuppressive regimens, and effectively manage post-transplant complications have helped HT remain a life-saving therapy that remains the standard of care in appropriately selected patients with advanced HF.

REFERENCES

1. Stehlik J, Edwards LB, Kucheryavaya AY, et al. The Registry of the International Society for Heart and Lung Transplantation: twenty-seventh official adult heart transplant report--2010. J Heart Lung Transplant. 2010;29(10):1089-103.
2. Stehlik J, Edwards LB, Kucheryavaya AY, et al. The Registry of the International Society for Heart and Lung Transplantation: Twenty-eighth Adult Heart Transplant Report--2011. J Heart Lung Transplant. 2011;30(10):1078-94.
3. (SRTR) OPaTNOaSRoTR. OPTN/SRTR 2010 Annual Data Report. Rockville, MD: Department of Health and Human Services, Health Resources and Services Administration, Healthcare Systems Bureau, Division of Transplantation;2011.
4. Hunt SA, Abraham WT, Chin MH, et al. 2009 Focused update incorporated into the ACC/AHA 2005 Guidelines for the Diagnosis and Management of Heart Failure in Adults A Report of the American College of Cardiology Foundation/American Heart Association Task Force on Practice Guidelines Developed in Collaboration With the International Society for Heart and Lung Transplantation. J Am Coll Cardiol. 2009;53(15):e1-90.
5. Jhund PS, Macintyre K, Simpson CR, et al. Long-term trends in first hospitalization for heart failure and subsequent survival between 1986 and 2003: a population study of 5.1 million people. Circulation. 2009;119(4):515-23.
6. Fonarow GC, Albert NM, Curtis AB, et al. Associations between outpatient heart failure process-of-care measures and mortality. Circulation. 2011;123(15):1601-10.
7. Roger VL. The heart failure epidemic. International journal of environmental research and public health. 2010;7(4):1807-30.
8. Aaronson KD, Schwartz JS, Chen TM, et al. Development and prospective validation of a clinical index to predict survival in ambulatory patients referred for cardiac transplant evaluation. Circulation. 1997;95(12):2660-7.
9. Parikh MN, Lund LH, Goda A, et al. Usefulness of peak exercise oxygen consumption and the heart failure survival score to predict survival in patients >65 years of age with heart failure. Am J Cardiol. 2009;103(7):998-1002.
10. Goda A, Lund LH, Mancini D. The Heart Failure Survival Score outperforms the peak oxygen consumption for heart transplantation selection in the era of device therapy.J Heart Lung Transplant. 2011;30(3):315-25.

11. Goda A, Lund LH, Mancini DM. Comparison across races of peak oxygen consumption and heart failure survival score for selection for cardiac transplantation. Am J Cardiol. 2010;105(10):1439-44.
12. Perrotta L, Ricciardi G, Pieragnoli P, et al. Application of the Seattle Heart Failure Model in patients on cardiac resynchronization therapy. Pacing Clin Electrophysiol. 2012;35(1):88-94.
13. Levy WC, Mozaffarian D, Linker DT, et al. The Seattle Heart Failure Model: prediction of survival in heart failure. Circulation. 2006;113(11):1424-33.
14. Gorodeski EZ, Chu EC, Chow CH, et al. Application of the Seattle Heart Failure Model in ambulatory patients presented to an advanced heart failure therapeutics committee. Circ Heart Fail. 2010;3(6):706-14.
15. Kalogeropoulos AP, Georgiopoulou VV, Giamouzis G, et al. Utility of the Seattle Heart Failure Model in patients with advanced heart failure. J Am Coll Cardiol. 2009; 53(4):334-42.
16. Goda A, Williams P, Mancini D, et al. Selecting patients for heart transplantation: comparison of the Heart Failure Survival Score (HFSS) and the Seattle heart failure model (SHFM). J Heart Lung Transplant. 2011;30(11):1236-43.
17. Mancini DM, Eisen H, Kussmaul W, et al. Value of peak exercise oxygen consumption for optimal timing of cardiac transplantation in ambulatory patients with heart failure. Circulation. 1991;83(3):778-86.
18. Mancini D, Lietz K. Selection of cardiac transplantation candidates in 2010. Circulation. 2010;122(2):173-83.
19. Guazzi M, Adams V, Conraads V, et al. Clinical recommendations for cardiopulmonary exercise testing data assessment in specific patient populations. Circulation. 2012;126(18):2261-74.
20. Balady GJ, Arena R, Sietsema K, et al. Clinician's Guide to cardiopulmonary exercise testing in adults: a scientific statement from the American Heart Association. Circulation. 2010;122(2):191-225.
21. Arena R, Myers J, Guazzi M. The clinical and research applications of aerobic capacity and ventilatory efficiency in heart failure: an evidence-based review. Heart Fail Rev. 2008;13(2):245-69.
22. Milani RV, Lavie CJ, Mehra MR. Cardiopulmonary exercise testing: how do we differentiate the cause of dyspnea? Circulation. 2004;110(4):e27-31.
23. Ferreira AM, Tabet JY, Frankenstein L, et al. Ventilatory efficiency and the selection of patients for heart transplantation. Circ Heart Fail. 2010;3(3):378-86.
24. Mehra MR, Kobashigawa J, Starling R, et al. Listing criteria for heart transplantation: International Society for Heart and Lung Transplantation guidelines for the care of cardiac transplant candidates--2006. J Heart Lung Transplant. 2006;25(9):1024-42.
25. Costanzo MR, Dipchand A, Starling R, et al. The International Society of Heart and Lung Transplantation Guidelines for the care of heart transplant recipients. J Heart Lung Transplant. 2010;29(8):914-56.
26. Patel ND, Weiss ES, Nwakanma LU, et al. Impact of donor-to-recipient weight ratio on survival after heart transplantation: analysis of the United Network for Organ Sharing Database. Circulation. 2008;118(14 Suppl):S83-8.
27. Lower RR, Shumway NE. Studies on orthotopic homotransplantation of the canine heart. Surg forum. 1960;11:18-9.
28. Traversi E, Pozzoli M, Grande A, et al. The bicaval anastomosis technique for orthotopic heart transplantation yields better atrial function than the standard technique: an echocardiographic automatic boundary detection study. J Heart Lung Transplant. 1998;17(11):1065-74.

29. Meyer SR, Modry DL, Bainey K, et al. Declining need for permanent pacemaker insertion with the bicaval technique of orthotopic heart transplantation. Can J cardiol. 2005;21(2):159-63.
30. Parry G, Holt ND, Dark JH, et al. Declining need for pacemaker implantation after cardiac transplantation. Pacing clin electrophysiol. 1998;21(11 Pt 2):2350-2.
31. Costanzo M, Dipchand A, Starling R, et al. The international society of heart and lung transplantation guidelines for the care of heart transplant recipients. Task Force 1: Perioperative Care of the Heart Transplant Recipient. 2010. Accessed December 2, 2012.
32. Lindenfeld J, Miller GG, Shakar SF, et al. Drug therapy in the heart transplant recipient: part I: cardiac rejection and immunosuppressive drugs. Circulation. 2004; 110(24):3734-40.
33. Taylor D, Meiser B, Webber S, et al. The international society of heart and lung transplantation guidelines for the care of heart transplant recipients. Task Force 2: Immunosuppression and Rejection. 2010. Accessed December 2, 2012.
34. Yanagida R, Czer LS, Reinsmoen NL, et al. Impact of virtual cross match on waiting times for heart transplantation. Ann Thorac Surg. 2011;92(6):2104-10.
35. Pham MX, Teuteberg JJ, Kfoury AG, et al. Gene-expression profiling for rejection surveillance after cardiac transplantation. N Engl J Med. 2010;362(20):1890-900.
36. Chih S, Chruscinski A, Ross HJ, et al. Antibody-mediated rejection: an evolving entity in heart transplantation. J Transplant. 2012;2012:210210.
37. Stewart S, Winters GL, Fishbein MC, et al. Revision of the 1990 working formulation for the standardization of nomenclature in the diagnosis of heart rejection. J Heart Lung Transplant. 2005;24(11):1710-20.
38. Lindenfeld J, Miller GG, Shakar SF, et al. Drug therapy in the heart transplant recipient: part II: immunosuppressive drugs. Circulation. 2004;110(25):3858-65.
39. Teuteberg JJ, Shullo M, Zomak R, et al. Aggressive steroid weaning after cardiac transplantation is possible without the additional risk of significant rejection. Clin Transplant. 2008;22(6):730-7.
40. Kobashigawa JA, Miller LW, Russell SD, et al. Tacrolimus with mycophenolate mofetil (MMF) or sirolimus vs. cyclosporine with MMF in cardiac transplant patients: 1-year report. Am J Transplant. 2006;6(6):1377-86.
41. Topilsky Y, Hasin T, Raichlin E, et al. Sirolimus as primary immunosuppression attenuates allograft vasculopathy with improved late survival and decreased cardiac events after cardiac transplantation. Circulation. 2012;125(5):708-20.
42. Shah KB, Parameshwar J. Advances in heart transplantation: the year in review. J Heart Lung Transplant. 2011;30(3):241-6.
43. Kobashigawa J, Miller L, Renlund D, et al. A randomized active-controlled trial of mycophenolate mofetil in heart transplant recipients. Mycophenolate Mofetil Investigators. Transplantation. 1998;66(4):507-15.
44. Page RL, Miller GG, Lindenfeld J. Drug therapy in the heart transplant recipient: part IV: drug-drug interactions. Circulation. 2005;111(2):230-9.
45. Raichlin E, Bae JH, Khalpey Z, et al. Conversion to sirolimus as primary immunosuppression attenuates the progression of allograft vasculopathy after cardiac transplantation. Circulation. 2007;116(23):2726-33.
46. Eisen HJ, Tuzcu EM, Dorent R, et al. Everolimus for the prevention of allograft rejection and vasculopathy in cardiac-transplant recipients. N Engl J Med. 2003;349(9):847-58.
47. Mancini D, Pinney S, Burkhoff D, et al. Use of rapamycin slows progression of cardiac transplantation vasculopathy. Circulation. 2003;108(1):48-53.

CHAPTER 14

Heart Failure

Anne P Canny

INTRODUCTION

There have been tremendous advances made in the treatment of heart failure (HF). There is a large body of research that supports the therapies that are commonly used to manage HF. These therapies have demonstrated that evidence-based medicine decreases mortality and morbidity in HF patients. However, despite these tremendous gains, the rate of HF hospitalizations, especially readmissions, remains high. Various studies have demonstrated that interventions utilizing a combination of patient education and close follow-up after discharge can decrease readmission rates.

The goals of HF management may vary from patient to patient. In some cases, goals will focus on medical management that prolongs life, with treatments ranging from medications to defibrillators to evaluation for heart transplant. In other cases, goals may focus more on symptoms reduction and improved quality of life. At later stages, treatment may include medications to provide comfort and the withdrawal of some therapies to allow patients a more peaceful death.

The successful management of HF depends on collaboration between patients and their healthcare providers. Care is complex, requiring patient adherence to a daily regimen of medications, dietary restrictions, exercise, daily weights, and symptom recognition and management. Financial constraints, family obligations, work schedules, transportation issues, and insurance limitations all present potential barriers to adherence. A team approach, incorporating physicians, nurses, pharmacists, social workers, case managers, physical therapists, and nutritionists is an effective way to manage HF. Various members of the healthcare team work closely with patients providing education and follow-up, helping them to adhere to prescribed medical regimens and overcome barriers to care. This sort of close medical follow-up has also been shown to improve patient outcomes and decrease readmissions for HF.

HEART FAILURE CENTERS

The HF center usually consists of a group of healthcare providers including physicians, registered nurses and/or nurse practitioners, pharmacists, social workers and nutritionists who have a background in HF management. Care focuses on the establishment of long-term collaborative relationships with patients, the optimization of medications, and cardiac devices based on established HF guidelines, the coordination of medical care with other disciplines, and extensive patient education.[1]

The goals of the HF center are improving clinical outcomes through close medical follow-up, improving symptom recognition and management, thereby increasing well-being and quality of life, and recognizing and correcting factors that may lead to worsening HF. The patients who may benefit most are those with recent HF hospitalizations, those with persistent New York Health Associations Class III or IV symptoms, those with poor social support or with financial issues, those who have had difficulty adhering to a treatment regimen in the past, and those with comorbidities, such as diabetes or chronic kidney disease.[1] However, due to the complexity of HF management, all patients benefit. In fact, some of the patients who have benefitted most from the HF center are those who have been previously labeled as noncompliant. A combination of close medical follow-up and nursing support, coupled with intensive education, makes it easier for these patients to follow their complex treatment regimens where previously they had failed.

Comprehensive patient and family/caregiver education and counseling are the cornerstones of HF management. The ultimate goal of education is improved self-care of the patient. Patients are taught to recognize the signs and symptoms of worsening HF and how to manage them. As they become more aware of their symptoms, they are able to spot subtle changes more quickly and address problems earlier, leading to prompt medical management and better outcomes. Patients are instructed to call with any changes in symptoms, especially weight gain, a decrease in functional capacity, worsening dyspnea, or paroxysmal nocturnal dyspnea (PND). Patients may sometimes be taught to self-regulate their diuretics based on weight changes and symptoms; however, they are always instructed to notify their healthcare provider if they are not responding to diuretics or are requiring increased doses on a more frequent basis.

Heart failure nurse coordinators play an integral role in the HF center. They triage phone calls from patients and help to manage their symptoms, deciding when medications can be adjusted at home versus arranging an urgent office visit or sending the patient to the emergency department. Nurses work hard to form close relationships with patients and encourage them to call with any changes from their baseline. Sometimes they will set up regularly scheduled phone calls just to check in and have patients report weights and symptoms to help establish a relationship and guide them in symptom recognition. Several studies have demonstrated that interventions with nursing phone calls to patients reduce HF readmissions.[2-6]

Additionally, nurses in the HF center help to regulate medications. A beta-blocker might be initiated at a low dose at an office visit and then titrated up every 2 weeks by a nurse after discussing blood pressures, weights, and symptoms with the patient over the phone. An aldosterone inhibitor may be started in the office and the dose adjusted by the nurse over the phone after laboratory results are checked. Doses of angiotensin converting enzyme inhibitors (ACEIs) can also be adjusted by nurses over the phone. Nurses routinely adjust potassium and magnesium supplements based on laboratory results. They also help to manage diuretic doses over the phone according to patient symptoms, weights and laboratory results. A study by Steckler et al. demonstrated that telephonic titration of ACEIs and beta-blockers by nurses was safe and helped patients to achieve target doses.[7] Additionally, all of these phone interactions further help to establish close relationships between patients and healthcare providers, resulting in improved compliance and follow-up.

Nurses in the HF clinic can also help patients deal with social and economic issues by directing them to the appropriate resources. Health insurance and prescription coverage is becoming more and more confusing and it is often difficult for patients to navigate the system. Nurses can help to obtain prior authorizations from insurances for noncovered medications, or direct patients to more affordable generic or formulary medications when appropriate. They can refer patients to social workers as needed to help with questions about medical disability or insurance changes. Nurses and/or social workers can also direct patients to services in the community that provide assistance with transportation.

One last role of the HF clinic is to enhance communication and provide collaboration between all the healthcare providers caring for HF patients. Many patients with HF have concomitant diseases and it is extremely important for all providers to communicate with one another.

Fonarow et al. followed 214 patients after hospital discharge who were listed for transplant and followed at a comprehensive HF and transplant center.[8] Patients and families received extensive education from a HF center nurse specialist regarding medications, diet, daily weights, exercise, prognosis, and worsening HF symptoms and other medical complications. Patients were followed closely after hospital discharge both with frequent clinic visits and phone calls. The education program was reinforced at each visit, medications were optimized, and symptoms were reviewed and addressed. Six months later, there was an overall improvement in functional status and a decrease in hospital readmissions. Thus, a combination of patient education provided in a setting which reinforces that education over a prolonged period of time and offers frequent clinical follow-up and patient support is shown to improve patient outcomes.

HEART FAILURE EDUCATION

Patient education is an essential component of HF management. The purpose of HF patient education is to improve self-care behavior and thus, hopefully promote compliance with the prescribed medical regimen. However, several studies have demonstrated that education alone does not lead to improved self-care.[9-10] This might be because the education and knowledge base required for managing HF is complex. Therefore, it is important for educational topics to be repeated and discussed and reinforced over time by nurses and other healthcare providers.

Edwardson's and Stromberg's reviews of the literature demonstrated that many patients with HF are not able to define their condition, identify their medications, and/or do not weigh themselves daily.[11-12] The educational topics that patients viewed as most important included general HF information, medications, prognosis, risk factors, and signs and symptoms of HF. The most appropriate time to do extensive teaching with patients is after discharge when the patient is home and adapting to medications and lifestyle changes.

SYMPTOM RECOGNITION AND EDUCATION

A general overview of HF pathophysiology is important so patients can have a basic understanding of how the heart works normally and how the weakened heart affects their health. This education provides the building blocks of symptom recognition, especially signs of fluid retention, including weight gain, increasing shortness of breath, and edema. The role of daily weights and the results of excess sodium consumption all tie into this lesson. The ability to recognize fluid retention at an early stage is extremely important in the self-management of HF. Patients should weight themselves daily after awakening and before eating. They should record their weight and pay close attention to their trends. If their weight increases by more than 2–3 pounds overnight or 5 pounds in a week, they should call their healthcare provider or adjust diuretics if they have been instructed to do so.[13]

DIETARY EDUCATION

Also tying into fluid retention is the sodium restricted diet. Again, in basic terms, HF patients should be taught that excess sodium consumption will likely result in fluid retention. A 2 g sodium diet is usually recommended. Patients should learn to read food labels and recognize common foods that are high in sodium, such as fast foods, canned soups and sauces, and frozen dinners. It is also important to realize that often the serving size listed on a food label is less than the amount that a patient might actually eat. Patients need to combine their sodium-restricted diet with daily weights, especially if they stray from their diets on occasion. Patients should understand that if they eat a meal that is saltier than usual, they should be especially diligent with checking their weight the next day and if it has increased, either adjust their diuretic dose as directed or call their healthcare provider. Patients should not ignore a dietary indiscretion, especially if it results in fluid retention, and healthcare providers should scold gently as to not discourage patients from calling in the future. Interestingly, Edwardson found that patients view dietary information as less important than other educational topics while nurses rate it as being very important.[11] Often, patients believe that they are adhering to a low-sodium diet by abstaining from added salt and do not consider the sodium that is already present in foods they eat. Therefore, it is important that dietary education is ongoing and reinforced over time.

Patients should pay close attention to the amount of fluid they consume. Often, patients who take diuretics have the mistaken perception that they need to drink lots of fluid to flush out their kidneys. Again referring to basic pathophysiology, patients should be instructed that excess fluid consumption may cause them to retain fluid and that they may need to restrict fluid intake, particularly if they require large doses of diuretics to control their symptoms. In these cases, a fluid restriction of 2 L is usually recommended.[13]

EXERCISE AND ACTIVITY EDUCATION

It is important that patients remain as active as possible. Even modest amounts of exercise will help to increase functional capacity and improve well-being.[13] Also, paying close attention to how they feel while exercising helps patients monitor their symptoms and helps guide healthcare providers as to how well therapies are working. Outpatient cardiac rehabilitation is a good option for patients, combining supervised and monitored exercise with nursing support and education; however, it often is not covered by health insurance for the primary diagnosis of HF. Education regarding exercise and activity should focus on aerobic exercise as tolerated, limiting exercise in extreme temperatures, and the avoidance of heavy lifting and isometric exercises. Patients with ICDs should learn to monitor their heart rate and limit exercise to levels that keep their pulse well below the ICD therapy range.

MEDICATION EDUCATION

Heart failure education should also include basic information about medications. Patients are encouraged to carry an accurate list of their medications; this list should include the name, dose, and frequency of all medicines. Patients should also be taught the basic purpose of each medication and common side effects. Since many of the cardiac medications lower blood pressure, patients should learn to change position slowly to avoid sudden episodes of lightheadedness. Patients who take many medications may need to stagger the doses to avoid taking several medicines that lower blood pressure at once. When a new medication is started or existing medication is adjusted, patients should be informed of potential effects and when to notify their physician. Medications, dosages, and frequency should be carefully reviewed at each office visit. Patients should be encouraged to share any medication difficulties they might be experiencing with their healthcare provider, including financial barriers, complex dose schedules, or side effects. An ongoing discussion of medications between patients and their healthcare providers will aid in compliance and improve patient outcomes.

RESOURCES FOR PATIENT EDUCATION

There are many educational resources available for patients and their families that provide good information about HF management. The HF Society of America publishes 11 HF education modules, dealing with subjects from diet and medications to advance care planning. All are written specifically for patients and are intended to provide information and help foster communication between patients and their healthcare providers. The American Association of Heart Failure Nurses also has educational information for patients on their website. Topics include symptoms, daily weights, diet and tips for partnering with a healthcare team. There is also a HF education phone hotline. Both of these sources provide reliable and accurate information that may be used to supplement the information and education provided by patients' healthcare providers.

DISCHARGE PLANNING AND READMISSIONS

Heart failure is one of the most common diagnoses for Medicare beneficiaries and it is the most common diagnosis associated with 30-day readmissions.[14] Readmission rates have been shown to be as high as 13% 15 days after discharge, 25% at 30 days, and 45% at 6 months.[15] In July 2009, The Center for Medicare and Medicaid Services (CMS) began publicly reporting 30-day readmission rates for patients discharged with HF. This focus on readmission is an effort by CMS to promote healthcare quality and efficiency, identifying repeated heart failure admissions as potential indicators of poor care and a need for better coordinated care, especially after discharge. HF readmissions within 30 days of discharge receive less than usual reimbursement from CMS. This reporting and decrease in reimbursement has led to a renewed effort by hospitals to come up with plans to reduce readmission rates for HF.

Part of the reason for high HF readmission rates is inadequate follow-up after discharge. Hernandez followed 30,136 HF patients from 225 hospitals and found that those who had early physician follow-up after discharge had lower rates of readmission within 30 days.[14] It is recommended that patients follow-up with a healthcare provider within 7–10 days of discharge.[1,16] Ideally, appointments should be established and reviewed with patients prior to discharge rather than instructing them to call for an appointment themselves and these appointments should be clearly stated in the patient discharge instructions.

Hernandez found that establishing transitional care helped to ensure the coordination and continuity of care between the inpatient and outpatient settings.[14] This is extremely important since it is common for patients to have inpatient care provided by a different healthcare team than the physicians who will follow them as outpatients. Transitional care typically includes communication between all physicians caring for a patient, preparing the patient for what to expect at the postdischarge visit, reconciling medications, following up on any outstanding tests needed to be done as an outpatient, and helping the patient learn to monitor signs and symptoms of worsening HF. For example, patients may follow up with a primary care physician who is not aware of a recent hospitalization and ensuing treatment changes. Therefore, it is helpful for patients to bring a copy of their discharge instructions to all appointments and ideally, physicians caring for hospitalized patients should communicate with patients' healthcare providers at time of discharge. A faxed copy of patient discharge instructions, listing the reasons for the hospitalization, diagnostic testing results, medications and prescribed follow up, is adequate.

All patients should be taught to recognize the basic signs and symptoms of worsening HF prior to discharge. Additionally, they should have a plan as to how to handle worsening symptoms or any other problems they might encounter after discharge, such as difficulty obtaining medications or trouble making their follow-up appointment. This can be especially problematic if patients encounter difficulties prior to their first follow-up appointments. It is, therefore, important that patients have someone they could contact with any issues after discharge, whether it be the doctor who cared for them in the hospital, their own physician (who has knowledge of the recent hospitalization), or a designated nurse case manager or HF nurse coordinator.

Hanson et al. reviewed 43 studies aimed at reducing HF readmission rates.[17] Predischarge interventions included patient education, medication reconciliation, discharge planning, and scheduled follow-up appointments made prior to discharge. Postdischarge interventions included follow-up phone calls, home visits, hotlines for patients to call with questions or problems, early follow-up appointments, and communication between inpatient and outpatient providers. Bridging or transitional interventions included physician continuity across the inpatient and outpatient settings, transition coaches, and patient-centered discharge instructions. He found no single intervention that by itself significantly decreased HF readmissions. However, most of the studies he reviewed that did decrease HF readmissions included the interventions of patient centered discharge instructions and telephone follow-up. Patient-centered discharge instructions engage patients in their discharge and follow-up, and help them to become more active participants in their own healthcare. This might include an individualized notebook or folder with

HF signs and symptoms, dietary tips, a chart for daily weights, a list of their current medications, and names and phone numbers for all their healthcare providers. Patients would be encouraged to bring this information to all appointments and share it with their healthcare providers.

Several studies have demonstrated that close follow-up after hospital discharge reduce HF readmissions.[3,5,18] These studies utilized a combination of intensive patient education and postdischarge follow-up by nurses. Interventions consisted primarily of office visits and follow-up phone calls, and in some cases, patients also received home nursing visits. Heart failure education was reinforced during all interactions, medications were reviewed, and any changes in symptoms were discussed. In the case of worsening symptoms, nurses either adjusted medications according to a prescribed algorithm or they referred patients to their health care provider. All results demonstrated a significant decrease in readmissions for HF. Phillips et al. performed a meta-analysis of 18 studies concerning HF patients who received extensive discharge planning and postdischarge support versus usual care.[4] The results show that comprehensive discharge planning and close follow-up during the postdischarge phase resulted in decreased readmissions for HF and importantly, did not increase costs.

One other intervention that Hanson et al. identified in their review is the role of a transition coach.[17] A transition coach is usually a nurse with specialized HF training who interacts with the patient throughout his or her hospitalization and continues to follow them for a period of time after discharge, either via telephone and/or home or office visits. This nurse would review signs and symptoms of worsening HF, help to monitor daily weights, review medications and potential side effects, and ensure that the patient has a timely follow-up with his or her healthcare provider. This role is very similar to that of a HF nurse coordinator. A heart failure nurse coordinator follows patients during their hospitalizations alongside physicians, provides HF education and discharge instructions, helps to coordinate care with all physicians at discharge, ensures that patients understand medication changes and are able to obtain their medications after discharge, helps to arrange home care as needed, and follows up on blood work and other testing that may be required after hospitalization. Additionally, because HF coordinators follow patients also in the outpatient setting, they are often able to offer insight as to problems that were occurring at home and treatment changes made prior to hospital admission.

Naylor et al. followed 239 patients aged 65 and older from the time of their admissions for HF through 3 months after hospital discharge.[19] The intervention group received daily hospital visits from HF advanced practice nurses, followed by intermittent home visits and telephone availability by nurses on a daily basis. The nurses evaluated patients' symptoms and responses to medical therapy and collaborated with their physicians in establishing guidelines for care and follow-up. At 1 year, the intervention group had fewer hospital readmissions and there were fewer total costs accrued. Although the nurses in this study performed home visits, they otherwise served a similar role to HF nurse coordinators in a HF center, teaching patients to recognize and evaluate symptoms, and coordinating care between patients and physicians.

CONCLUSION

The effective management of patients with chronic HF requires a multidisciplinary team approach. Physicians, nurses, pharmacists, social workers, nutritionists, physical therapists, and case managers all help to contribute to the successful management of HF patients. Management should bridge both the inpatient and outpatient settings so that patient care is fluid and consistent. Communication between all members of the healthcare team is essential.

Heart failure patients are expected to adhere to a complex medical regimen which is often difficult to follow. Patients who have a basic understanding of HF and its management, including symptom recognition, medications, dietary restrictions, and exercise goals are more likely to have good compliance with their medical regimen. A close relationship between healthcare providers and patients helps to establish realistic goals of care. These goals may change over time reflecting the patient's current health status.

As patients' heart failure progresses, medical management may focus more on palliation and comfort if other advanced therapies, such as transplant or VAD are not viable options. It is important to discuss with patients their wishes and goals of therapy. For patients whose symptoms are very difficult to control despite optimal medical therapy, it may be reasonable to consider home IV inotropes as a way to improve quality of life and reduce hospitalizations. Patients may also benefit from periodic IV diuretics given at home if oral diuretics are inadequate. As patients' goals of care focus more on palliation and comfort, it is also important to help patients make decisions regarding end-of-life care. In these cases, it may be prudent to discuss code status and the deactivation of defibrillators. Hospice care is also a reasonable option. These are often difficult topics for patients to discuss and it is important for them to have the guidance and support of their healthcare providers when making these decisions.

The care of HF patients is complicated, both because of the medical complexity of HF itself, other contributing comorbidities, limitations of care due to cost and/or insurance coverage, and patients' individual lifestyles and other limiting factors. Patients should always be encouraged to play an active role in their healthcare and discuss any impediments to this care with their healthcare team. This, in turn, should result in better overall management of patients with HF and a presumed reduction in hospital admissions and healthcare costs. However, it is best to remember that in all cases, the ultimate goal of HF medical care and management is maintaining and improving the patient's quality of life.

REFERENCES

1. Hauptman PJ, Rich MW, Heidenreich PA, et al. The heart failure clinic: a consensus statement of the Heart Failure Society of America. J Card Fail. 2008;14:801-15.
2. Dunagan WA, Littenberg B, Ewald GA, et al. Randomized trial of a nurse-administered, telephone-based disease management program for patients with heart failure. J Card Fail. 2005;11:358-65.
3. Krumholz HM, Amatruda J, Smith GL, et al. Randomized trial of an education and support intervention to prevent readmission of patients with heart failure. J Am Coll Cardiol. 2002;39:83-9.
4. Phillips CO, Wright SM, Kern DE, et al. Comprehensive discharge planning with post-discharge support for older patients with congestive heart failure: a meta-analysis. JAMA. 2004;291:1358-67.
5. Rich MW, Beckham V, Wittenberg C, et al. A multidisciplinary intervention to prevent the readmission of elderly patients with congestive heart failure. N Engl J Med. 1995;333:1190-5.
6. Riegel B, Carlson B, Kopp Z, et al. Effect of a standardized nurse case-management telephone intervention on resource use in patients with chronic heart failure. Arch Intern Med. 2002;162:705-12.
7. Steckler AE, Bishu K, Wassif H, et al. Telephone Titration of Heart Failure Medications. J Cardiovasc Nurs. 2011;26:29-36.
8. Fonarow GC, Stevenson LW, Walden JA, et al. Impact of a comprehensive heart failure management program on hospital readmission and functional status of patients with advanced heart failure. J Am Coll Cardiol. 1997;30:725-32.
9. Powell LH, Calvin JE, Richardson D, et al. Self-management counseling in patients with heart failure: The heart failure adherence and retention randomized behavioral trial. JAMA. 2010;304:1331-8.
10. Yehle KS, Plake KS. Self-efficacy and educational interventions: a review of the literature. J Cardiovasc Nurs. 2010;25:175-88.
11. Edwardson SR. Patient education in heart failure. Heart Lung. 2007;36:244-52.
12. Stromberg A. The crucial role of patient education in heart failure. Eur J Heart Fail. 2005;7:363-9.
13. Grady KL, Dracup K, Kennedy G, et al. Team management of patients with heart failure: a statement for healthcare professionals from the Cardiovascular Nursing Council of the American Heart Association. Circulation. 2000;102:2443-56.
14. Hernandez AF, Greiner MA, Fonarow GC. Relationship between early physician follow-up and 30-day readmission among Medicare beneficiaries hospitalized for heart failure. JAMA. 2010;303:1716-22.
15. Ross JS, Chen J, Lin ZQ, et al. Recent trends in readmission rates after heart failure hospitalization. Circ Heart Fail. 2010;3:97-103.
16. Gheorghiade M, Peterson ED. Improving postdischarge outcomes in patients hospitalized for acute heart failure syndromes. JAMA. 2011;305:2456-7.
17. Hansen LO, Young RS, Hinami K, et al. Interventions to reduce 30-day rehospitalization: a systematic review. Ann Intern Med. 2011;155:520-8.
18. Kasper EK, Gerstenblith G, Hefter G, et al. A randomized trial of the efficacy of multidisciplinary care in heart failure outpatients at high risk of hospital readmission. J Am Coll Cardiol. 2002;39:471-80.
19. Naylor MD, Brooten DA, Campbell RL, et al. Transitional care of older adults hospitalized with heart failure: a randomized, controlled trial. J Am Geriatr Soc. 2004;52:675-84.

Index

Page numbers followed by f refer to figure and t refer to table

D

E

F

G

S

T

U

V